Common Problems in

Pediatric Gastroenterology and Nutrition

CONTRIBUTORS

William G. Bithoney, M.D.
Assistant Professor of Pediatrics
Harvard Medical School
Director of Primary Care Clinic
The Children's Hospital
Boston, Massachusetts

Cheryl J. Bunker, M.D.
Instructor in Medicine
Harvard Medical School
Fellow in Gastroenterology
Beth Israel Hospital
Boston, Massachusetts

Tien-Lan Chang, M.D.
Instructor in Pediatrics
Harvard Medical School
Assistant in Pediatrics
Massachusetts General Hospital
Boston, Massachusetts

George Christopoulous, M.D.
Visiting Scientist
Division of Gastroenterology and
  Nutrition
The Children's Hospital
Boston, Massachusetts

Joaquin Cortiella, M.D., M.P.H.
Fellow in Gastroenterology
The Children's Hospital
Boston, Massachusetts

Mounif El-Youssef, M.D.
Fellow in Gastroenterology
The Children's Hospital
Boston, Massachusetts

Daniel M. Epstein, M.D.
Instructor in Pediatrics
Harvard Medical School
Assistant in Psychiatry
The Children's Hospital
Boston, Massachusetts

Victor L. Fox, M.D.
Instructor in Pediatrics
Harvard Medical School
Assistant in Gastroenterology
The Children's Hospital
Boston, Massachusetts

Talyn Hanissian, M.D.
Fellow in Gastroenterology
The Children's Hospital
Boston, Massachusetts

Stephen C. Hardy, M.D.
Resident in Pediatrics
Massachusetts General Hospital
Boston, Massachusetts

Paul Harmatz, M.D.
Assistant Professor of Pediatrics
Harvard Medical School
Assistant Pediatrician
Massachusetts General Hospital
Boston, Massachusetts

Kristy Hendricks, R.D., D.Sc.
Instructor in Pediatrics
Harvard Medical School
Assistant in Nutrition (Pediatrics)
Massachusetts General Hospital
Boston, Massachusetts

Barry Z. Hirsch, M.D.
Fellow in Gastroenterology
The Children's Hospital
Boston, Massachusetts

Esther Jacobowitz Israel, M.D.
Instructor in Pediatrics
Harvard Medical School
Assistant in Pediatrics
Massachusetts General Hospital
Boston, Massachusetts

Ronald E. Kleinman, M.D.
Associate Professor of Pediatrics
Harvard Medical School
Pediatrician
Massachusetts General Hospital
Boston, Massachusetts

Alan M. Leichtner, M.D.
Assistant Professor of Pediatrics
Harvard Medical School
Associate in Gastroenterology
The Children's Hospital
Boston, Massachusetts

Craig W. Lillehei, M.D.
Instructor in Surgery
Harvard Medical School
Assistant in Surgery
The Children's Hospital
Boston, Massachusetts

Clifford W. Lo, M.D., M.P.H., Sc.D.
Instructor in Pediatrics
Harvard Medical School
Assistant in Nutrition
The Children's Hospital
Boston, Massachusetts

Eric S. Maller, M.D.
Instructor in Pediatrics
Harvard Medical School
Assistant in Gastroenterology
The Children's Hospital
Boston, Massachusetts

S.R. Martin, M.D., F.R.C.P. (C)
Fellow in Gastroenterology
The Children's Hospital
Boston, Massachusetts

Tracie L. Miller, M.D.
Fellow in Gastroenterology
The Children's Hospital
Boston, Massachusetts

Anne Munck, M.D.
Visiting Scientist
The Children's Hospital
Boston, Massachusetts

M. Stephen Murphy, M.D.
Fellow in Gastroenterology
The Children's Hospital
Boston, Massachusetts

Samuel Nurko, M.D.
Instructor in Pediatrics
Harvard Medical School
Assistant in Gastroenterology
The Children's Hospital
Boston, Massachusetts

Veronique A. Pelletier, M.D.
Fellow in Nutrition
The Children's Hospital
Boston, Massachusetts
Research Fellow
Clinical Research Center
Applied Biological Sciences
Massachusetts Institute of Technology
Cambridge, Massachusetts

Richard H. Sandler, M.D.
Fellow in Gastroenterology
The Children's Hospital
Boston, Massachusetts
Research Fellow
Clinical Research Center
Massachusetts Institute of Technology
Cambridge, Massachusetts

Benjamin Shneider, M.D.
Resident in Medicine
The Children's Hospital
Boston, Massachusetts

Richard A. Schreiber, M.D.C.M., F.R.C.P.(C)
Fellow in Gastroenterology
The Children's Hospital
Boston, Massachusetts

Robert C. Shamberger, M.D.
Assistant Professor of Surgery
Harvard Medical School
Assistant in Surgery
The Children's Hospital
Boston, Massachusetts

Nancy Sheard, Sc.D., R.D.
Instructor in Pediatrics
Harvard Medical School
Associate Director
Nutrition Support Service
The Children's Hospital
Boston, Massachusetts

John D. Snyder, M.D.
Assistant Professor of Pediatrics
Harvard Medical School
Associate in Gastroenterology
Combined Program in Pediatric
* Gastroenterology and Nutrition*
The Children's Hospital
Boston, Massachusetts

Joseph P. Vacanti, M.D.
Assistant Professor of Surgery
Harvard Medical School
Assistant in Surgery
The Children's Hospital
Boston, Massachusetts

W. Allan Walker, M.D.
Chief, Combined Program in Pediatric
* Gastroenterology and Nutrition*
Professor of Pediatrics
Harvard Medical School
Boston, Massachusetts

Barry K. Wershil, M.D.
Instructor in Pediatrics
Harvard Medical School
Assistant in Gastroenterology
The Children's Hospital
Boston, Massachusetts

Harland S. Winter, M.D.
Assistant Professor in Pediatrics
Harvard Medical School
Associate in Gastroenterology
The Children's Hospital
Boston, Massachusetts

FOREWORD

It is hard to believe that it is only 18 years since the first textbook in pediatric gastroenterology was published. Since that time there has been a steady expansion in the literature in this field, which reflects the remarkable growth of knowledge concerning diseases of the gastrointestinal tract and the liver that affect children. This expansion in knowledge can almost be regarded as an explosion, and it relates to the safe application of new diagnostic techniques and technology to these disorders. This volume aims to provide a practical approach to pediatric gastroenterology, by guiding students, residents, pediatricians, and other care providers, as well as the subspecialist clinician in a case-oriented fashion. The clinical material has been taken from recent cases seen in the Combined Program in Gastroenterology and Nutrition at Children's and Massachusetts General Hospitals in Boston. These cases provide accounts of specific disease states such as cystic fibrosis and celiac disease; they also address symptom complexes such as acute and chronic diarrhea, emphasizing pathophysiological mechanisms. The book also provides an account of gastroenterological manifestations of systemic disease, including the latest scourge, AIDS. The nutritional implications of gastrointestinal disease are also covered, accompanied by a practical guide to the nutritional management of affected children.

The authors have included more than 50 tables, which summarize data on the evaluation, differential diagnoses, treatment recommendations, and recent literature related to the cases presented. In addition, many chapters contain photographs of radiographic and histologic findings or figures of surgical interventions or schemas for evaluation and diagnosis.

It is, therefore, a pleasure for me to introduce this important addition to the literature of pediatric gastroenterology.

John A. Walker-Smith, M.D, F.R.C.P., F.R.A.C.P.
Professor of Paediatric Gastroenterology
University of London
St. Bartholomew's Hospital and Queen Elizabeth Hospital for Children
London, England

PREFACE

This book was written to provide a case-oriented practical guide for clinicians, house officers, students, gastroenterologists, and nutritionists to pediatric patients with disorders of the gastrointestinal (GI) tract. The case-oriented approach—a departure from the standard textbook format—was chosen to involve the reader in the thought processes used in evaluating and treating children and adolescents with GI disease. Colleagues from surgery, gastroenterology, and nutrition have added their perspectives.

Each chapter includes an actual case seen in the Combined Program in Gastroenterology and Nutrition at Children's and Massachusetts General Hospitals. These cases represent typical, and at times atypical, presentations of the disorders discussed.

In addition to the case presentations, almost all chapters are structured to provide general background information, including epidemiologic features, pathophysiology, clinical features, diagnosis, and treatment. Many chapters contain tables that summarize important clinical findings and approaches to management or treatment. Photographs of radiographic, surgical, and histologic features have also been included. The references have been chosen to provide a concise listing that emphasizes the most recent relevant literature as well as classic descriptions and definitive reviews.

We hope that our readers will find this to be a helpful and instructive resource in their assessment and management of children with gastroenterologic and nutritional disorders. If so, we will feel that the book has been a success.

Many people beyond the authors listed contributed to this effort. We gratefully acknowledge the contributions of all of our colleagues—students, residents, fellows, nursing staff, and physicians—who helped us care for and learn from the patients whose cases are presented here. We also wish to extend special thanks to Joy Rocke and Stacia Langenbahn for their expert technical assistance.

John D. Snyder, M.D.
W. Allan Walker, M.D.

CONTENTS

PART III: THE LIVER   *193*

PART IV: THE PANCREAS   *285*

PART V: SYSTEMIC CONDITIONS AFFECTING THE GASTROINTESTINAL TRACT   *303*

PART ONE

The Esophagus

1 Esophageal Atresia and Tracheoesophageal Fistula

George Christopolous, M.D.

This 16-year-old boy had been the full-term product of an uncomplicated pregnancy. Shortly after birth he was noted to have increased salivation, and when he was offered a bottle feeding, he developed coughing and cyanosis. An attempt to pass a feeding tube to the stomach was unsuccessful, and a chest x-ray film with the tube in place showed the tip to be arrested at the thoracic inlet (Fig 1–1), and air was present within the intestinal loops. These findings confirmed the diagnosis of esophageal atresia with distal tracheoesophageal fistula, and these defects were repaired on the second day of life. The fistula was divided and a primary end-to-end esophageoesophageal anastomosis was performed. The postoperative course was uneventful.

At 4 years of age the child presented with dysphagia and failure to thrive and was found to have a stenosis at the level of the esophageal anastomosis that required repeated bougienage or pneumatic dilatations. Despite this therapy, a barium swallow examination showed moderate dilatation of the proximal esophagus and a tight stricture extending from the level of the carina to 8 cm distally. Long-term intensive medical therapy with antacids and cimetidine did not result in improvement of the stricture. He continued to complain of dysphagia and poor weight gain and eventually developed a complete stricture of his esophagus in spite of intermittent dilatations. Therefore, a Nissen fundoplication was performed at age 12 years. Subsequently he was admitted on several occasions for incomplete intestinal obstruction, which was treated conservatively.

His overall course following the fundoplication was improved, and he was able to eat a regular diet and gain some weight, although he remained very thin. He denied dysphagia, nausea, or vomiting but radiologic and endoscopic evidence of his stricture persisted, necessitating repeated pneumatic balloon dilatations. An esophageal biopsy performed during endoscopy 2.5 years after his fundoplication showed mild esophagitis, and he was maintained on cimetidine and antacids. He also underwent a series of pneumatic dilatations as well as a home dilatation program. During this period he continued to deny any symptoms attributable to the stricture. Despite his home dilation program he was found on follow-up examination 4 years after his surgery to have a 5-cm long stricture of the midesophagus that could not be negotiated by the endoscope. He is currently on a program of repeated pneumatic dilatations, antacids, and ranitidine.

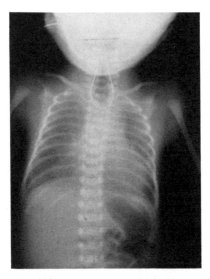

FIG 1–1.
Plain radiograph demonstrating curling of
the nasogastric tube at the level of the
fourth thoracic vertebra corresponding to
the bottom of the proximal pouch. The air
in the stomach and small bowel loops is
evidence for a distal tracheoesophageal
fistula.

DISCUSSION

Esophageal atresia with or without tracheoesophageal fistula is a congenital anomaly that occurs with a frequency of about 1:3,000 to 1:4,500 live births.[1] The
most common type, termed C in Gross's classification,[2] is a blind proximal pouch
with a distal tracheoesophageal fistula (Fig 1–2), accounting for about 85% of the
cases.[3–5] Tracheoesophageal fistula is frequently associated with other congenital
anomalies, including cardiac defects (37%), imperforate anus (13%), and other gastrointestinal (GI) anomalies (8.5%).[6] A particular group of anomalies has been given
the eponym VATER and includes vascular or vertebral, anal, tracheoesophageal,
and radial or renal malformations.[4]

Waterston, in 1962, correlated operative survival in children with tracheoesophageal fistula with birth weight, prematurity, and associated anomalies.[3] He distinguished three different prognostic categories (Table 1–1) associated with increasing

risk for operative morbidity and mortality. His overall survival following surgery was 59% and was heavily influenced by a very high mortality in patients in his category C.[3] As shown in Table 1–1, prognosis has since greatly improved, reaching an overall survival of 65% to 90%, mainly because of the improved quality of today's neonatal intensive care.[6–8] Category C with severe prematurity, severe coexistent anomalies, and severe pneumonia still has the worst prognosis in all series.

Clinical Features

This patient initially presented with a fairly typical history for a child with a blind esophageal pouch and a distal tracheoesophageal fistula (see Fig 1–2), (type C). As is very often the case, an uncomplicated pregnancy preceded a normal birth. Polyhydramnios can be encountered[4] and may provide a clue to the possible diagnosis, although other congenital malformations are more frequently associated with this condition. Increased salivation, caused by regurgitation of saliva from the atretic proximal pouch, gives the first hint to the diagnosis. Abdominal distention may be present if enough air passes through a distal tracheoesophageal fistula to the stomach and the intestines. Symptoms are precipitated, as in this case, by the first feedings and include choking, coughing, cyanosis, and pneumonia due to aspiration.

Diagnosis

An important diagnostic clue is provided by the inability to pass a feeding tube to the stomach, although a false sense of security can be caused by the use of a soft

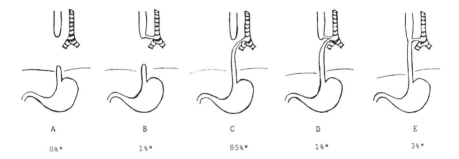

| A | B | C | D | E |
| 8%* | 1%* | 85%* | 1%* | 3%* |

FIG 1–2.
Schematic drawing of the types of esophageal atresia and tracheoesophageal fistula following the classification of Gross.[2] Not included is type F, which represents congenital stenosis.
*Frequencies derived from Waterson,[3] Osimek et al.,[4] and Holder.[5]

TABLE 1–1.
Operative Survival According to Waterston's Risk Categories*

Risk Category	Birth Weight, lb (kg)	Interfering Conditions	Median Operative Survival, % (Range)
A	>5.5 (>2.5)	None	97 (94–100)
Ba	3.7–5.5 (1.7–2.5)	None	
b	>5.5 (>2.5)	Moderate pneumonia and congenital anomaly	81 (53–97)
Ca	<3.7 (<1.7)	None	
b	>3.7 (>1.7)	Severe pneumonia and congenital anomaly	68 (6–88)

*Adapted from Waterston,[3] Grosfeld and Ballantine,[6] Touloukian,[7] and McKneally et al.[8]

catheter, which can be advanced easily only to coil up in the atretic pouch. If the diagnosis is suspected, an upright chest x-ray film should be obtained, preferably with the nasogastric tube in place to demonstrate the bottom of the atretic pouch, which can be visualized by injecting a small amount of air through the tube. Contrast examinations are rarely needed and increase the risk for aspiration. The distance from the tip of the catheter to the bifurcation of the trachea also gives a rough estimate of the distance between the proximal and distal esophageal segment. Further preoperative diagnostic studies should be performed only to rule out other suspected congenital anomalies.

Management

Once the diagnosis is established, aspiration should be avoided by elevating the child's head and applying continuous suction through a catheter in the proximal pouch. Other general measures include the use of an infant warmer, oxygen, parenteral nutrition, and antibiotic treatment. Immediate yet elective surgical repair is indicated for Waterston's category A patients (see Table 1–1). For category B infants a delayed primary repair is advocated after the child's condition has been stabilized. In addition to the general recommendations previously mentioned, a gastrostomy tube should be placed to aspirate gastric contents and prevent their regurgitation through the tracheoesophageal fistula. When postoperative complications, coexistent anomalies, or prematurity preclude oral feedings, this gastrostomy may be important for feeding these infants. Category C infants are managed by a staged repair giving priority to the correction of the most serious and life-threatening conditions.

With the improved quality of today's neonatal intensive care facilities, the prognosis following surgery is usually very good, particularly for Waterston categories A and B. The majority of deaths is attributable to associated congenital defects or to prematurity with its attendant complications. The surgical repair has a number of potential complications, including stricture (23%), anastomotic leak (5%–6%), recurrent tracheoesophageal fistula (4%), pneumothorax, scoliosis, as well as functional sequelae such as esophageal dysmotility with resulting gastroesophageal reflux.[1, 9, 10]

Outcome

Stricture formation is the most common complication following repair of tracheoesophageal fistula and may be related to a significant extent to technical aspects of the operation. Extensive stretching of the pouch with resulting tension on the anastomosis caused by compromised blood supply will greatly favor stricture formation.[3, 11] Such tension can often be avoided by performing circular myotomies on the proximal pouch,[12] thus gaining up to 2 to 3 cm. Leakage and the resulting inflammation around the area of the anastomosis can also favor scarring and subsequent stenosis.[8, 11] However, these factors do not fully account for strictures that are as resistant to therapy and dilatations as was the case with this patient, nor do they account for the dysphagia of which many patients complain in absence of identifiable significant anatomic stenosis.

Another major factor predisposing to stricture formation appears to be impaired esophageal motility, which is almost always present in patients with tracheoesophageal fistula.[13] This abnormal motility may even cause dysphagia in some patients without identifiable significant anatomic stenosis.[13] Among the first to use functional studies to demonstrate esophageal dysfunction, Orringer et al. found varying abnormalities in 21 of 22 patients,[14] and this high frequency of abnormalities has been confirmed by others.[13, 15] Findings include an abnormally low lower esophageal sphincter (LES) pressure, abnormal peristalsis in the midportion or in the distal esophagus, but normal peristalsis in the cervical esophagus.[13, 15] The low LES pressure and the impaired esophageal motility may frequently result in gastroesophageal reflux and influence the development of a stricture.[13–16] Reflux esophagitis is common in these patients, and as many as 35% of patients eventually undergo fundoplication.[11, 14–16]

In this respect this patient is a rather common example. His stenosis was greatly influenced by gastroesophageal reflux and necessitated a fundoplication, which, however, did not abolish reflux. As a result his stricture continued to progress, causing his symptoms to improve because gastric contents were prevented from reaching inflamed parts of the esophagus.

The specific etiology of esophageal dysmotility and gastroesophageal reflux in patients with tracheoesophageal fistula is unknown. Manipulations during the operation may be one contributing factor, especially extensive mobilization of the lower esophageal pouch.[8, 14] Excessive tension on the anastomosis has also been correlated with a higher incidence of gastroesophageal reflux.[11] Whether this is the result of interference with the blood supply or severance of vagal branches to the body of the esophagus has not been clarified. In addition, mobilization may also alter the angle of His and shorten the intraabdominal part of the LES, thus promoting reflux.[8, 11, 13] Another factor contributing to the esophageal dysmotility may be congenital motility disturbance; patients with H-type fistula have been demonstrated to have similar motor disturbances prior to surgery.[15] Inadvertent nerve damage may also be a factor because complete bilateral cervical vagotomy high in the neck has produced a similar condition without alteration of LES function.[15] Children with esophageal resection for benign stricture have not experienced similar dysmotility after surgery. These findings suggest that congenital factors contribute to esophageal dysmotility, although surgical manipulations may also play a role.

Medical management of gastroesophageal reflux consists principally of oral antacids at a dose of 0.5 to 1.0 ml/kg or H_2 blockers (20–40 mg of cimetidine kg/ day divided in four doses or, in older children, 150 mg of rantidine twice daily), aiming at abolishing the acidity of the refluxing gastric contents. In addition, metoclopramide (0.1–0.2 mg/kg dose, given four times daily) may also be used in selected cases to promote GI motility and increase LES tone. Although the motility disturbance is present for life,[14, 16] many patients seem to improve with age[17] or medical treatment.[8] However, an increased incidence of recurrent reflux postoperatively has been documented,[14] which, as in this patient, may create problems including worsening of an existing stricture. Unfortunately, no criteria exist to identify which patients will require fundoplication. Each patient should therefore be assessed carefully, and surgery should be considered only if intensive medical management fails to control symptoms or complications.[15]

A problem that has received little attention in patients with tracheoesophageal fistula is their nutritional status and its effect on later development and growth. Factors that should be considered include birth weight, prematurity, length of hospitalization, coexisting congenital anomalies, degree of dysmotility, gastroesophageal reflux, and the development of stenosis. Cohen and Greecher found that 24% of 108 patients undergoing surgery (including 16 for tracheoesophageal fistula repair) remained below the fifth percentile for height and weight at 5 years of follow-up.[18] However, Andrassy et al.[19] and Rickham[20] showed that unless such factors as coexisting congenital anomalies or postoperative complications are involved, prognosis of physical development in patients after tracheoesophageal fistula repair is excellent. When nutritional problems occur, a gastrostomy placed during the initial phase of management may prove a very valuable route for feeding. If enteral feedings are precluded, hyperalimentation may be life saving until enteral feedings can be instituted.

SUMMARY

Restoration of esophageal continuity and repair of the tracheoesophageal fistula have resulted in the survival of many neonates but have solved only the primary problem for infants with this anomaly. The associated problems of other congenital anomalies, prematurity, the immediate complications of surgery, nutritional problems, and esophageal dysmotility with its attendant gastroesophageal reflux and stricture formation often have great impact on the quality of the child's life. The long-term assessment and management of these attendant problems provide a continuing challenge to the clinician.

REFERENCES

1. Randolph JG: Esophageal atresia and congenital stenosis, in Welch KJ, Randolph JG, Ravitch MM, (eds): *Pediatric Surgery.* Yearbook Medical Publishers, Chicago, 1986 pp 682–693.
2. Gross RE: Atresia of the esophagus, in *The Surgery of Infancy and Childhood: Its Principles and Techniques.* Philadelphia, WB Saunders Co, 1953, pp 75–102.
3. Waterston DJ: Esophageal atresia: Tracheoesophageal fistula. A study of survival in 218 infants. *Lancet* 1962; 1:819–822.
4. Osimek CD, Cromson RC, Alysworth AS: An epidemiologic study of tracheoesophageal fistula and esophageal atresia in North Carolina. *Teratology* 1982; 25:53–59.
5. Holder TM, et al: Esophageal atresia and tracheoesophageal fistula: A survey of its members by the surgical section of the American Academy of Pediatrics. *Pediatrics* 1964; 34:542.
6. Grosfeld JL, Ballantine TVL: Esophageal atresia and tracheoesophageal fistula: Effect of delayed thoracotomy on survival. *Surgery* 1978; 84:394–402.
7. Touloukian RJ: Long-term results following repair of esophageal atresia by end-to-side anastomosis and ligation of the tracheoesophageal fistula. *J Pediatr Surg* 1981; 16:983–988.
8. McKneally MF, Britton LW, Scott JR, et al: Surgical treatment of congenital esophageal atresia. *Ann Thorac Surg* 1984; 38:606–610.
9. Dudley NE, Phelan PD: Respiratory complication in long-term survivors of esophageal atresia. *Arch Dis Child* 1976; 51:279–282.
10. Strodel WE, Coran AG, Kirsch MM, et al: Esophageal atresia. A 41 year experience. *Arch Surg* 1979; 114:523–527.
11. Jolley SG, Johnson DG, Roberts CC, et al: Patterns of gastroesophageal reflux in children following repair of esophageal atresia and distal tracheoesophageal fistula. *J Pediatr Surg* 1980; 15:857–862.
12. Livaditis A: End-to-end anastomosis in esophageal atresia. A clinical and experimental study. *Scand J Thorac Cardiovasc Surg* 1969 (suppl 2):7 20.
13. Werlin SL, Dodds WJ, Hogan WJ, et al: Esophageal function in esophageal atresia. *Dig Dis Sci* 1981; 26:796–800.
14. Orringer MB, Kirsch MM, Sloan H: Long-term esophageal function following repair of esophageal atresia. *Ann Surg* 1977; 186:436–443.
15. Parker AF, Christie DL, Cahill JL: Incidence and significance of gastroesophageal reflux following repair of esophageal atresia and tracheoesophageal fistula and the need for antireflux procedures. *J Pediatr Surg* 1979; 14:5–8.
16. Fonkalsrud EW: Gastroesophageal fundoplication for reflux following repair of esophageal atresia. Experience with nine patients. *Arch Surg* 1979; 114:48–51.
17. Shepard R, Fenn S, Sieber WK: Evaluation of esophageal function in postoperative esophageal atresia and tracheoesophageal fistula. *Surgery* 1966; 59:608–617.
18. Cohen IT, Greecher CP: Nutritional status following surgical correction of congenital gastrointestinal anomalies. *J Pediatr Surg* 1979; 14:386–389.
19. Andrassy RJ, Patterson RS, Ashley J, et al: Long-term nutritional assessment of patients with esophageal atresia and/or tracheoesophageal fistula. *Pediatr Surg* 1983; 18:431–435.
20. Rickham PP: Infants with esophageal atresia weighing under 3 pounds. *J Pediatr Surg* 1981; 16(suppl 1):595–598.

2 Gastroesophageal Reflux

Harland S. Winter, M.D.

A 14-year-old boy insidiously developed dysphagia at the age of 11 years. At that time, a barium swallow revealed an esophageal stricture, which was dilated without further evaluation. Six months later another dilatation was performed. One year later, his symptoms returned. A third dilatation was successfully completed, and he was referred for further evaluation of esophageal function. He had no previous history of regurgitation in infancy or heartburn during childhood.

The barium swallow radiographic study demonstrated a proximal narrowing. A continuous intraesophageal pH probe study was performed with one probe in the distal esophagus above the gastroesophageal junction and a second probe near the stricture. Prolonged acid clearance time was demonstrated by both probes. The longest episode of acid reflux at the distal probe lasted 11 minutes; however, the proximal probe detected acid for as long as 31 minutes, suggesting that the area of stricture had severe dysmotility. A motility study confirmed a diffuse motility disorder involving the smooth muscle (lower) portion of the body of the esophagus, whereas the lower esophageal sphincter (LES) pressure was normal. Esophageal biopsies cephalad and caudad to the stricture revealed severe, active esophagitis with infiltration of eosinophils. In addition, basal zone hyperplasia was present distal to the stricture.

At this point it was difficult to determine whether the dysmotility caused the reflux esophagitis or if esophagitis resulted in dysmotility. The patient was treated with an H_2 antagonist for 3 months. Following therapy, the esophageal motility returned to normal, and there was no evidence for delayed acid clearance by pH probe study. However, subsequent biopsies of the esophageal mucosa demonstrated active inflammation. Because he remained asymptomatic, he elected to discontinue medical therapy.

DISCUSSION

This case illustrates many of the problems encountered by pediatricians in evaluating reflux. The biopsies suggested that this child had had acid reflux long before clinical symptoms were noted. No exceptional history of colic or vomiting was elicited during infancy, suggesting that pathologic reflux may be "silent" until symptoms of a stricture become evident. The clinician is faced with the difficult problem of determining which clinical criteria reliably predict pathologic reflux.

Pathophysiology

An accurate definition that clearly distinguishes physiologic gastroesophageal reflux from pathologic reflux is difficult to establish. Instinctively, the clinician would expect pathologic reflux to lead to tissue injury or clinical symptoms, whereas physiologic reflux would be tolerated by the individual without evidence for esophageal damage. Physiologic reflux commonly occurs in infants in the first year of life but may also occur in adults.[1] The point at which reflux changes from physiologic to pathologic is unknown, but there is likely a continuum between physiologic and pathologic reflux determined by acid clearance time and the duration of ongoing reflux. The exact etiopathogenesis of esophageal injury is unknown but may be related to a combination of esophageal sphincter dysfunction, abnormal peristalsis, delayed gastric emptying, or inability to adequately neutralize acid.[2] Identifying which of these factors is abnormal in a patient aids in guiding specific therapy.

Clinical Features

The signs and symptoms of gastroesophageal reflux can vary by age and are especially common in young children.[1] In the first year of life vomiting (especially postprandial) is the most common complaint, but irritability or abdominal pain can also be seen. If the regurgitation is severe, failure to thrive may result. Pulmonary symptoms including aspiration and reactive airway disease can also occur.[1] Esophagitis with blood loss can result in hematemesis, melena, and anemia.

In addition to these manifestations, older children, who are better able to verbalize their complaints, can describe heartburn, which may be associated with a bitter taste or water brash, dysphagia, and chest pain.[2] Small amounts of emesis may be found on the pillow or bed sheets, and episodes of regurgitation can occur when the patient is bending over or during valsalva maneuvers.[1] Gastroesophageal reflux may also be associated with rumination, finger clubbing, reactive airway disease, Sandifer's syndrome (contortions of the head and neck), and possibly sudden infant death syndrome.[2] As was demonstrated by this patient, pathologic gastroesophageal reflux can be silent and can be associated with stricture formation.

Diagnosis

An approach to the diagnostic evaluation of reflux is outlined in Table 2–1. First, one must decide when to investigate symptoms. Criteria are listed in Table 2–2. Vomiting or regurgitation alone is not an indication to initiate an evaluation in a child unless symptoms persist beyond 15 months of age. Associating gastroesophageal reflux with symptoms may be difficult.[1–3] Part of the confusion relates to the terminology used to define reflux. An individual who regurgitates gastric contents into the esophagus does not, a priori, have reflux that will result in esophageal injury. In adults, more than three episodes of an intraesophageal pH of less than 4 lasting longer than 5 minutes is considered to be prolonged.[4] In normal infants, two to three episodes of pH less than 4 in 24 hours are common, and episodes of pH less than 4 lasting as long as 10.5 minutes have been noted.[5] In older children, some have

TABLE 2–1.

Evaluation of Reflux

Question	Test(s)
1. Does pathologic reflux exist?	pH probe
2. What is the etiology of the pathologic reflux?	Upper gastrointestinal (GI) series, esophageal motility, technetium 99m scintiscan
3. What are the sequelae of pathologic reflux?	Upper GI series, esophageal biopsy

TABLE 2–2.

Indications for Evaluation of Pathologic Reflux

<15 mo of Age	>15 mo of Age
1. GI blood loss (anemia, hemetemesis, hematochezia)	1. Rumination
2. Recurrent pneumonia	2. Recurrent vomiting
3. Failure to thrive	3. GI blood loss
	4. Recurrent pneumonia
	5. Failure to thrive
	6. Stricture formation

considered an episode of acid reflux that lasts longer than 4 minutes to be abnormal.[6] These differences indicate that large, prospective studies are needed to provide better criteria to define normal and abnormal probes.

Although variation exists among studies regarding the definition of abnormal acid clearance, the pH probe study can quantitate acid clearance time and may identify those children with "pathologic" reflux who may need more extensive evaluation. In contrast, children with "physiologic" reflux have normal acid clearance times. In the patient presented, the pH probe study confirmed pathologic acid reflux. However, other diagnostic studies were needed to determine the cause and sequelae of pathologic reflux.

As part of the initial evaluation of pathologic reflux in children, one should attempt to identify whether an anatomic abnormality such as malrotation, annular pancreas, or duplication is present.[1] These conditions are best assessed by barium swallow and upper GI radiographic series.

The relationship between lower esophageal sphincter pressure and pathologic reflux is controversial. As this case illustrates, children with normal sphincter pressures may develop esophagitis and stricture if the ability of the esophagus to clear acid is impaired. In general, motility studies add little clinical information that affects therapy. Two exceptions to this dictum are children with dysphagia, as in this case, and children who are being evaluated for fundoplication. If surgical intervention is being considered, motility studies are very useful in demonstrating that peristaltic activity is normal. In children with severe motor problems of the esophagus, a fundoplication may enhance the delay in acid clearance and further complicate management. The demonstration that this patient's dysmotility reverted to normal after medical therapy suggests that the esophagitis led to abnormal peristalsis.

The gastric scintiscan may be indicated if delayed gastric emptying or aspiration is suspected. Diabetes mellitus and other disorders such as connective tissue disease affecting smooth muscle activity may be associated with a delay in gastric emptying. Cerebral palsy and other neurologic diseases may cause incoordinated swallowing and aspiration. Because these problems did not relate to this patient, a scintiscan was not performed. Therapeutic intervention for patients with a delay in gastric emptying may include medications that enhance antral contractility such as metoclopramide or domperidone.

Histologic changes may indicate the severity and duration of pathologic reflux that are difficult to assess solely by esophageal function testing or by endoscopic observation alone.[7] Intraepithelial eosinophils in the esophagus, one of the earliest histologic manifestations of gastroesophageal reflux, may be seen alone or in association with other features of esophagitis.[6] However, histologic criteria reported in adults such as basal zone hyperplasia, papillary lengthening, and neutrophilic infiltration may not be present in children.[6] Eosinophils are not specific for acid injury alone and may also be found in other conditions, including alkaline (or bile) reflux or allergic gastroenteritis.[8] Thus, in the appropriate clinical setting, intraepithelial eosinophils are a marker for ongoing reflux and should be considered an early sign of esophagitis. The time needed for intraepithelial eosinophils to appear following injury is not known, but they are rarely found in esophageal biopsies in children less than 1 year of age unless the child has a concomitant esophageal motility disorder.[6] Factors such as duration of reflux and acid clearance time determine the tempo of the injury.

Treatment

A child who does not meet the criteria in Table 2–2 for evaluation, but whose symptoms require intervention, may respond to conservative management (Table 2–3). The prone position with the head elevated minimizes the frequency of reflux.[9] In contrast, those infants with pathologic reflux (delayed acid clearance) frequently require more than conservative therapy. The therapy is guided by determining which pathophysiologic factors may be playing a role in the patients' disease: inability to adequately neutralize acid, low gastroesophageal sphincter pressure, or delayed gastric emptying. Medications such as antacids, H_2 blockers, bethanechol,[10] metoclopramide,[11] and domperidone[12] may be beneficial. If esophagitis exists, H_2 blockers such as cimetidine or ranitidine may be used. Their superiority over antacids has not been demonstrated.

TABLE 2–3.
Conservative Management for Reflux

1. Small, frequent feedings
2. Prone position after eating, with head and chest elevated
3. Thickened feedings
4. Sleeping position: prone, head of bed elevated

Decreased gastroesophageal sphincter pressure and delayed gastric emptying can be treated by metoclopramide, which may increase LES pressure and decrease gastric residual.[11] Domperidone, currently an investigational drug related to metoclopramide, has similar effects on the stomach and esophagus but may not cross the blood-brain barrier. The early experience with domperidone indicates that it may have a lower incidence of CNS side effects than metoclopromide.

SUMMARY

Gastroesophageal reflux in children may be a self-limited or progressive disorder with troublesome sequelae. Fortunately, most children's symptoms resolve early in childhood without lasting problems. However, as this case illustrates, difficulties may develop insidiously without obvious clinical manifestations. Objective evidence of prolonged acid clearance time, mucosal injury, progressive pulmonary dysfunction, or poor growth are important criteria that will identify most children at risk for long-term problems.

REFERENCES

1. Berquist WE: Gastroesophageal reflux in children: A clinical review. *Pediatr Ann* 1982; 11:135–42.
2. Herbst JJ: Gastroesophageal reflux. *J Pediatr* 1981; 98:859–870.
3. Richter JE, Castell DO: Gastroesophageal reflux: Pathogenesis, diagnosis and therapy. *Ann Intern Med* 1982; 97:93–103.
4. Johnson LF, Demeester TR: Twenty-four hour pH monitoring of the distal esophagus. *Am J Gastroenterol* 1974; 62:325.
5. Vandelplas Y, Sacre-Smits L: Continuous 24-hour esophageal pH monitoring in 285 asymptomatic infants 0–15 months old. *J Pediatr Gastroenterol Nutr* 1987; 6:220.
6. Winter HS, Madara JL, Stafford RJ, et al: Intrapithclial cosinophils—a new diagnostic criterion for reflux esophagitis. *Gastroenterology* 1982; 83:118–123.
7. Biller JA, Winter HS, Grand RJ, et al: Are endoscopic changes predictive of histological esophagitis in children? *J Pediatr* 1983; 103:215–218.
8. Tummala V, Barwick KW, Sontag SJ, et al: The significance of intraesophageal eosinophils in the histologic diagnosis of gastroesophageal reflux. *Am J Clin Pathol* 1986; 87:43–48.
9. Orenstein SR, Whitington PF, Orenstein DM: The infant seat as treatment for gastroesophageal reflux. *N Engl J Med* 1983; 309:760.
10. Orenstein SR, Lofton SW, Orenstein DM: Bethanechol for pediatric gastroesophageal reflux: A prospective, blind, controlled study. *J Pediatr Gastroenterol Nutr* 1986; 5:549.
11. Hyams JS, Leichtner AM, Zamett LO, et al: Effect of metoclopramide on prolonged intraesophageal pH testing in infants with gastroesophageal reflux. *J Pediatr Gastroenterol Nutr* 1986; 5:716.
12. Grill BB, Hillemeyer AC, Semeraro LA, et al: Effects of domperidone therapy on symptoms and upper gastrointestinal motility in infants with gastroesophageal reflux. *J Pediatr* 1985; 106:311–316.
13. Randolph J: Experience with the Nissen fundo-publication for the correction of gastroesophageal reflux in infants. *Ann Surg* 1983; 198:579.

3 Achalasia

M. Stephen Murphy, M.B., B.Ch., M.R.C.P.

The patient was a 10-year-old boy who 9 months prior to admission began to complain of food sticking in his throat and then developed recurrent episodes of vomiting. Over the succeeding months he complained of worsening dysphagia, and his appetite progressively decreased. For 3 months he had pain that was localized to the central chest and epigastrium and was unrelated to meals. On closer questioning he was found to have a history of cough for several years, which was especially pronounced during the night.

At the time of admission he was having great difficulty in swallowing solid foods and liquids. He commented that he frequently had froth in his mouth, especially when running or lying down, and he had begun to notice gurgling sounds in his chest. He vomited undigested food many times throughout each day and, on occasion, had found regurgitated food on his pillow after sleeping. During this period of his illness his weight had decreased by 11 lb (5 kg).

He had previously been well, and there was no relevant history of illness among his relatives. His parents described him as a very anxious child and had attributed his symptoms to this in the early stages of his illness.

On physical examination he was cooperative but was distressed and wept frequently. His height and weight were on the 75th and 25th percentiles, respectively. The examination was otherwise unremarkable. His abdomen was soft, nontender, and nondistended, and no masses were palpable. His rectal examination was normal. There were no abnormalities on neurologic examination.

His laboratory evaluation was normal and included a hemoglobin value of 14.4 gm/dl. A chest radiogram was normal, but a barium swallow demonstrated marked dilatation of the esophagus, and smooth tapering to a "beaked" distal esophagus suggestive of achalasia (Fig 3–1). Esophagoscopy demonstrated a slightly capacious esophagus, but no evidence of esophagitis or stricture and the endoscope was passed easily through the lower esophageal sphincter (LES). Manometric studies failed to demonstrate any peristaltic waves in the body of the esophagus, and there was no drop in LES pressure with swallowing. The diagnosis of achalasia was thus confirmed.

He underwent pneumatic dilatation of the LES, and this produced a satisfactory initial result. His dysphagia improved, and within 6 months his weight was close to the 75th percentile. He has had several subsequent exacerbations of symptoms that have been treated with pneumatic dilatation. Both he and his parents are strongly opposed to surgery.

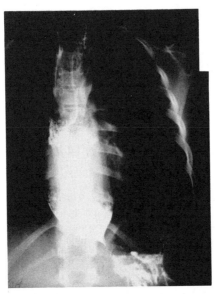

FIG 3–1.
Barium esophagogram showing narrowed
distal esophagus ("beak-like" appearance)
and dilated proximal esophagus.

DISCUSSION

Achalasia is a primary motility disorder of the foregut, which is characterized by an absence of peristalsis in the distal two thirds of the esophagus and a failure of relaxation of LES in response to swallowing.[1] In addition, esophageal emptying is delayed, the resting tension in the LES is often increased, there may be hypertrophy of the circular smooth muscle of the esophageal body, and the esophagus may become greatly dilated.[1]

It is a relatively uncommon condition, occurring in less than 1 in 100,000 individuals per year.[2] Only 5% of cases in a large reported series had symptoms before 14 years of age.[3] Because of the rarity of achalasia in childhood, it may not be considered in the differential diagnosis of dysphagia and consequently undue delay in diagnosis or inappropriate treatment may occur.

Pathophysiology

The etiology of achalasia is unknown. The best established histopathologic finding is a marked deficiency or absence of ganglion cells in the esophageal myenteric plexus, although this finding is not uniform.[4] Neuromuscular pathologic changes have also been demonstrated at various levels from the brain stem to the esophageal smooth muscle cells. Loss of cells in the dorsal motor nucleus of the vagus and the caudal portion of the nucleus ambiguous have been reported, but the number of patients studied were small, and the significance of these findings is uncertain.[5] The abnormalities seen in the smooth muscle cells are nonspecific, and electron microscopic examination has revealed ultrastructural changes that are consistent with denervation rather than a primary muscle disorder.[6]

Although there is still uncertainty with regard to the site and nature of the primary lesion, there is increasing evidence that the physiologic abnormalities in achalasia may be explained by the absence or impaired function of nonadrenergic, noncholinergic inhibitory nerve fibers supplying the esophagus.[1] These fibers, for which the inhibitory neurotransmitter has not yet been identified, are known to have a role in both contraction of esophageal body circular muscle fibers and relaxation of the LES.[1] Smith[4] has demonstrated an absence of a subgroup of argyrophilic myenteric ganglion cells in achalasia, and it has been speculated that these argyrophilic cells are the ganglion cells of the nonadrenergic noncholinergic inhibitory system.[1]

The contribution of genetic factors to achalasia is unclear. There are occasional reports of achalasia in siblings,[7] but these are very much the exception. Although environmental factors might explain the occurrence of familial cases, a genetic component is supported by the occurrence of achalasia in association with familial glucocorticoid deficiency and alacrima.[8]

Clinical Features

The clinical presentation in childhood is similar to that in adults (Table 3–1),[3, 9, 10] although younger children may present with severe failure to thrive as the prominent feature.[11] Boys and girls are affected in approximately equal numbers. The onset of symptoms may occur at any age, although cases presenting in early infancy are exceptional.[12] There may be a delay of several years from onset to diagnosis,[9] and, indeed, symptoms are often insidious and intermittent in the early stages of the disease.[3]

TABLE 3–1.
Clinical Features of Achalasia*

Dysphagia	85%
Regurgitation of undigested food	80%
Failure of growth	73%
Substernal chest pain	50%
Pulmonary symptons (asthma, pneumonia, chronic bronchitis, chronic productive cough)	27%

*Adapted from Moersch,[3] Azizkhan et al.,[9] and Lemmer et al.[10]

The commonest presenting symptoms in children are regurgitation and dysphagia. As in this case, regurgitation is often described as vomiting; the food has an undigested appearance, and food particles on the child's pillow in the morning may provide a clue to diagnosis.[3] Affected children are noted to eat more slowly than other family members. Liquids usually cause as much swallowing difficulty as solids, although some children find that the passage of solid food can be facilitated by drinking copious fluids.[3] Dysphagia may fluctuate greatly in severity even during the course of a single meal. Most children complain of food lodging under the lower end of the sternum, but in others the discomfort is felt in the throat; some undiagnosed cases have undergone tonsillectomy in an attempt to relieve this symptom.[3] Retrosternal pain is not uncommon and may occasionally be the presenting complaint.[9] The pain is sometimes severe, and it may not be related to meals.[10] As a consequence of poor nutritional intake, weight loss may occur, and impaired growth is common.[9]

Patients with achalasia may suffer from recurrent pulmonary infections as a result of aspiration of esophageal contents, and this complication appears to be more frequent and more severe in children.[11] Nocturnal cough is often reported, and aspiration may occur mostly during sleep. In some children chronic pulmonary symptoms are the presenting feature.[13]

Diagnosis

The radiologic features in achalasia are often highly suggestive of the condition.[14] A plain chest radiograph may demonstrate mediastinal widening with a prominent shadow to the right of the cardiac silhouette. This is due to the dilated esophagus, and a lateral view shows that the shadow is in the posterior mediastinum. Chest radiography may also reveal an air-fluid level within the esophagus, the absence of a gastric air bubble, and the presence of secondary changes of pulmonary disease. A barium swallow may merely show poorly coordinated peristalsis and a slight delay in the passage of barium through the LES, or, as in this case, there may be marked dilatation of the esophagus with evidence of retained food, absence of peristalsis, uncoordinated esophageal contractions, and failure of LES relaxation. The dilated esophagus tapers smoothly at its distal end resulting in a highly characteristic "beaked" appearance.

Esophageal manometry provides the definitive diagnosis.[1] It confirms the absence of peristalsis, the failure of LES relaxation during swallowing, and perhaps also the presence of raised LES pressure. Administration of methacholine, which does not alter peristalsis in the normal esophagus, markedly worsens the disordered motility pattern of achalasia and so may be helpful diagnostically.[10]

Upper gastrointestinal (GI) endoscopy is routinely done and can rule out other causes of esophageal obstruction such as severe esophagitis and stricture. Endoscopy may demonstrate a dilated esophagus with retained food and secretions.

The combination of food refusal, severe weight loss, and "vomiting" has on occasion led to a mistaken diagnosis of anorexia nervosa,[16] and the patient presented here was believed to have symptoms related to psychologic factors in the early stages of his illness. Other disorders must also be considered in the differential diagnosis. Although achalasia has been reported in the neonate,[12] transient "cardiospasm" may also occur, which is indistinguishable radiologically but which recovers within a few days.[17] Achalasia must be distinguished from other causes of esophageal obstruction in childhood, including strictures, vascular rings, and foreign bodies, and other disorders associated with esophageal dysmotility, such as familial dysautonomia, scleroderma, dermatomyositis, polymyositis, and idiopathic intestinal pseudobstruction. The combination of endoscopic, radiologic, and manometric studies will differentiate achalasia from these conditions.[6] Very rarely diffuse esophageal spasm may occur in childhood,[18] and because intermediate forms of this disorder exist, difficulty could be encountered in distinguishing this condition from achalasia.[1]

Treatment

Even in adult patients with achalasia no consensus has been achieved with regard to the optimal approach to treatment. Partial destruction of the LES is often successful in improving esophageal emptying and so relieving the symptoms of the disease. This may be done surgically or by forcibly dilating the sphincter. The usual surgical procedure used is a modification of Heller's cardiomyotomy, in which the LES muscle is divided down to the mucosa.[10] Temporary relief may be obtained by the passage of a dilator through the cardia. For lasting results forceful dilatation of the LES is needed, and this may be done by pneumatic dilatation using a bag of fixed diameter filled with air under pressure.[19] Because of the difficulties inherent in measuring the success of either method, and because different centers use different modifications of the techniques, there is no compelling evidence in favor of either method. The success rate with pneumatic dilatation may be somewhat less than with esophagomyotomy, and a small percentage of patients suffer an esophageal perforation. However, for many patients dilatation avoids the need for surgery, and the incidence of posttreatment reflux esophagitis and stricture formation appears to be lower than is seen following esophagomyotomy.[20] For this reason it may be argued that surgery should be reserved for those who have not responded satisfactorily to a trial of dilatation.[20]

There is even greater uncertainty about the optimal management of achalasia in children. Many have favored the use of a modified Heller's myotomy, with or without a combined antireflux procedure.[10, 11] Experience in the use of pneumatic dilatation in children is limited, and because the success rate appears less than with surgery, it has been argued that early esophagomyotomy is to be preferred.[10] However, Azizkhan et al.[9] and, more recently, Nakayama et al.[21] have reviewed their experience with both methods over 20-year periods and have recommended an initial trial of pneumatic dilatation in children more than 9 years of age. In those who fail to respond or relapse quickly, they favor proceeding to surgery rather than repeating the dilatation.

In recent years pharmacologic agents that might improve esophageal emptying and eliminate the need for dilatation or esophagomyotomy have been sought. Both isosorbide dinitrate and the calcium channel blocking agent nifedipine can be effective in relieving dysphagia, and though isosorbide dinitrate is not well tolerated because of side effects, nifedipine may have a role in the management of selected patients or in those awaiting a definitive procedure.[22]

Treatment for achalasia is palliative, and even after relief of the distal obstruction, some degree of esophageal stasis usually persists. Although the association has been disputed, there is a widely held view that achalasia is associated with the later development of esophageal carcinoma, and this complication has even been reported many years after an apparently successful esophagomyotomy.[23] Information about this long-term outlook for children with achalasia is very limited. A long-term follow up study of adults for periods of between 9 months and 25 years (mean 8.3 years) following esophagomyotomy found no evidence that the result of the operation tended to deteriorate with time.[24] There was, however, a strong association between poor outcome and a long history of symptoms before surgery, and most surgeons agree that results in patients with a greatly dilated esophagus are less satisfactory.[19] Early diagnosis of achalasia in childhood may be important, therefore, not only in preventing the immediate morbidity associated with the condition but also in improving the long-term prognosis.

SUMMARY

Achalasia, an important cause of regurgitation and dysphagia in children, is caused by disordered motility of the distal two thirds of the esophagus and a failure of relaxation of the LES in response to swallowing. The diagnosis is suspected clinically and radiographically and confirmed by manometric testing. Many patients improve with dilatation therapy, with surgical intervention reserved for those who fail this treatment.

REFERENCES

1. Christensen J: Foregut motility, in Baron JH, Moody FG (eds): *Gastroenterology, Foregut.* New York, Butterworths, 1981, vol 1, pp 241–271.
2. Roth JLA: Achalasia and other motor disorders of the esophagus, in Bockus HL (ed): *Gastroenterology.* Philadelphia, WB Saunders Co, pp 191–246. 1974.
3. Moersch HJ: Cardiospasm in infancy and childhood. *Am J Dis Child* 1920; 38:294–298.
4. Smith B: Achalasia of the cardia, in Smith B (ed): *The Neuropathology of the Alimentary Tract.* London, Edward Arnold, pp 25–34. 1972.
5. Casella RR, Brown AL, Sayre GP, et al: Achalasia of the esophagus: Pathologic and etiologic considerations. *Ann Surg* 1946; 160:474–486.
6. Vantrappen G, Helemans J: Esophageal motility disorders, in van der Reis L (ed): *The Oesophagus. Frontiers of Gastrointestinal Research.* Basel, S. Karger AG, 1978, pp 49–75.
7. Stoddard CJ, Johnson AG: Achalasia in siblings. *Br J Surg* 1982; 69:84–85.
8. Allgrove J, Clayden GS, Grant DB: Familial glucocorticoid deficiency with achalasia of the cardia and deficient tear production. *Lancet* 1978; 1:1284–1286.
9. Azizkhan RG, Tapper D, Eraklis A: Achalasia in childhood: A 20 year experience. *J Pediatr Surg* 1980; 15:452–456.
10. Lemmer JH, Coran AG, Wesley JR, et al: Achalasia in children: Treatment by anterior esophageal myotomy (modified Heller operation). *J Pediatr Surg* 1985; 20:333–338.

11. Ballantine TVN, Fitzgerald JF, Grosfeld JL: Transabdominal esophagomyotomy for achalasia in children. *J Pediatr Surg* 1980; 15:457–461.
12. Asch MJ, Liebman W, Lachman RS, et al: Esophageal achalasia: Diagnosis and cardiomyotomy in a newborn infant. *J Pediatr Surg* 1974; 9:911–912.
13. Schultz EH: Achalasia in children as a cause of recurrent pulmonary disease. *J Pediatr* 1961; 59:522–528.
14. McLellan M, Clarke EA: Radiological case of the month. Achalasia. *Am J Dis Child* 1986; 140:813–814.
15. Kramer P, Ingelfinger FJ: Esophageal sensitivity to mecholyl in cardiospasm. *Gastroenterology* 1951; 19:242–253.
16. Smith MS, Christie DL: An adolescent with vomiting and weight loss. *J Adolesc Health Care* 1984; 5:279–282.
17. Sorsdahl OA, Gay BB: Achalasia of the esophagus in childhood. *Am J Dis Child* 1965; 109:141–146.
18. Fontan JP, Heldt GP, Heyman MB, et al: Esophageal spasm associated with apnea and bradycardia in an infant. *Pediatrics* 1984; 73:52–55.
19. Vantrappen G, Hellemans J: Treatment of achalasia and related motor disorders. *Gastroenterology* 1980; 79:144–154.
20. Vantrappen G, Janssens J: To dilate or to operate? That is the question. *Gut* 1983; 24:1013–1019.
21. Nakayama DK, Shorter NA, Boyle JT, et al: Pneumatic dilatation and operative treatment of achalasia in children. *J Pediatr Surg* 1987; 22:619–622.
22. Maksimak M, Perlmutter DH, Winter HG: The use of nifedipine for the treatment of achalasia in children. *J Pediatr Gastroenterol Nutr* 1986; 5:883–886.
23. Heiss FW, Tarshis A, Ellis FH: Carcinoma associated with achalasia. Occurrence 23 years after esophagostomy. *Dig Dis Sci* 1984; 29:1066–1069.
24. Goulbourne IA, Walbaum PR: Long term results of Heller's operation for achalasia. *J R Coll Surg Edinb* 1985; 30:101–103.

PART TWO

The Stomach and Intestine

4 Upper Gastrointestinal Tract Bleeding

John D. Snyder, M.D.

A 14-year-old girl had been perfectly well until 2 days before admission when she developed a fever of 38.0°C, nausea, abdominal cramps, and diarrhea. The day before admission she developed nonbilious vomiting without rash, abdominal distention, or urinary tract complaints. On the day of admission she had resolution of her fever, abdominal pain, and diarrhea but vomited bright red blood and was brought to the emergency room. Further questioning revealed that she had no prior history of peptic disease, esophagitis, nasal congestion or irritation, bleeding problems, liver disease, melena, hematochezia, alcohol or aspirin ingestion, and no family history of ulcer disease or vascular malformations.

On physical examination she was found to be at the 50th percentile for height and weight. She was tachycardic and had a 20 mm Hg drop in her blood pressure when moved from supine to a sitting position. She was anicteric, pale, and had no skin lesions. Her head, ear, eye, nose, and throat; pulmonary; and cardiac examination results were normal. Her abdomen was soft, mildly tender in the epigastrium, and without masses or hepatosplenomegaly. Dark brown, Hematest-positive stool but no other abnormalities were found on rectal examination. The remainder of the examination was unremarkable. Initial laboratory values included hemaglobin 12.2 mg/dl, and normal peripheral smear, white blood cell count, platelet count, urinalysis, liver function tests, prothrombin time, and partial thromboplastin time.

While she was being evaluated in the emergency room, she vomited 150 ml of bright red blood and gastric fluid. A large-bore intravenous (IV) line was started, and she was given 10 mg of vitamin K intravenously. Two liters of Ringer's lactate was given with resolution of her postural hypotension; her repeat hemoglobin value was 9.5 mg/dl. After the patient was stabilized, an esophagogastroduodenoscopy was performed that revealed two 1-cm long superficial tears of the distal esophageal mucosa; no other lesions were identified. She had no further bleeding from her Mallory-Weiss tears and was discharged on the following day.

DISCUSSION

Upper gastrointestinal (GI) bleeding refers to blood loss from a site proximal to the ligament of Treitz. The list of diagnostic possibilities is extensive and can vary

TABLE 4–1.

Diagnostic Possibilities for Upper Gastrointestinal Bleeding in Children by Age

Age	Condition
Neonates and infants	Hemorrhagic disease of the newborn
	Swallowed maternal blood
	Hemorrhagic gastritis
Children	Mallory-Weiss tear
	Esophageal varices
All ages	Swallowed blood
	Esophagitis
	Stress ulcer
	Peptic disease
	Foreign body
	Vascular malformation
	Gastropancreatic duplication
	Gastritis

according to the age of the patient (Table 4–1).[1-3] The incidence of the various etiologies also varies by age, although precise determination of incidence is difficult, given the paucity of studies that quantify the causes of upper GI tract bleeding in the pediatric age group. The incidence of peptic ulcer disease appears to be rising, although this may actually reflect the increased use of fiberoptic endoscopy, which permits more accurate diagnosis of upper GI mucosal lesions.[4] As more mucosal lesions are found, the percentage of cases caused by esophageal varices has fallen.[4]

Clinical Features

The history and physical examination of the child with upper GI bleeding can greatly aid in limiting the diagnostic possibilities. Hematemesis almost always localizes the lesion to a site above the ligament of Treitz. Exceptions to this generalization include high jejunal obstructions, enterogastric fistula, and gastrocolic fistulas.[5] The effortless regurgitation of bright red blood suggests bleeding from esophageal varices. Melanotic stools can be seen with either upper or lower GI bleeding, but bright red or dark red blood in the stools is much more likely to be caused by a distal small intestinal or colonic lesion.[5] However, rapid upper GI bleeding from esophageal varices (see Chapter 44) or an ulcer eroding into an artery can yield bright red blood per rectum. Streaking of blood on the stools indicates an anal or rectal mucosal lesion.

Careful questioning about epistaxis, coughing, hemoptysis, or genitourinary symptoms is potentially very helpful in identifying the source of bleeding. A history of vomiting before the onset of bleeding raises the possibility of a Mallory-Weiss tear, as seen in this case. Evidence for unusual stresses, including trauma, burns or CNS disease, should be sought because they can predispose to secondary ulcers (see Chapter 5); a family history of peptic ulcer disease is often found. Dizziness or loss of consciousness can be critical signs of significant blood loss.

A careful history of medication or drug use, especially for nonsteroidal anti-inflammatory agents, steroids, and alcohol, should always be obtained. These drugs have all been associated with the development of ulcers.[6] The dietary history is important to obtain since red stools can be caused by food coloring, beets, Kool-Aid, gelatin dessert, and antibiotic syrups, whereas black stools can be caused by iron preparations, bismuth subsalicylate (Pepto-Bismol), and spinach.[3]

The physical examination begins with careful attention to the vital signs. Postural changes in pulse and blood pressure indicate significant volume depletion, as can tachycardia and hypotension. After examination of the skin, the nasopharynx should be carefully examined to look for a source of bleeding. The examiner should also seek signs of portal hypertension, including splenomegaly and ascites, as well as jaundice and spider nevi. The rectal examination is an essential part of the evaluation.

Diagnosis

The first step in evaluating a patient with suspected GI blood loss is to document that the patient has bled. Since several foods and medicines can make the stools or emesis red or black, the presence of heme should be confirmed. Stools may be tested with either Hemoccult or Hematest methods.[7] Gastric fluid may interfere with the accuracy of these tests, so emesis may be tested with the new Gastroccult (Smith Klein Corporation) slide test.[8] In neonates an Apt test should be performed to determine whether the blood is maternal in origin.

The peak age of onset varies for the different etiologies listed (see Table 4–1), but age alone cannot exclude the possibility that a specific condition is the cause of bleeding.[3] An approach to evaluation of upper GI bleeding is found in Table 4–2. The most important of the initial diagnostic tests is nasogastric intubation; detection of blood usually indicates that the site of bleeding is proximal to the ligament of Treitz, although irritation from passage of the tube itself may cause a small amount of bleeding. The absence of blood does not completely rule out an upper GI bleeding source but essentially eliminates the possibility of an active ongoing hemorrhage. Several laboratory tests may be of help, including a complete blood count, reticulocyte count, peripheral smear, coagulation studies, liver function tests, and a urinalysis.

The advent of fiberoptic endoscopy permits the diagnosis of many more cases of upper GI bleeding, but the importance of endoscopy in upper GI bleeding is controversial. Initially, endoscopy to identify the source of bleeding was thought to direct and improve therapy and prognosis.[9] However, numerous studies have documented that the mortality rate, number of transfusions, need for surgery, and duration of hospitalization are not improved by emergency endoscopy.[9, 10] This lack of benefit is attributed to the fact that the great majority of patients with upper GI bleeding stabilize with conservative medical management.[9] In one series in adults, 94% of patients stabilized with conservative management, and rebleeding occurred in only 24%.[10] No similar data are available in children, but our clinical experience indicates that comparable or better results are seen.

Our policy is to observe and support a child who is hemodynamically stable, who has no signs of chronic illness, and who is not having active, ongoing bleeding. If the child has lost enough blood to have unstable vital signs or has evidence for chronic liver disease, an endoscopy is done after initial efforts at stabilization have been made. When endoscopy is performed, preparations are made to undertake sclerotherapy of varices or bipolar electrocautery of a bleeding ulcer if they are present. Endoscopy can also be helpful in directing therapy if a visible vessel in an ulcer crater is found indicating an increased risk of bleeding recurrence.[11] If electrocautery is not successful, the endoscopist's findings can guide the surgeon's intervention.

Radiographic contrast studies are of little benefit in the setting of an acute upper GI bleed. However, an abdominal flat plate radiograph can demonstrate obstruction that could cause more distal intestinal bleeding. An ultrasound can be helpful in evaluating the liver and its vascular supply in a patient suspected of having portal hypertension. Angiography or radiolabeled red blood cell (RBC) scans are rarely required for diagnosis in an upper GI bleed but can be helpful if the lesion is beyond the endoscopist's reach.

Treatment

The treatment is obviously dependent on the nature and severity of the bleeding site. General guidelines for acute management are included in Table 4–3. If bleeding is severe, the first efforts are directed at acute stabilization of the patient. The patient is placed in a semisitting position with legs elevated and given 5 to 10 mg of vitamin K intravenously as soon as the initial laboratory tests are obtained. Volume replacement, if required, is given as normal saline or Ringer's lactate until blood products are available.

Gastric lavage is instituted using saline, although the ability of lavage to stop bleeding has never been clearly documented.[12] Lavage can be helpful in determining the rate of continuing bleeding and should be done with room temperature saline, which is as effective as iced saline.[13] Although hypothermia may reduce gastric blood flow, recent studies suggest that coagulation is impaired,[14] and iced solutions can cause hypothermia in small children. No data are available to support the use of vasoconstrictors or antacids in the gastric lavage.

Infusion of packed RBCs, whole blood, and platelets, if indicated, are used to maintain the hemodynamic equilibrium. If these methods are not successful in con-

TABLE 4–2.

Initial Evaluation of Hematemesis or Melena

History and physical examination
Nasogastric intubation
Initial laboratory tests
    Stool guaiac
    Serial hematocrits (if bleeding continues)
    Blood urea nitrogen value, serum creatinine
    Prothrombin and partial thromboplastin times,
      platelet count
    Apt test (if neonate)

TABLE 4–3.
Management of Upper Gastrointestinal Bleeding

Initial assessment
History and physical examination
Laboratory determinations (see Table 4–2)
Acute stabilization (concurrent with assessment)
Semi-sitting position
IV vitamin K (5–10 mg)
Volume replacement (normal saline or Ringer's lactate, followed by blood products)
Saline lavage
IV cimetidine
Continued bleeding
Continued infusion of blood products
IV vasopressin (0.1–0.4 units/1.73 m²/min)
Interventional endoscopy
Sclerotherapy
Electrocautery
Angiography with selective embolization
Balloon tamponade
Surgery

trolling the bleeding, interventional endoscopy is undertaken to determine the cause. The endoscopist should be prepared to do electrocautery of a bleeding ulcer or sclerotherapy of esophageal varices if they are found.

If bleeding persists, a continuous IV infusion of vasopressin (0.1–0.4 units/1.73 m²/minute or a bolus of 20–40 units/1.73 m²) is used to try to control the bleeding. Intravenous vasopressin has been found to be as effective as intrarterial vasopressin and is the method of choice because of fewer severe side effects.[15]

Angiography can also be considered to identify the upper GI bleeding site and selective infusion of vasopressin or embolization with an absorbable gelatin sponge (Gelfoam) can be undertaken.[16] Balloon tamponade of esophageal varices has been associated with high morbidity and mortality and is being supplanted by the more successful use of endoscopic sclerotherapy.[7] If the bleeding continues despite these measures, surgical intervention is required.

When the bleeding has stopped, antacids or cimetidine should be started. Antacids have been shown to be particularly helpful in preventing stress ulcers in an intensive care unit setting and should be titrated to keep the pH above 5.0.[17]

Prognosis

The prognosis depends on the nature and severity of the underlying illness. Fortunately, upper GI bleeding in most children can be controlled in the acute setting. Even bleeding from esophageal varices in children is likely to stop spontaneously.[14]

Mortality in children is related to an initial hemoglobin value of less than 7 mg/dl, a transfusion requirement of more than 85 ml/kg of blood without surgical intervention, the presence of a coagulation disorder, or the coexistence of another life-threatening disease.[1]

SUMMARY

Upper GI bleeding in children, defined as bleeding from a location above the ligament of Treitz, can be caused by a wide variety of lesions (see Table 4–1). The diagnostic evaluation is greatly aided by a careful history and physical examination and should always include passage of a nasogastric tube (see Table 4–2). The advent of fiberoptic endoscopy has greatly improved the ability to identify the bleeding site. The management depends on the cause and severity of the bleeding, but general guidelines for assessment and management can be applied to each patient (see Table 4–3).

REFERENCES

1. Cox K, Ament ME: Upper gastrointestinal bleeding in children and adolescents. *Pediatrics* 1979; 63:408–413.
2. Oldham KT, Lobe TE: Gastrointestinal hemorrhage in children: A pragmatic update. *Pediatr Clin North Am* 1985; 32:1247–1263.
3. Roy CC, Morin CL, Weber AM: Gastrointestinal emergency problems in pediatric practice. *Clin Gastroenterol* 1981; 10:225–254.
4. Christie DL, Ament ME: Upper gastrointestinal fiberoptic endoscopy in pediatric patients. *Gastroenterology* 1977; 72:1244–1248.
5. Bynum TE: Axioms on gastrointestinal bleeding. *Hosp Pract* 1977; 12:52–69.
6. Silverstein FE, Feld AD, Gilbert DA: Upper gastrointestinal tract bleeding: Predisposing factors, diagnose and therapy. *Arch Intern Med* 1981; 141:322–327.
7. Hyams JS, Leichtner AM, Schwartz AN: Recent advances in diagnosis and treatment of gastrointestinal hemorrhage in infants and children. *J Pediatr* 1985; 106:1–9.
8. Rosenthal P, Thompson J, Singh M: Detection of occult blood in gastric juice. *J Clin Gastroenterol* 1984; 6:119.
9. Conn HO: To scope or not to scope. *N Engl J Med* 1981; 304:967–969.
10. Peterson WL, Barnett CC, Smith HJ, et al: Routine early endoscopy in upper-gastrointestinal-bleeding: A randomized, controlled trial. *N Engl J Med* 1981; 304:925–929.
11. Storey DW, Bown SG, Swain CP, et al: Endoscopic prediction of recurrent bleeding in peptic ulcers. *N Engl J Med* 1981; 305:915.
12. Gilbert DA, Saunders DR, Peoples J: Failure of iced saline lavage to suppress hemorrhage from experimental bleeding ulcers. *Gastroenterology* 1979; 76:1138A.
13. Ponsky JL, Hoffman M, Swayngin DS: Saline irrigation in gastric hemorrhage: The effect of temperature. *J Surg Res* 1980; 28:204–205.
14. Waterman NG, Walker JL: The effect of gastric cooling on hemostasis. *Surg Gynecol Obstet* 1973; 137:80–82.
15. Johnson WC, Widrich WC, Ansell JE, et al: Control of bleeding varices by vasopressin: A prospective randomized study. *Ann Surg* 1977; 186:369.

16. Filston HL, Jackson DC, Johnsrude IS: Arteriographic embolization for control of recurrent severe gastric hemorrhage in a 10-year-old boy. *J Pediatr Surg* 1981; 14:276.
17. Hastings RL, Skillman JJ, Bushnell LS, et al: Antacid titration in the prevention of acute gastrointestinal bleeding: A controlled randomized trial in 100 critically ill patients. *N Engl J Med* 1978; 298:1041–1045.

5   Peptic Ulcer Disease in Children

Barry Z. Hirsch, M.D.

A 17-year-old previously healthy girl presented to the emergency room with a 2-week history of dull, continuous epigastric pain and anorexia. The pain was worse when supine, frequently awakened her at night, and was not associated with meals or weight loss. Her only medication was an oral contraceptive, and she denied use of aspirin, corticosteroids, or alcohol but did smoke a fourth of a pack of cigarettes per day and smoked marijuana several times per week. Her past medical history was significant for an appendectomy at age 11 years and two suicide attempts at age 14 years. The family history was positive for peptic ulcer disease (PUD) in the maternal grandmother. On physical examination she was a well-appearing, cooperative adolescent who had a very flat affect. Her vital signs were normal; she weighed 140.2 lb (63.6 kg). The head, ear, eye, nose, and throat; chest; and cardiovascular examination results were within normal limits. The abdominal examination revealed subxiphoid tenderness without rebound or costovertebral discomfort; bowel sounds were normal in pitch and frequency. There were no masses or hepatosplenomegaly. Rectal examination revealed no anal lesions, and guaiac-positive brown stool was present in the vault. The pelvic examination findings were normal. Laboratory evaluation revealed a hemoglobin value of 13 mg/dl, a normal white blood cell count, platelet count, erythrocyte sedimentation rate, urinalysis, alanine aminotransferase (ALT), aspartate aminotransferase (AST), alkaline phosphatase, amylase, and electrolyte values. Cultures from the throat, rectum, and cervix were negative. A presumptive diagnosis of peptic ulcer disease was made, and she was started on a regimen of 15 ml of Mylanta 30 minutes before meals and at bedtime. The patient was not seen again until 8 months later when she presented with epigastric pain and hematemesis and admitted to noncompliance with her medications. A nasogastric tube was passed, and guaiac-positive coffee ground material was aspirated. A repeat complete blood count revealed a stable hematocrit value and mean corpuscular volume. An esophagogastroduodenoscopy revealed a single 5-ml bulbar duodenal ulcer (Fig 5–1). The patient did well on a 6-week course of ranitidine.

DISCUSSION

Peptic ulcer disease refers to one or more circumscribed areas of mucosal erosion

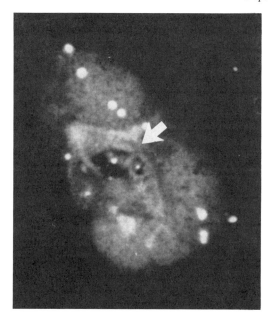

FIG 5–1.
Endoscopic view of ulcer crater
(arrow).

involving the esophagus, stomach, or small intestine that can vary in depth from superficial to clear perforation of the bowel wall.[1, 2] The lesions are characterized by their size, depth, location, healing stage, and etiology.[2]

The true incidence of PUD in children is unknown. A recent review reported an incidence of 4.4 cases per 10,000 inpatient admissions.[1] The rising incidence of PUD in children is probably influenced by the increasing utilization of endoscopic evaluations in the pediatric population.

Boys have a much higher incidence of PUD than do girls.[2] When all types of ulcers are grouped together, boys outnumber girls 2:1. When considering primary ulcers alone or ulcers in children more than 12 years of age, the incidence is closer to 3:1.[2]

Pathogenesis

Little is known about the etiology of peptic ulcers, which have traditionally been classified as either primary or secondary. The two groups appear to have a different epidemiology, clinical presentation, and course.[3] However, this classification may be too broad since each category encompasses different types of PUD, each with its own characteristics.

Primary peptic ulcers are defined as those that occur in patients without known predisposing illnesses or medications.[2] Primary ulcers are much more common than secondary ones in older children and adults but are rarely seen in young children.[1] By adolescence the ratio of primary to secondary ulcers is 4:1.[2] A similar relationship applies to the location of the ulcers. Gastric ulcers are much more common in the younger age groups; however, by 6 to 18 years of age duodenal ulcers are almost five times more common.[3]

Peptic ulcers are located in areas of the alimentary tract exposed to pepsin and hydrochloric acid (HCl), and there is much supporting evidence that at least some primary ulcers are a consequence of the action of these compounds.[5] However, there is great overlap in the basal and maximal acid output of children with ulcers and normal children, indicating that other factors must be involved.[4, 5] The strongest evidence available to support a role for acid and pepsinogen is the response of patients to medication that either neutralizes or prevents the secretion of acid.

More recent work has focused less on the action of pepsin and HCl and more on the importance of the integrity of the mucosal mucous-bicarbonate barrier that maintains an H^+ gradient between lumen and tissue.[5] Ulcerogenic agents can cause alterations in this barrier, including changes in the luminal electrolyte concentrations, electrical potential difference, gastric content of histamine, and gastric blood flow.[6] Prostaglandins appear to play a key role in mucosal defense because they stimulate mucous and alkali secretion, and their production appears to be impaired in PUD patients.[5]

Several other factors have been hypothesized to play a role in PUD, including personality traits and psychologic stresses.[2, 5] Studies have attempted to characterize an ulcer personality in children consisting primarily of unexpressed hostility related to bereavement, separation, or inadequacy.[2, 5] The evidence supporting these theories is inconclusive at this point. The role of diet is also controversial. At present there is no rational basis for eliminating any aspect of the diet except alcohol.[3] Smoking, however, has been shown not only to increase the incidence of PUD but to decrease the response to medication and increase the relapse rate.[7]

There may also be a genetic component to PUD because monozygotic twins have a 50% concordance rate, with the ulcers occurring in identical sites.[2] Family history is positive in 26% to 70% of affected children vs. 5% to 15% in controls.[2] Attempts at identifying an HLA marker for PUD have been unrewarding; however, there is a known association between blood type O and duodenal ulcers.[2]

Secondary ulcers occur in patients with an underlying illness or who are on medications that can cause PUD.[8] They are also known as stress ulcers and appear to be more frequent in patients who have sustained serious trauma, severe burns, or who have intracranial disease. Boys and girls are affected equally, and the rate of occurrence in the stomach and duodenum is similar.[5]

The only medications associated with PUD are the nonsteroidal anti-inflammatory agents and corticosteroids.[5] There has been much debate about the link between corticosteroids and ulcers, and it is generally agreed that the risk becomes significant only when a cumulative dose of greater than 1 gm is used.[9]

One of the newest factors considered in the etiology of ulcers is *Campylobacter pylori*. This organism has been isolated from patients with gastritis and associated gastric or duodenal ulcers and is also often found in patients with PUD resistant to therapy.[10] The organism appears to be sensitive to bismuth subsalicylate (Pepto-Bismol, Denol) as well as a number of antibiotics.[10] Although *C. pylori* has been reported in association with ulcer disease in children, the true incidence is not known.[11] At this point it is unclear what role, if any, this organism plays in the etiology of PUD.[10]

Clinical Features

Classically, ulcer pain in adults presents as a burning or gnawing sensation in the epigastrium, usually in the fasting state, and is often improved by eating. However, this presentation is neither sensitive nor specific in diagnosing PUD in children.[8, 12] In fact, infants and children are much more likely to present with vomiting, and pain, if present, is often atypical.[8] A combination of factors that have proved helpful in predicting which children will have PUD includes epigastric pain, pain related to the intake of food, vomiting, melena, and a positive family history.[12] In young children PUD is more likely to present as a catastrophic illness with vomiting, abdominal distention, and perforation.[1]

Diagnosis

The evaluation of patients with suspected PUD should begin with a thorough consideration of other diagnostic possibilities. Since there are no pathognomonic points in the history or physical examination, the physician is often faced with an enormous differential diagnosis, including many of the causes of abdominal pain, vomiting, and occult blood in the stools. All patients should receive a complete blood cell count to document a stable hematocrit. A liver profile as well as serum amylase may also be drawn since diseases of the biliary tract can cause similar symptoms. Other components of the evaluation should be individualized based on the patient's symptoms.

The two most important tools in the diagnosis of PUD are the upper gastrointestinal (GI) contrast study and esophagogastroduodenoscopy (EGD). The upper GI study can detect 25% to 50% of gastric ulcers and 50% to 89% of duodenal ulcers compared with those found at endoscopy.[13, 14]

Patients with characteristic histories and physical examinations who do not appear severely compromised by their symptoms often receive a therapeutic trial of medication before an extensive workup is begun. If a patient does not improve or his or her symptoms worsen, further diagnostic evaluation is indicated.

Treatment

The treatment of PUD is directed toward protecting the ulcerated mucosal barrier. The categories of medical therapy include antacids, H_2 antagonists, and coating agents (Table 5-1).

Oral antacids have been shown to be as efficacious as other forms of therapy for PUD, are inexpensive, and have a long record of safety. Their major disadvantage is noncompliance secondary to their relative unpalatability and the need to take seven doses daily. They are primarily composed of magnesium or aluminum hydroxide. Magnesium has the advantage of rapid neutralization of acid but has the unfortunate side effect of causing diarrhea.[15] Aluminum-containing agents can cause constipation and are often used in an alternating regimen with magnesium-containing antacids to maintain a normal stooling rate. The usual duration of therapy is 4 to 6 weeks. Antacids are also available in a pill form, but these have only about 10% of the neutralizing capacity of 15 ml of the liquid form.[15]

Calcium carbonate has also been used and has the greatest neutralizing capacity of any of the antacids. However, calcium appears to cause a rebound increase in acid secretion.[15]

The second major category is the H_2 antagonists, which block the histamine receptor responsible for acid secretion in the GI tract.[16] The success of H_2 blockers is similar to that of antacids and results in an approximately 80% healing rate after a 6-week course.[17] Although antacids are commonly prescribed in addition to H_2 blockers, there are no data indicating improved outcome, and antacids can inhibit the absorption of cimetidine.[18]

A third form of therapy for PUD is the coating compound sucralfate, the polyaluminum hydroxide salt of sucrose sulfate. When exposed to an acid environment, it forms negatively charged polyvalent bridges to necrotic tissue proteins preventing contact with HCl and pepsin.[19] There is little binding to normal tissues, but the drug will bind to food and some medications. The drug also buffers acid, inhibits the action of pepsin, and absorbs bile salts.[19] Sucralfate appears to be at least as effective as antacids and H_2 blockers and more effective in preventing relapse in patients who smoke.[7] The drug has very little absorption, thereby eliminating the need for precise adjustments for weight and age. Since sucralfate requires an acid environment, the drug should not be given with antacids.

The newest drug currently being investigated is omeprazole. This drug appears to block the final step in the common pathway of a number of stimulants for acid

TABLE 5–1.
Drug Therapy for Peptic Ulcer Disease*

Medication	Dose	Major Side Effects
Antacids		
$Mg(OH)_2$	1 ml/kg/dose orally up to 30 cc 30 min before and 1 hr after each meal and at bedtime	Diarrhea
$Al(OH)_3$	Same	Constipation
Al-Mg hydroxide	Same	Diarrhea
H_2 antagonists		
Cimetidine	20–40 mg/kg/day(up to 300 mg/ dose) orally or intravenously in 4 doses	Thrombocytopenia, neutropenia, gynecomastia, impotence, hepatic and cerebral toxicity
Ranitidine	4 mg/kg/day(up to 150 mg/dose) orally in 2 doses (give one half of the dose intravenously)	Leukopenia, thrombocytopenia, gynecomastia, hepatic, cardiac and cerebral toxicity
Coating agents		
Sucralfate	1 gm twice daily (adult)	Constipation

*Adapted from Peterson et al.,[15] McGuigan,[16] Collin-Jones et al.,[17] Steinberg et al.,[18] Nagashima,[19] and Clissold and Campoli-Richards.[20]

secretion, and recent studies indicate that it may be highly effective.[20] Currently no data are available in children.

Appropriate therapy may not have a significant impact on symptoms, and patients treated with placebo often have a similar resolution of pain as those treated with medication.[15] Patients who continue to demonstrate signs or symptoms of disease after an empiric trial of medication often have an EGD performed to document the presence of an ulcer. In those with a previously documented ulcer, an alternative medication or long-term prophylactic therapy may be required.

Patients with recurrent PUD should be evaluated for Zollinger-Ellison syndrome in which gastric hypersecretion is caused by a gastrinoma located either in the pancreas, stomach, or duodenum. The diagnosis is suspected in patients with recurrent or intractable PUD and is confirmed by finding an elevated fasting serum gastrin level.[3] If no ulcer can be demonstrated in patients with characteristic symptoms, an alternative etiology for the symptoms should be sought.

Surgical management of children with PUD is usually reserved for major complications of uncontrolled bleeding, gastric outlet obstruction, and perforation. Although there is limited experience in pediatric patients, the preferred surgery appears to be vagotomy and a pyloroplasty.[21]

Prognosis

The prognosis for PUD is quite variable. Primary ulcers have been reported to have a high recurrence rate, and a recent report of adults who had PUD as children revealed that only one third spontaneously became free of symptoms for a prolonged period without surgery.[22] Recurrent duodenal ulcers increase the risk of complications from hemorrhage, perforation, and obstruction. Therefore, prophylactic therapy using H_2 blockers or sucralfate is recommended. These drugs have been shown to prevent recurrence in 75% of adult patients for up to 1 year.[23]

SUMMARY

Peptic ulcer disease is increasingly recognized as a disease of infants and children. The clinical symptoms often include atypical pain and vomiting. Three modes of treatment appear to be effective, including antacids, H_2 blockers, and surface-coating agents. The long-term outcome is usually good, although recurrent episodes are not uncommon.

REFERENCES

1. Tolia V, Dubois RS: Peptic ulcer disease in children and adolescents. *Clin Pediatr* 1983; 22:665–669.
2. Byrne WJ: Diagnosis and treatment of peptic ulcer disease in children. *Pediatr Rev* 1985; 159:63–66.
3. Silverman A, Roy CC: Disorders of stomach and duodenum, in *Pediatric Clinical Gastroenterology,* ed 3. St Louis, CV Mosby Co, 1983; p 164.

4. Euler AR, Byrne WJ, Campbell MF: Basal and pentagastrin stimulated gastric acid se-cretory rates in normal children and in those with peptic ulcer disease. *J Pediatr* 1983; 103:766–768.
5. Nord KS: Peptic ulcer disease in the pediatric population. *Pediatr Clin North Am* 1988; 35:117–140.
6. Ritchie WP: Pathogenesis of acute gastric mucosal injury. *Viewpoint Dig Dis* 1983; 15:17–20.
7. Lam SK, Hui WY, et al: Sucralfate overcomes adverse effect of cigarette smoking on duodenal ulcer healing and prolongs subsequent remission. *Gastroenterology* 1987; 92:1193–1201.
8. Deckelbaum RJ, Roy CR, et al: Peptic ulcer disease: A clinical study in 73 children. *Can Med Am J* 1974; 3:225–228.
9. Conn HO, Blitzer BL: Nonassociation of adrenocorticosteroid therapy and peptic ulcer. *N Engl J Med* 1976; 294:473–479.
10. Dooley CP, Cohen H: The clinical significance of *Campylobacter pylori. Ann Intern Med* 1988; 108:70–79.
11. Drumon B, Sherman P, Cutz E, et al: Association of *Campylobacter pylori* on the gas-tric mucosa with antral gastritis in children. *N Engl J Med* 1987; 316:1557–1561.
12. Tomomasa T, Hsu JY, et al: Statistical analysis of symptoms and signs in pediatric patients with peptic ulcer. *J Pediatr Gastroenterol Nutr* 1986; 5:711–715.
13. Nord KS, Rossi TM, Lebenthal E: Peptic ulcers in children: The predominance of gas-tric ulcers. *Am J Gastroenterol* 1981; 75:153–157.
14. Ament ME, Christie DL: Upper gastrointestinal fibrotic endoscopy in pediatric patients. *Gastroenterology* 1977; 72:1244–1248.
15. Peterson WL, Sturdevant MD, et al: Healing of duodenal ulcer with an antacid regi-men. *N Engl J Med* 1977; 297:341–345.
16. McGuigan JE: A consideration of the adverse effects of cimetidine. *Gastroenterology* 1981; 80:181–192.
17. Collin-Jones DG, et al: Reducing overnight secretion of acid to heal duodenal ulcers. Comparison of standard divided dose of ranitidine with a single dose administered at night. *Am J Med* 1984; 77(suppl 5B):116–122.
18. Steinberg WM, Lewis JH, Katz DM: Antacids inhibit absorption of cimetidine. *N Engl J Med* 1982; 306:400–404.
19. Nagashima R: Mechanisms of sucralfate. *J Clin Gastroenterol* 1981; 3(suppl 2): 117–127.
20. Clissold SP, Campoli-Richards DM: Omeperazole: A preliminary review of its pharma-codynamic and pharmacokinetic properties, and therapeutic potential in peptic ulcer dis-ease and Zollinger-Ellison syndrome. *Drugs* 1986; 32:15–47.
21. Ravitch MM, Duremides GD: Operative treatment of chronic duodenal ulcer in child-hood. *Ann Surg* 1970; 171:641–646.
22. Murphy MS, Eastham EJ: Peptic ulcer disease in childhood: Long-term prognosis. *J Gastroenterol Nutr* 1987; 6:721–724.
23. Strum WB: Prevention of duodenal ulcer recurrence. *Ann Intern Med* 1986; 105:757–761.

6   Pyloric Stenosis

Joaquin Cortiella, M.D.

A 12-day-old boy presented to the emergency room because of vomiting for 3 days. The child was the 7.6 lb (3.5 kg) product of a full-term gestation born by cesarean section because of fetal distress to a 21-year-old primigravida woman. There were no complications during the pregnancy, labor, or delivery. The Apgar scores were 7 at 1 minute and 9 at 5 minutes. The patient was breast-fed until the day of admission and had normal yellowish stools without mucus, blood, or melena. The child had been doing well until 3 days prior to admission, when he began to vomit after every other feed. Two days prior to admission, he began to vomit after every feeding, yet appeared happy and alert. One day prior to admission, the child became irritable, continued to have nonbilious, nonprojectible vomiting, was afebrile and had no change in his stools. On the day of admission, the child was afebrile and hemodynamically stable, and his height, weight, and head circumference were at the 50th percentile. He had normal skin; head, ear, eye, nose, and throat; pulmonary; and cardiac examinations. His abdominal examination revealed no palpable masses. The rectal examination was normal, and his stool was Hematest negative. His laboratory results included normal electrolyte values, BUN valve creatinine level, white blood cell count, differential cell count, and urinalysis; his hemoglobin value was 13.3 mg/dl. While in the emergency room, the child was observed to have projectile vomiting, and an upper gastrointestinal (GI) series showed an elongated, narrow pyloric canal (string sign) consistent with pyloric stenosis (PS) (Fig 6–1). He was taken to the operating room, where PS was confirmed and a pyloromyotomy was done. Postoperatively the child did well and was sent home with no further vomiting.

DISCUSSION

Pyloric stenosis (PS), which was first described in 1717, is the commonest cause of intestinal obstruction in infants.[1] The incidence is 1 in 500 live births, and boys are affected four to five times more commonly than girls.[2] Pyloric stenosis is seen more frequently in earlier births and is often seen in firstborn boys.[1] Family clusters of cases are common.[1] Socioeconomic status, race, or feeding with breast milk or formula do not appear to be significant risk factors.[2]

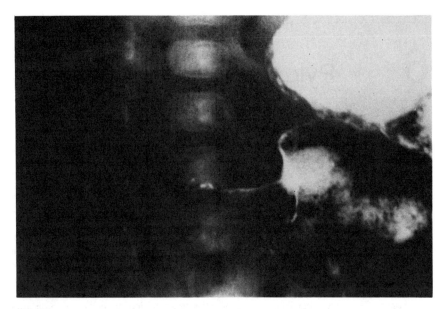

FIG 6–1.
Upper GI radiographic series showing an elongated, narrow pyloric canal (string sign).

Pathophysiology

The pathogenesis of PS is unknown, but since PS rarely occurs before 2 weeks or later than 4 to 6 months of life, some combination of developmental factors likely play a role. Among the factors that have been considered are heredity, diet, acid secretion, mucosal function, muscular anatomy, GI hormones, neuronal function, and gastric motility patterns, but the specific mechanism is still not understood.[3] Pyloric stenosis is usually classified as a congenital disorder, but several pieces of information indicate that it may be an acquired lesion. The vomiting in PS typically begins at 2 to 4 weeks of age and is rarely seen in the first 2 weeks of life.[4, 5] Supportive evidence for an acquired etiology also comes from a series of 1,000 normal male newborns, all of whom had a normal upper GI radiographic series soon after birth; 5 of these infants later developed PS.[6] In addition, PS has rarely been reported in autopsy findings of stillborn infants.[3]

A genetic predisposition likely plays a role in the development of PS.[1] A family history of PS is found in about 5% of cases.[7, 8] Only conflicting evidence is available on the possible role of such factors as diet, acid secretion, and hormonal or neuronal influences. One currently popular unproved conceptual model is that immaturity of the myenteric plexus or pyloric spasm accounts for the inability of the pylorus to open. The gastric musculature propels gastric contents against the closed pylorus, producing edema and narrowing of the canal.[9] Concomitant hypertrophy of the pyloric and gastric musculature then sets up a vicious cycle that can progress to a high-grade obstruction. Further research into the pathogenetic mechanisms is obviously needed.

Clinical Features

The hallmark of the clinical presentation of PS is nonbilious vomiting (Table 6–1). Classically, the child has a history of previous good health, as had the child presented here, but develops persistent vomiting that eventually occurs after every feeding. Some patients may present with poor weight gain and, in severe cases, can present with failure to thrive. The emesis is nonbilious but may contain blood. Typically, these infants are extremely hungry and irritable and want to be fed frequently. The vomiting can lead to dehydration, loss of skin turgor, irritability, and eventually to listlessness. Jaundice can also be seen. The positive physical findings in PS are usually confined to the abdomen, where distention and visible gastric peristaltic waves, passing from the left upper quadrant across to the right, are often found. The classical finding of a small, firm, moveable midabdominal mass, or olive-sized tumor, to the right of the umbilicus is more likely to be appreciated after the child has vomited. The "olive" is found in about 50% of cases,[5] as in this patient.

A number of abnormal laboratory values are found in patients with PS. Because of the persistent vomiting, a hypochloremic metabolic acidosis, hyperphosphatemia, concentrated urine, and hemoconcentrated hemoglobin and hematocrit values may be found. An unconjugated hyperbilirubinemia is also seen in 1% to 2% of patients[5] similar to that seen in other patients with proximal small bowel obstruction.

Diagnosis

The diagnosis of PS is often made on clinical criteria in a child with a history of progressive, nonbilious vomiting who has abdominal distention, gastric peristaltic waves, and an olive-sized abdominal mass to the right of the umbilicus. The diagnosis is usually confirmed with an upper GI series or an abdominal ultrasound. The upper GI study shows an elongated narrowing of the gastric antrum (see Fig 6–1), or "string sign," and may also show an indentation of both the duodenal bulb and the gastric antrum by the pyloric mass. The upper GI study is also helpful in ruling out other causes of upper GI obstruction. The abdominal ultrasound provides an effective noninvasive way to evaluate the length and diameter of the pyloric muscle.[10] Teele and Smith have identified specific criteria to assess the hypertrophied width of the

TABLE 6–1.
Typical Clinical Presentation of Pyloric Stenosis

Features	Findings
Age	2–4 weeks, classically
Sex	Boys 4:1, often firstborn
Signs and symptoms	Nonbilious vomiting
	Gastric fluid wave
	Olive-sized tumor
Laboratory findings	Hypochloremic alkalosis
	Hemoconcentration
	Hyperbilirubinemia (unconjugated)

pyloric muscle and elongation of the central canal for PS[10]; a width greater than 4.0 cm and length greater than 1.5 cm are considered abnormal.

The differential diagnosis list should include the many other causes of vomiting, including neurologic, infectious, anatomical, and metabolic etiologies. Increased intracranial pressure must be ruled out and sepsis or infection (especially of the urinary tract) should be sought. The upper GI series will help to rule out other anatomical causes such as malrotation, Ladd's bands, a duplication, or an antral web. It may also demonstrate an antral ulcer that can cause swelling and pyloric obstruction with subsequent hypertrophy. Eosinophilic gastroenteritis, which can cause gastric outlet obstruction, has recently been reported to cause a PS-like picture in infants.[11] Metabolic causes should also be sought if an acidosis that does not respond quickly to fluid and electrolyte therapy is present.

The pathologic finding in PS is a thick, firm, and swollen pyloric muscle. The concentric hypertrophy causes elongation and obstruction of the pyloric channel.

Treatment

The definitive treatment for PS is pyloromyotomy. Surgery is undertaken as soon as any sodium, chloride, potassium, and water losses are corrected. The operative procedure involves incision and rupture of the full length of the circular muscle of the tumor.[12]

Medical management is still used successfully in Europe and Japan, especially in less severe cases of PS.[13, 14] Medical treatment for PS includes methscopolamine nitrate to reduce the gastric waves and administration of small volume or transpyloric feedings. Ten percent to 40% of patients treated medically have eventually required surgical intervention.[13, 14]

The most common complication of the surgery is postoperative vomiting; one large series reported vomiting in 65% of the patients following surgery.[5] In patients who continue to vomit after successful pyloromyotomy, evaluation of eosinophilic gastroenteritis should be considered.[11]

SUMMARY

Pyloric stenosis must always be considered in the infant who presents with nonbilious vomiting, especially between 2 to 4 weeks of age. A higher suspicion should be present for firstborn boys and those with a positive family history. The usual outcome in children with PS treated with pyloromyotomy is excellent. Most children will enjoy a complete recovery, as did the child presented here.

REFERENCES

1. Ravitch MM: The story of pyloric stenosis. *Surgery* 1962; 48:1117–1143.
2. Knox EG, Armstrong E, Haynes R: Changing incidence of infantile hypertrophic pyloric stenosis. *Arch Dis Child* 1983; 58:582–585.

3. Markowitz RI, Wolfson BJ, Huff DS, et al: Infantile hypertrophic pyloric stenosis—congenital or acquired? *J Clin Gastroenterol* 1982; 4:39–44.
4. Meekes CS, DeNicola RR: Hypertrophic pyloric stenosis in a newborn infant. *J Pediatr* 1948; 33:94–97.
5. Scharli A, Sieber WK, Kieslivitter WB: Hypertrophic pyloric stenosis at Children's Hospital of Pittsburgh from 1912 to 1967. A critical review of current problems and complications. *J Pediatr Surg* 1964; 4:108–114.
6. Wallgren A: Preclinical stage of infantile hypertrophic pyloric stenosis. *Am J Dis Child* 1946; 72:371–376.
7. Berglund G, Rabo E: A long-term follow-up of patients with pyloric stenosis-with special reference to heredity and later morbidity. *Acta Paediatr Scand* 1972; 62:130–132.
8. McKeown T, MacMahon B: Infantile hypertrophic pyloric stenosis in parent and child. *Arch Dis Child* 1955; 30:497–500.
9. Lynn H: The mechanism of pyloric stenosis and its relationship to preoperative preparation. *Arch Surg* 1960; 81:453–459.
10. Teele RL, Smith EH: Ultrasound in the diagnosis of idiopathic hypertrophic pyloric stenosis. *N Engl J Med* 1977; 296:1149–1150.
11. Snyder JD, Rosenblum N, Wershil B, et al: Pyloric stenosis and eosinophilic gastroenteritis in infants. *J Pediatr Gastroenterol* 1987; 6:543–547.
12. Benson CD: Infantile hypertrophic pyloric stenosis in Welch KJ, et al; *Pediatric Surgery*, ed 4. Chicago, Year Book Medical Publishers, 1986, pp 811–815.
13. Mellin GW, Santulli TV, Altman HS: Congenital pyloric stenosis. A controlled evaluation of medical treatment utilizing methyl-scopolaminenitrate. *J Pediatr* 1965; 66:649–57.
14. Jacoby NM: Pyloric stenosis: Selective medical and surgical treatment. A survey of 16 years' experience. *Lancet* 1962; 1:119–121.
15. Yamashiro Y, Mayama H, Yammamoto K, et al: Conservative management of infantile pyloric stenosis by nasoduodenal feeding. *Eur J Pediatr* 1981; 136:187–192.

7   Foreign Body Ingestion

John D. Snyder, M.D.

A 12.5-year-old boy was well until the day of admission when he ingested a 7.6-cm hat pin while playing with a homemade blowgun. He felt no immediate discomfort and had no respiratory distress, hematemesis, or fever. The patient's physical examination was completely normal; no oral cavity bleeding was found. A radiograph of the stomach (Fig 7–1) demonstrated the presence of the needle in the upper intestinal tract. Removal of the pin using fiberoptic endoscopy was attempted, but the pin had already passed beyond the stomach. The patient was sent home and returned for serial radiographs to follow the transit of the pin. The pin was excreted in his stool on the fourth day after ingestion. He remained free of abdominal pain, distention, or hematochezia.

DISCUSSION

Foreign body ingestions continue to be a common clinical problem, especially in younger children. The majority of children who have gastrointestinal (GI) foreign body ingestions are younger than this patient and are in the age group from birth to 4 years.[1] The foreign bodies most commonly ingested include coins, bones, food debris, pins, and razor blades but can include a wide variety of radiopaque and nonradiopaque objects of various sizes and shapes from glass fragments to bedsprings or scissors.[2, 3] When a foreign body becomes lodged in the esophagus, it requires immediate attention.

Esophageal Foreign Bodies

Esophageal foreign bodies are usually found at the cricopharyngeal level but can also become lodged in the middle and lower third of the esophagus.[3] Symptoms of an esophageal foreign body include chest or throat discomfort, gagging, retching, retrosternal pain, increased salivation, and respiratory distress. Removal is required because foreign bodies that become lodged in the esophagus can cause ulceration that may lead to perforation. The great majority of patients who have esophageal foreign body ingestions have no evidence of previous esophageal abnormality.[1]

Conservative management of esophageal foreign bodies has utilized several

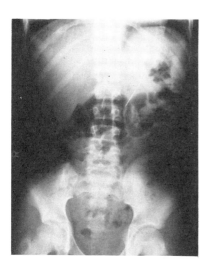

FIG 7–1.
Abdominal radiograph showing hat pin in proximal small intestine.

medications to help aid passage. Glucagon can relax the esophageal and lower esophageal sphincter smooth muscle and allow normal peristalsis to push the foreign body through.[4] Gas-forming agents can produce carbon dioxide in the esophagus and help to push food into the stomach.[5] Digestive enzymes such as papain have also been used for meat ingestions,[6] but are used less frequently now because they may cause mucosal erosion, increasing the risk for complications from endoscopy if it is required later.[7]

Removal of esophageal foreign bodies can be accomplished by endoscopy, insertion of a Foley catheter, or, rarely, surgery. Endoscopic removal is usually performed under general anesthesia to provide total relaxation of the patient and to protect the airway. Forceps, a wire loop, a grasper, or a retrieval basket (Fig 7–2) can be passed through a flexible fiberoptic endoscope to secure the object for removal. A rigid endoscope can be used to permit the passage of larger removal instruments. Foley catheters are also used to aid in smooth foreign body removal. In this technique, the catheter is passed into the stomach, pulled back into the distal esophagus, filled with radiopaque contrast material, and pulled back under fluoroscopic guidance.[8] The procedure should be done by an experienced fluoroscopist to minimize the risk of aspiration. Surgery is required only if there is danger of a perforation.

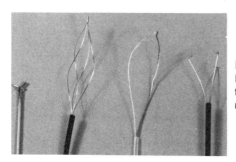

FIG 7–2
Forceps, retrieval basket, wire loop, and three-pronged grasper used in endoscopic removal of foreign bodies.

Gastric and Intestinal Foreign Bodies

Foreign bodies that have reached the stomach are usually managed conservatively since 80% to 90% will be passed spontaneously without difficulty.[2, 3] The size, configuration, or number are not helpful in predicting whether a particular ingested object will pass spontaneously.[2] However, chicken bones and toothpicks have been reported to place the patient at greater risk for perforation.[2] As evidenced by this patient, even long, sharp objects can pass through the intestinal tract without causing harm.

Serial radiographs are obtained to follow the progress of the foreign body because a small percentage can be held up in transit at the level of the pylorus, the junction of the second and third portions of the duodenum, the ligament of Treitz, and the ileocecal region.[3] Pressure necrosis can then occur, leading to hemorrhage or perforation.[2]

Surgical intervention is required if evidence for possible perforation is present or if the object fails to progress through the intestine. Generally, an ingested object is allowed 2 to 3 weeks to pass through the intestinal tract. Ingested objects in children routinely take 4 to 7 days to pass.[3] Objects that contain lead or mercury should be removed sooner if lodged in the stomach because they could potentially cause poisoning.

Button Battery Ingestions

Button battery ingestions deserve special mention since they have received a great deal of attention in recent years because of their increasing frequency.[9-11] Injury from the batteries can be caused by direct corrosive action, low-voltage burns, and pressure necrosis,[12] and cases of perforation, especially of the esophagus, and death have been reported.[10] However, if the battery passes the esophagus, the chance for harmless passage through the GI tract is excellent.[11] Current recommendations are based on the results of the National Button Battery Ingestion Study (Table 7–1).[11] Because of the potentially grave consequences of batteries lodged in the esophagus, immediate removal is required.[11] In the absence of impaction in the esophagus or signs and symptoms of bowel perforation, close follow-up is essential, but endoscopic or surgical retrieval are unnecessary.[11]

TABLE 7–1.

Button Battery Ingestion Protocol*

1. Obtain an initial x-ray film to confirm ingestion and location.
2. If it is lodged in the esophagus, use endoscopic retrieval.
3. If it is past the esophagus, follow it clinically; intervene if fever, vomiting, or hematochezia develop.
4. Obtain a follow-up x-ray film in 4 days.

*Adapted from Litovitz TL: Battery ingestions: Product accessibility and clinical course. *Pediatrics* 1985; 75:469–476.

Complications

Although most patients have an uneventful course, as our patient did, complications from foreign body ingestions can occur. The most serious complication is perforation, which occurs in less than 1% of ingestions.[13] Because of this potentially serious complication, the progress of passage of the foreign body must be carefully monitored, and parents are instructed to observe all stools. The diet should not be changed because no foods will protect the intestinal lining from possible trauma.[3] Cathartics should be avoided because active peristalsis may increase the risk for traumatic injury.

SUMMARY

Prevention continues to be the best treatment for foreign body ingestions. Esophageal foreign bodies require removal, whereas gastric or intestinal foreign bodies will usually pass uneventfully if conservative management is used. Button batteries lodged in the esophagus must be removed immediately.

REFERENCES

1. Brooks JW: Foreign bodies in the air and food passages. *Ann Surg* 1972; 175:720–732.
2. Selivanov V, Sheldon GF, Cello JP, et al: Management of foreign body ingestion. *Ann Surg* 1984; 199:187–191.
3. Spitz L: Management of ingested foreign bodies in childhood. *Br Med J* 1971; 4:469–472.
4. Trenkner SW, Maglinte DDT, Lehman G, et al: Esophageal food impaction: Treatment with glucagon. *Radiology* 1983; 149:401–403.
5. Rice BT, Spiegel PK, Dombrowski PJ: Acute esophageal food impaction treated by gas-forming agents. *Radiology* 1983; 146;299–301.
6. Chaikhouni A, Kratz JM, Crawford FA: Foreign bodies of the esophagus. *Am Surg* 1985; 51:173–179.
7. Cavo JW, Koops HJ, Grybowski RA: Use of enzymes for meat impactions in the esophagus. *Laryngoscope* 1977; 87:630–634.
8. Brown EG, Hughes JP, Koenig HM: Removal of foreign bodies lodged in esophagus by a Foley catheter without endoscopy: Success with two cases. *Clin Pediatr* 1972; 11:468–471.
9. Temple DM, McNeese MC: Hazards of battery ingestion. *Pediatrics* 1983; 71:100–103.
10. Litovitz TL: Button battery ingestions. *JAMA* 1983; 249:2495–2500.
11. Litovitz TL: Battery ingestions: Product accessibility and clinical course. *Pediatrics* 1985; 75:469–476.
12. Katz L, Cooper MT: Danger of small children swallowing hearing aid batteries. *J Otolaryngol* 1978; 7:467.
13. Maleki M, Evans WE: Foreign-body perforation of the intestinal tract. *Arch Surg* 1970; 101:475–477.

8   Caustic Ingestion

John D. Snyder, M.D.

A 22-month-old boy had been in excellent health until the day of admission when he was found on the bathroom floor next to an opened bottle of a liquid lye compound. The clear viscous fluid was on his face, his clothes, and the floor. His mother called the poison control center, which advised her to give milk, not to induce vomiting, and to bring the child to the hospital for evaluation. On examination the child was playful and alert and was not drooling. His examination was unremarkable except for two 5-mm erosions on his buccal mucosa. He had no stridor or dyspnea. Because he refused to take fluids, an intravenous (IV) line was started, and he was observed overnight. On the following day, a fiberoptic endoscopic examination was performed, and the child's duodenum, stomach, and esophagus were free of injury. The child took fluids without difficulty after the procedure and was discharged later that day.

DISCUSSION

Caustic ingestions are common occurrences in children and can lead to severe injuries, including stricture or perforation.[1] The group at greatest risk for accidental ingestion is children less than 5 years old.[1]

The great majority of injuries caused by caustic ingestions are due to alkali or acids.[1, 2] In a recent large study of childhood ingestions, 86% of the children ingested alkali, and 14% ingested an acid.[2] Bleach is also a commonly ingested compound but fortunately results in far less morbidity than ingestion of acids or alkali.

Pathogenesis

The pathogenesis of injury is related to the corrosive nature of the ingested substance, its quantity and concentration, and the duration of time in contact with the mucosa.[3, 4] Acid injuries cause coagulation necrosis and are more likely to occur in the stomach and spare the esophagus.[5] Because an eschar usually forms, some protection is provided against deeper injury. Alkaline agents cause liquefaction necrosis with saponification of fats and proteins and vascular thrombosis leading to further cellular necrosis and degeneration.[5] Full thickness injuries often occur after alkaline ingestions and can result in perforation.[5] When the initial lesions caused by acid or alkali ingestion are less severe, the child may be asymptomatic after the episode, but silent strictures due to cicatrization may still form.

Clinical Features

The clinical presentation of ingestion is often similar to that seen with this patient. The actual ingestion event is often not observed, but the caretaker has suggestive evidence for the event because of an opened bottle or container near the child. This child had two small oral lesions, which indicated that an ingestion had indeed occurred, but was otherwise asymptomatic. Signs and symptoms do not predict the presence or severity of an intestinal lesion following an ingestion; no difference was found in the occurrence of esophageal lesions in symptomatic and asymptomatic patients.[2] Vomiting, dysphagia, increased salivation, abdominal pain, and refusal to drink occurred in only 20% to 33% of the patients who had significant burns.[2] Similarly, the absence of oral lesions is no guarantee that damage has not occurred to the esophagus or stomach. Oropharyngeal burns were absent in about 25% of children who had esophageal lesions.[2]

Although the clinical signs and symptoms previously mentioned do not indicate the presence or severity of an esophageal lesion, substernal pain, back pain, and abdominal rigidity are important clues that mediastinitis or peritonitis may have occurred. Hoarseness, stridor, aphonia, and dyspnea suggest that epiglottic or laryngeal injury have occurred.[5]

Laboratory data are obtained primarily to help manage the complications of ingestion. The most helpful diagnostic study is endoscopy, which permits direct visualization of the stomach and esophagus to determine the presence and extent of injury. Earlier endoscopic studies using rigid endoscopes did not progress beyond the level of the first lesions for fear of causing perforation,[6] but more recent studies using the new small-diameter, flexible fiberoptic endoscopes indicate that panendoscopy can be safely done.[7, 8] Examination of the stomach as well as the esophagus is essential because the presence of esophageal burns does not correlate with gastric burns.[5] Once the patient has been stabilized, an early endoscopic evaluation will determine whether esophageal or gastric lesions exist and whether further evaluation and therapy will be needed.

Radiographic studies are also useful in the evaluation of caustic ingestions. In patients who have esophageal and gastric lesions, follow-up contrast studies can demonstrate scarring, strictures, and outlet obstruction.[9] Chest and abdominal radiographs must be obtained in a patient suspected of perforation.

Treatment

The initial therapy of a patient with a caustic ingestion is centered on stabilization of the patient by providing replacement fluids, electrolytes, and blood.[5] The condition of the airway must be assessed immediately and intubation performed if the airway is compromised. Evidence for esophageal or gastric perforation indicates the likely need for early surgical intervention.

Most children who ingest caustic agents have little or no evidence for injury,[2] as was the case in our patient. Because there were no esophageal or gastric lesions and the patient tolerated fluids and food, he was discharged to his parents' care to be seen in follow-up in 2 weeks.

In patients who have evidence of injury, controversy surrounds the choice of proper management. Steroids and antibiotics are frequently used, although their use has never been evaluated in a controlled study.[5] The rationale for steroid use is based on animal studies that have demonstrated decreased collagen formation, fibroplasia, and subsequent stricture formation.[10] Antibiotics are used in conjunction with steroids because of the increased risk of infection. The major potential complication of steroids in addition to infection is the risk of perforation of a severely damaged viscus because of the attendant slower wound healing.[6]

The current recommendations for the treatment of caustic ingestions are found in Table 8–1.[3, 11] Despite the risks of steroid use and the lack of controlled clinical trials proving their efficacy, steroids are often administered in high doses (1–2 mg/kg) for 2 to 3 weeks and then tapered.[3] Ampicillin or a similar antibiotic is also often given.

Complications

The two major complications of caustic ingestions are stricture formation and the development of esophageal carcinoma (especially after lye ingestion).[5] A stricture can develop in 10% to 20% of patients with evidence for burns,[1, 3, 11] and an upper gastrointestinal (GI) radiographic series should be done at 1 month following the insult. The risk of developing esophageal cancer is increased in persons who ingest a caustic substance. In one series of more than 2,400 patients with carcinoma of the esophagus, 2.6% had a history of lye ingestion as children.[12] Thus, children who have ingested a caustic agent should be thoroughly evaluated if dysphagia develops at a later time.

TABLE 8–1.
Recommendations for Treating a Caustic Ingestion*

1. Dilute immediately with water or milk. Do *not* give emetics.
2. Perform endoscopy early to decide whether therapy will be required.
3. If esophageal or gastric lesions are found at endoscopy:
   a. Prednisone (1–2 mg/kg) and ampicillin (100–200 mg/kg/day) or a similar antibiotic are given for 2 to 3 weeks, although their effect has not been documented.
   b. Obtain upper GI series at 1 month and later, if dysphagia occurs.

*Adapted from Moore[3] and Postlethwait.[11]

SUMMARY

Caustic ingestions continue to be a common and potentially serious problem in children. Early evaluation using a fiberoptic endoscopy hastens the diagnosis and permits timely institution of therapy. Close follow-up is required for any child with evidence of caustic lesions. Steroids and antibiotics are often given, although their efficacy has not been documented.

REFERENCES

1. Hawkins DB, Demeter MJ, Barnett TE: Caustic ingestion: Controversies in management. A review of 214 cases. *Laryngoscope* 1980; 90:98–108.
2. Gauderault P, Parent M, McGuigan MA, et al: Predictability of esophageal injury from signs and symptoms: A study of caustic ingestion in 378 children. *Pediatrics* 1983; 71:767–769.
3. Moore WR: Caustic ingestions: Pathophysiology, diagnosis, and treatment. *Clin Pediatr* 1986; 25:192–196.
4. Citron BP, Pincus IJ, Geobas MC, et al: Chemical trauma of the esophagus and stomach. *Surg Clin North Am* 1968; 48:1303–1311.
5. Goldman LP, Weigert JM: Corrosive substance ingestion: A review. *Am J Gastroenterol* 1984; 79:85–90.
6. Kirsh MM, Ritter F: Caustic ingestion and subsequent damage to the oropharyngeal and digestive passage. *Ann Thorac Surg* 1976; 21:74–82.
7. Chung RSK, DenBesten L: Fiberoptic endoscopy in treatment of corrosive injury of the stomach. *Arch Surg* 1975; 100:725–728.
8. Sugarva C, Mullins RJ, Lucas CE, et al: The value of early endoscopy following caustic ingestion. *Surg Gynecol Obstet* 1981; 153:553–556.
9. Johns TT, Thoeni RF: Severe corrosive gastritis related to Drano: an unusual case. *Gastrointest Radiol* 1983; 8:25–28.
10. Webb WR, Koutros P, Ecker RR, et al: An evaluation of steroids and antibiotics in caustic burns of the esophagus. *Ann Thorac Surg* 1970; 9:95–102.
11. Postlethwait RW: Chemical burns of the esophagus. *Surg Clin North Am* 1983; 63:915–924.
12. Appleqvist P, Salmo M: Lye corrosion and carcinoma of the esophagus: A review of 63 cases. *Cancer* 1980; 45:2655–2658.

9 Diagnosis of Inflammatory Bowel Disease

Barry Z. Hirsch, M.D.

A 15-year-old boy was in excellent health until 3 weeks prior to admission when he noticed shortness of breath while playing football. One week later he developed crampy lower abdominal pain immediately after meals and began having three to four watery stools per day. His stools were described as dark brown but without melena or blood. He denied nausea, vomiting, fevers, arthralgias, photophobia, perianal problems, rashes, anorexia, use of antibiotics, or weight loss. His persistent fatigue, diarrhea, and abdominal pain resulted in a hospital admission for evaluation. On physical examination the patient appeared chronically ill and had a temperature of 38.4°C. His height and weight were at the 50th percentiles for age. The skin, head, ear, eye, nose, and throat; pulmonary; and cardiac examination results were unremarkable. There were no submandibular or cervical lymph nodes palpable. He had a soft, scaphoid abdomen without tenderness, masses, or hepatosplenomegaly. Rectal examination revealed normal sphincter tone and dark brown, Hemoccult-positive stool in the vault. The musculoskeletal and neurologic examinations were within normal limits. Results of his laboratory evaluation revealed the following: hematocrit 17 mg/dl, mean corpuscular volume (MCV) 61, reticulocyte count 4.4%, platelet count 416,000/mm^3, erythrocyte sedimentation rate (ESR) 70 mm/hour, total protein level 5.7 gm/dl, and albumin level 2.3 gm/dl. His white blood cell (WBC) count, liver profile, prothrombin time, and partial thromboplastin time were normal. A methylene blue stain of the stool revealed moderate numbers of poly-morphonuclear (PMN) leukocytes. Diagnostic tests in the hospital included negative stool examination for bacterial or parasitic pathogens, negative blood cultures, and a negative tuberculin skin test result. An upper gastrointestinal (GI) radiographic series with small bowel follow through was normal. A flexible sigmoidoscopy to the splenic flexure revealed focal areas of hemorrhage interspersed among normal-appearing mucosa with blood coming from above. No pseudopolyps, cobblestoning, or fistula formation was seen. Biopsy specimens from both normal- and abnormal-appearing areas showed a marked chronic inflammatory cell infiltrate of the lamina propria with focal crypt abscesses (Fig 9–1). No areas of normal mucosa were found in the 10 biopsy specimens submitted, and no granulomas or intranuclear inclusions were seen. Based on these clinical and pathologic findings, the patient was diagnosed as having ulcerative colitis.

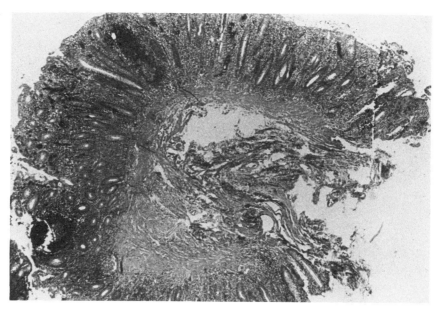

FIG 9–1.
Rectal biopsy showing diffuse colitis with inflammatory cell infitrate, mucin depletion, and altered crypt architecture (×50).

DISCUSSION

Inflammatory bowel disease (IBD) exists in two principal forms: ulcerative colitis (UC) and Crohn's disease. Ulcerative colitis refers to idiopathic chronic inflammatory disease characterized by a continuous involvement of the rectal and colonic mucosa and to a lesser extent the adjacent submucosa.[1] The muscularis interna and externa and the serosa are almost never involved except in the complication of toxic megacolon.[1] Crohn's disease (CD) is also a chronic inflammatory disorder, but it can affect any part of the GI tract from the mouth to the anus and causes inflammation in a transmural distribution.[1] A comparison of epidemiologic, clinical, and pathologic features of UC and CD is found in Table 9–1.

    The incidence of UC and CD is approximately 6/100,000 people, and recent studies have indicated that the incidence of CD is increasing compared with UC.[2–4] A twofold to fourfold higher incidence of IBD has been reported in persons of Jewish descent, and a fourfold higher incidence is reported in whites compared with nonwhites.[2] Most pediatric cases present between the ages of 10 and 19 years, with less than 2% of all cases of IBD occurring before the age of 10 years.[2] Despite the rarity of the disease in very young patients, there have been several case reports of IBD in infants.[5] Fifteen percent to 40% of patients have a family history of IBD.[6]

TABLE 9–1.
Comparison of Ulcerative Colitis and Crohn's Disease

Features	UC	CD
Epidemiologic		
Onset	Early peak 10–30 yr	Same
Sex	M = F	Same
Race	Especially whites	Same
Genetics	Family aggregation	Same
Clinical		
Abdominal pain	Less common	Common
Diarrhea	Common	Less common
Hematachezia	Common	Rare
Extraintestinal manifestations	Common	Common
Weight loss	25%–50%	65%–75%
Delayed growth	5%–10%	20%–30%
Rectum involved	Almost all	Less common
Pathologic		
Distribution	Mucosa	Transmural
	Continuous	Focal, segmental
	Colon	All bowel

Pathophysiology

Epidemiologic and histocompatibility surveys have indicated that genetic factors have a role in IBD.[1, 4, 7] The genetic factors probably establish susceptibility with disease actually precipitated by external factors such as infectious, dietary or environmental agents, and an altered immune system.[1] Numerous infectious organisms have received intensive scrutiny, including *Yersinia enterocolitica, Clostridium difficile, Campylobacter, Chlamydia,* L-forms, mycobacteria, *Escherichia coli,* and several viruses, but none has been found consistently in IBD patients.[1] Processed sugar and a long list of food additives have been studied, but no data exist to implicate any environmental agent in IBD.[8] Psychosomatic factors, once thought to play a major role in IBD, are now believed to be of minor importance.[9]

Immunologic causes are now the most popular mechanisms advanced to explain the pathophysiology of IBD. Although no consistent defects in humoral or cell-mediated immunity have been demonstrated as antecedents to the development of IBD, the identification of cytotoxic monocytes and tissue specific antibodies indicate that immune mechanisms may be of great importance.[1] A popular hypothesis of the pathogenesis of IBD describes UC and CD as parts of the spectrum of a single disease process with differing manifestations resulting from the site of the immunologic reaction, the nature of the initiating antigen, and genetic influences.[10] Immunologic priming of the gut by luminal organisms or environmental antigens could occur early in life with genetic factors determining those who are at risk to develop a hypersensitivity reaction later in life that results in IBD. Once the priming is established, any insult that increases intestinal mucosal permeability to enteric pathogens or environmental agents could precipitate an immunologic reaction in the bowel wall.[10] Clearly, much more basic research is required before the pathogenesis of IBD is completely understood.

Clinical Features

The clinical presentation of UC and CD in children have some important differences that are outlined in Table 9–1. Abdominal pain is almost always a feature of CD but is less common in UC. Conversely, diarrhea, hematochezia, and rectal involvement are much more commonly seen in UC than CD.[11] Growth faltering and weight loss are more often manifestations of CD (see Chapter 10). Some complaints like the extraintestinal manifestations of iritis, arthritis, rashes (erythema nodosum and pyoderma gangrenosum), and apthous stomatitis are seen with equal frequency in both diseases.[11] The interval between the onset of symptoms and the time of diagnosis is usually between 6 months and 1 year for UC and about 1.5 years for CD.[12]

Diagnosis

The findings from the clinical history and physical examination are of great importance in guiding the diagnostic evaluation. Because this patient had signs and symptoms of fatigue, diarrhea, abdominal pain, and blood in the stool, infectious, malignant, and autoimmune causes of colitis were sought (Table 9–2).

The enteric pathogens that cause infectious colitis act by either invasive or cytotoxic mechanisms. A tuberculin skin test should also be placed since enteric tuberculosis can present in a fashion very similar to CD.[13]

Intestinal lymphoma can occur in young persons, but the absence of lymph node, liver, or spleen enlargement made this diagnosis unlikely in this patient. In addition, there was no evidence from the CBC count to support the diagnosis.

Idiopathic colitis can also be associated with Henoch-Schönlein purpura (Chapter 46) and the hemolytic uremic syndrome (Chapter 47). The CBC count, peripheral smear, urinalysis, BUN value, and creatinine clearance are helpful in ruling out these diagnoses.

TABLE 9–2.
Initial Laboratory Evaluation of Inflammatory Bowel Disease

Blood tests*
CBC count, differential cell count, ESR, creatinine clearance, BUN, urine analysis
Albumin
Iron, total iron-binding capacity
(Liver function tests, amylase)
Stool tests
Fecal leukocytes
Culture (*Y. enterocolita, Salmonella, Shigella, Chlamydia, Campylobacter, E. coli*)
Toxin titer (*C. difficile*)
Ova and parasites (*Entamoeba histolytica*)
Tuberculin skin test

*CBC = complete blood cell; BUN = blood urea nitrogen.

When these initial tests do not yield a diagnosis, a sigmoidoscopic examination should be performed. This is usually done now by flexible sigmoidoscopy, which permits examination to the splenic flexure with only minor discomfort to the patient. Multiple sigmoidoscopic biopsies can provide histologic evidence of colitis and help in differentiating between UC and CD. The visual sigmoidoscopic findings in this case suggested the possibility of skip areas suggestive of CD: however, the biopsies revealed active continuous inflammation in all the specimens, consistent with UC. These findings emphasize the importance of multiple biopsies of abnormal- as well as normal-appearing areas. It is also crucial that a biopsy of the rectum be performed since this is an area that is usually spared in CD and is almost always involved in UC.[14]

The histologic findings are usually not diagnostic alone since many conditions may cause similar findings of increased inflammatory cells in the lamina propria, crypt abscesses, reduced number of goblet cells, epithelial destruction, branching of crypts, and frank ulcerations.[13, 14] The biopsies must be evaluated carefully for granulomas that would suggest CD or intranuclear inclusions suggestive of a viral infection. Recently histologic criteria that may help differentiate UC from acute self-limited colitis (usually infectious) have been reported.[15] The discriminating finding was plasmacytosis in the lamina propria extending to the mucosal base with mucosal distortion. However, to be diagnostic, the biopsy specimens had to be obtained within a few days of the onset of illness.

An upper GI radiographic study with small bowel follow through is done to determine whether small bowel involvement is present. A barium enema (or colonoscopy) may also be done as part of the initial evaluation to determine the extent of colonic involvement. Ulcerative colitis, which is confined to the colon, is marked by superficial ulcers, loss of haustration, shortening, and continuous involvement.[16] Crohn's disease, which may involve any segment of the GI tract, classically has serpiginous ulcers, thumb printing, skip areas, and the string sign.[16]

Using a combination of clinical, laboratory, radiologic, and histologic findings, CD can be differentiated from UC and in at least 80% of cases.[1] However, the need for close, long-term follow-up and reassessment of these patients is essential in confirming the diagnosis.

SUMMARY

Ulcerative colitis and CD are the two principal forms of idiopathic IBD. The pathophysiologic mechanisms of these diseases are unknown, but genetic and immunologic factors likely play important roles. The epidemiologic features of UC and CD are similar (see Table 9–1), but distinct clinical, radiologic, and histologic findings permit differentiation in at least 80% of cases. In the initial evaluation, infectious, malignant, and autoimmune causes of colitis must be ruled out.

REFERENCES

1. Kirsner JB, Shorter RG: Recent developments in ''nonspecific'' inflammatory bowel disease. *N Engl J Med* 1982; 306:775–785, 837–848.

2. Monk M, Mendeloff AI, Siegel CI, et al: An epidemiological study of ulcerative colitis and regional enteritis among adults in Baltimore: I. Hospital incidence and prevalence, 1960–1963. *Gastroenterology* 1968; 54:822–824.
3. Sedlack RE, Whistnant J, Elveback LR, et al: Incidence of Crohn's disease in Imstead County, Minnesota, 1935–1975. *Am J Epidemiol* 1980; 112:759–763.
4. Garland CF, Lilienfeld AM, Mendeloff AI, et al: Incidence rates of ulcerative colitis and Crohn's disease in fifteen areas of the United States. *Gastroenterology* 1981; 81:1115–1124.
5. Ein SH, Lynch MJ, Stephens CA: Ulcerative colitis in children under a year: A twenty year review. *J Pediatr Surg* 1971; 6:264–271.
6. Farmer RG, Michener WM, Mortimer EA: Studies of family history among patients with inflammatory bowel disease. *Clin Gastroenterol* 1980; 9:271–278.
7. Singer HC, Anderson JGD, Frischer H, et al: Familial aspects of inflammatory bowel disease. *Gastroenterology* 1971; 61:423–430.
8. Sherman RP, Zeeman MG: Immunologic alterations by environmental chemicals: Relevance of studying mechanisms versus effects. *J Immunopharmacol* 1980; 2:285–307.
9. Helzer JE, Chammos S, Norland CC, et al: A study of the association between Crohn's disease and psychiatric illness. *Gastroenterology* 1984; 86:324–330.
10. Shorter RG, Huizenga KA, Spencer RJ: A working hypothesis for the etiology and pathogenesis of non-specific inflammatory bowel disease. *Am J Dig Dis* 1972; 17:1024–1032.
11. Hamilton JR, Bruce GA, Abdourhaman M, et al: Inflammatory bowel disease in children and adolescents. *Adv Pediatr* 1979; 26:311–341.
12. Grand RJ, Homer DR: Approaches to inflammatory bowel disease in childhood and adolescence. *Pediatr Clin North Am* 1975; 22:835–850.
13. Richter JM, Dickerson GR: Case records of the Massachusetts General Hospital. *N Engl J Med* 1983; 309:96–104.
14. Admans H, Whorwell PJ, Wright R: Diagnosis of Crohn's disease. Dig Dis Sci 1980; 25:911–915.
15. Nostrant TT, Kumar NB, Appelman HD: Histopathology differentiates acute self-limited colitis from ulcerative colitis. *Gastroenterology* 1987; 92:318–328.
16. Laufer I, Hamilton J: The radiologic differentiation between ulcerative colitis and granulomatous colitis. *Am J Gastroenterol* 1976; 66:259–269.

10 Growth Failure in Inflammatory Bowel Disease

Esther Jacobowitz Israel, M.D.

A 14-year-old boy had been in good health until 2 weeks prior to his referral for evaluation of anemia and poor growth. At that time he was seen by his pediatrician for upper respiratory tract symptoms and was noted to be pale; his hematocrit was 29% with a low mean corpuscular volume (MCV) of 62. A closer review of the previous few months showed that he did have occasional epigastric pain of 1 minute's duration, relieved by eating. He had a normal stool pattern, but 1 day prior to his visit he had a stool with fresh blood. He had grown 2.5 cm in the last 17 months and had lost 4 lb (1.8 kg) during that time. There was no history of rash photophobia or joint pain, though he did complain of recurrent mouth ulcers. His energy level appeared to be decreased over the past month.

His past medical history showed that 3 years prior to evaluation, a microcytic anemia (hematocrit 34%, MCV 67) had been noted at a routine physical examination. His family history included an episode of gastrointestinal (GI) bleeding in his father at age 23 years secondary to a gastric ulcer. There was no history in the family of inflammatory bowel disease (IBD).

The physical examination showed a very thin, small boy. His weight was 74 lb (33.6 kg) (<5th percentile), and his height was 145 cm (<5th percentile). His oropharynx revealed an ulcer on the uvula. The abdomen was soft with normal bowel sounds, and there were no masses, liver, or spleen palpable. His pubertal development was Tanner stage II. There were two anal fissures, and the stool in the rectal vault was heme positive. Extremities showed clubbing of the fingernails.

Results of the laboratory evaluation were significant for an erythrocyte sedimentation rate of 50 mm/hour, a low serum iron level of 19 mg/dl with total iron-binding capacity of 207 μg/dl. The total protein level was 6.3 gm/dl, albumin level was decreased at 2.5 gm/dl. The platelet count was 445,000/mm³, and the reticulocyte count was 4.6%.

A barium enema examination demonstrated a segment of descending colon with aphthoid ulcers, suggesting IBD. The upper GI series showed thickened antral and duodenal folds, nodular thickening and narrowing of several jejunal loops, and a normal terminal ileum. An esophagogastroduodenoscopy showed erythema in the antrum and edema of the duodenal bulb. An antral biopsy revealed an epithelioid cell granuloma, consistent with Crohn's disease (Fig 10–1).

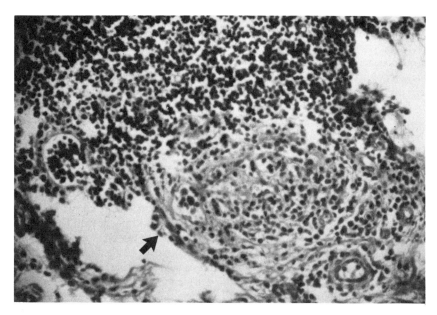

FIG 10–1.
Gastric antral biopsy (×100) containing an epitheliod granuloma *(arrow).*

DISCUSSION

Delayed growth and sexual maturation are reported to occur in 20% to 30% of children and adolescents with Crohn's disease and in about 5% to 10% of those with ulcerative colitis.[1] If patients who present in late pubertal development are eliminated, the number can be as high as 85%.[2] As in the patient presented here, growth failure can develop in a quiet and insidious manner and must be aggressively sought in each pediatric patient if it is to be found. Inflammatory bowel disease should always be considered in the differential diagnosis of growth failure in children and adolescents.

Growth failure is a serious problem of IBD of childhood and a difficult one to manage. The adolescent years are a period of dramatic growth and sexual development, and the occurrence of short stature and delayed pubescence may lead to serious adjustment problems for the adolescent. Recognition of this complication and prompt management is essential for the establishment of "catch-up growth." Before efforts to restore growth and maturation are initiated, however, an understanding of the factors that contribute to this complication is required.

Pathophysiology

Over the years, a multifactorial pathogenesis for the etiology of the growth failure in IBD has been suggested. The factors that have been implicated have been nutritional, endocrinologic, and iatrogenic (secondary to therapy).

Nutritional factors can be related to one of three problems: decreased intake, increased energy expenditure, and increased losses. Decreased nutrient intake has been documented in patients with Crohn's disease and growth failure, with the majority of patients taking in less than the recommended number of calories for age.[3] The decreased intake is believed mainly to be due to postprandial pain and anorexia. Low zinc levels seen in the plasma and hair of children with IBD have been correlated with decreased taste acuity and may play a role in the anorexia.[4] A major factor in the decreased caloric intake can be the low-fiber/milk-free diet often used in IBD that can result in deficiencies of certain essential nutrients and vitamins (calcium, folic acid, fat, protein, and B and D vitamins), particularly in growing children and adolescents. The efficacy of such dietary manipulation in the control of the IBD symptoms, however, has not been demonstrated and therefore should be discouraged, particularly in patients where a large portion of the caloric intake comes from milk-related products. The incidence of lactose intolerance in children with IBD, in fact, has been reported to be equal to a control population of children with chronic abdominal pain with normal GI x-ray films.[5] It is therefore prudent to obtain a lactose breath hydrogen test when lactose intolerance is suggested and to use commercially available formulations of lactase for those patients who are intolerant but whose primary source of protein is from dairy products.

Increased nutritional requirements are also present in patients with Crohn's disease. The increased requirement may result from inflammation, fever, and steroid use. Studies have shown that energy expenditure per unit weight is increased in IBD patients who are less than 90% of their ideal body weight.[6] However, other studies have not substantiated this finding.

Increased nutrient losses frequently occur and may be related to numerous factors such as mucosal inflammation, diarrhea, corticosteroid treatment, and malabsorption. Macronutrients, as well as vitamins and minerals, are affected. Abnormal D-xylose absorption has been demonstrated in 20% to 40% of patients indicating an altered intestinal mucosa.[9] Enteric protein loss occurs in 75% of patients with Crohn's disease.[9] This is a result of a leaky, inflamed mucosa and a deficiency of peptidases in injured jejunal mucosa that affect digestion and absorption adversely. Carbohydrate malabsorption also occurs and is related to altered small bowel integrity. Reduction of all disaccharidase along with decreased jejunal surface area has been described in patients who have no radiologic or histologic evidence of small bowel disease.[10] Steatorrhea occurs in 20% to 30% of patients with IBD,[11] at least in part due to ileal dysfunction with resultant bile salt malabsorption and bacterial overgrowth with consequent decreased micellar pool.

These factors can result in specific nutritional deficiency states. Iron deficiency occurs as a result of chronic intestinal blood loss and decreased iron uptake when the intestinal disease is active. Folate deficiency is present in as many as 50% of patients with Crohn's disease[12] and appears to be secondary to three different factors: poor diet, malabsorption due to jejunal dysfunction, and sulfasalazine therapy.[13] Vitamin B_{12} deficiency is reported in 40% of patients with Crohn's disease secondary to terminal ileal disease and resection as well as bacterial overgrowth.[8] Decreased levels of zinc in the serum, hair, and urine have been seen with Crohn's disease and is related to malabsorption, steatorrhea, and corticosteroid therapy. Zinc deficiency's relation to growth retardation, aside from its effects on taste acuity, is as yet unknown.

Endocrine abnormalities have long been sought to explain the growth deficits in IBD, but no abnormality has been documented.[3] Normal growth hormone levels and normal thyroid function have uniformly been found. The association of somatomedin C in the growth failure of IBD has recently received a great deal of attention.[14] Somatomedin C is thought to mediate the growth-promoting effects of growth hormone, but low levels are thought to reflect and not cause growth failure. Serial measurement of somatomedin C has been suggested as a tool for following the progress of patients with growth failure in IBD.[14]

Finally, the drug therapy of IBD can impair growth. The principal offender is corticosteroid treatment, the mainstay of therapy. Patients with active disease can often have an initial burst of growth when placed on steroid therapy, but chronic therapy suppresses growth.[11]

Clinical Features

Each patient with IBD and growth retardation requires a full assessment to determine which mechanism or combination of mechanisms is operational (Table 10–1). Proper evaluation of the patient with growth failure includes the need for old growth charts to assess growth velocity. A thorough nutritional assessment should include a good dietary history to determine the true caloric intake. A fall of greater than 0.8 in. (2.0 cm) from the previous height velocity prior to the pubertal growth spurt, a height velocity of less than 1.6 in. (4.0 cm)/year, or a fall in the height percentile all suggest true impairment of growth.[16] The weight/height ratio is helpful in assessing whether the nutritional complications of the disease are acute (low weight/height) or chronic (normal weight/height). Arm anthropometry should be done by an individual who is experienced in the technique. Pubertal staging and skeletal age determination (left wrist x-ray films) are done to provide an indication of the amount of time available for catch-up growth, which will influence the aggressiveness of the approach to the growth failure. Recently an assay for type I procollagen has been suggested as a biochemical marker of growth in children with IBD and repeated determinations may allow rapid assessment of the effects of various therapeutic interventions on growth.[17] As discussed earlier somatomedin C levels may also be used in a similar way. The laboratory evaluation should include an evaluation of the nutrients that might be affected. A stool examination for α_1-antitrypsin activity can be used to assess intestinal protein loss. The stool should also be examined for fat particles and blood. Serum albumin, iron, folate, vitamin B_{12}, zinc, calcium, and phosphorus values should also be measured. Malabsorption of specific nutrients can be assessed: breath tests for lactose and lactulose can determine lactose tolerance and bacterial overgrowth, respectively, and a Shilling test for vitamin B_{12} absorption helps to assess the functional capacity of the terminal ileum.

Therapy

The two key elements that allow for growth are control of disease activity and

TABLE 10–1.

Evaluation of Growth Failure in Inflammatory
Bowel Disease*

Dietary evaluation
   Caloric intake
   Activity level
Anthropometric evaluation
   Growth velocity
   Weight/height ratio
   Anthropometry
   Tanner developmental stage
   Bone age
Laboratory evaluation
   Protein status
   Total protein, albumin
   Biochemical markers of growth
      Procollagen type I
      Somatomedin C
   Vitamin/mineral/trace element status
      Ferritin
      Folate
      Calcium
      Magnesium
      Vitamin A
      Vitamin B_{12}
      Vitamin K (prothrombin time)
      Zinc
   Stool fat, blood, protein

*Adapted from Rosenthal et al.[15]

provision of adequate nutrition. The methods available for control of disease activity are limited. Corticosteroids remain the mainstay of therapy in Crohn's disease and often for ulcerative colitis. Growth frequently will improve initially when steroid treatment is begun, despite its growth retardive effects, probably because of reduced inflammation. Children with stable disease can continue to grow if steroids are administered on an alternate-day regimen.[18] Other pharmacologic agents used include sulfasalazine, metronidazole, and azathioprine (see Chapter 11). More recently, it has been recognized that total parenteral nutrition (TPN) and enteral nutrition can be helpful in controlling disease activity, and these therapeutic modalities are increasingly being used when standard pharmacologic management has failed to achieve a remission (Table 10–2).[3, 19, 21–26] Some practitioners have used TPN or elemental feedings as a primary treatment course as well.[18, 19] The duration of remission after the nutritional interventions are highly variable but generally short lived.

    The enteral formulations used to achieve disease control are referred to as "elemental diets" because they require little or no enzymatic hydrolysis for absorption and contain no fiber.[20–26] They are believed to act by reducing factors that could potentially perpetuate inflammation (e.g., dietary toxins and complex proteins), sup-

TABLE 10–2.
Daily Intakes That Reversed Growth Failure in IBD

Investigator	Caloric Intake	Nutritional Therapy
Layden et al.[21]	75 kcal/kg	TPN
Kelts et al.[3]	95 kcal/kg	TPN + regular diet
Strobel et al.[19]	60–80 kcal/kg	TPN + regular diet
Morin et al.[22]	80 kcal/kg	Nasogastric elemental + regular diet
Kirschner et al.[23]	2,200–3,000 kcal	Oral elemental + regular diet
Motil et al.[24]	93 kcal/kg	Nasogastric elemental + regular diet
O'Morain et al.[25]	50–75 kcal/day	Nasogastric elemental
Navarro et al.[26]	130–150% RDA*	Nasogastric elemental

*RDA = Recommended daily allowance.

plying adequate calories in a simple state, and altering bowel flora. These formulas are generally not palatable when taken orally, and the large amount of fluid required frequently results in bloating and discomfort. Therefore, they are usually administered via a nasogastric tube, often as an overnight infusion, allowing the patient to maintain a relatively normal lifestyle during the day. For patients who do not tolerate or improve on the enteral nutrition, TPN may be required.[19]

Surgery for IBD is generally employed for the complications of the disease, such as stricture, fistula formation, perforation, or abscess. However, poor growth not responsive to medical therapy is another indication for surgery. In adolescents approaching the closure of their epiphyseal growth plates, growth failure alone can be an indication for surgery in Crohn's disease.

Controlling disease activity, however, is only part of the battle to overcome in growth failure in IBD. The provision of adequate nutrition is also essential to reverse growth failure because higher caloric and nutrient requirements are frequently required compared to those in normal individuals.

Caloric needs may be estimated in a number of ways. In children whose weight for height is appropriate, this generally turns out to be approximately 70 to 80 kcal/kg/day.[3] However, an adjustment of the recommendations is necessary and is based on an individual patient's response. Calories may be administered using central venous alimentation, peripheral IV alimentation, elemental diets, or specialized formulas, and the results for growth can be good. When the disease activity is under control, the beneficial effects of good nutrition alone, rather than the manner in which it is delivered, appears to stimulate growth (Table 10–2). This table summarizes the range of caloric intakes and routes of administration recommended by various investigators. The easiest way to provide nutritional supplementation is to just increase dietary intake with standard table foods. When the disease is active, however, such a diet may exacerbate the symptoms. Oral supplementation, therefore, with a commercially available liquid formula can then be attempted. If satiety becomes a problem and the patient is unable to increase the total caloric intake, nasogastric feedings or parenteral alimentation can be used.

SUMMARY

Growth failure in IBD can be an extremely difficult problem to overcome, but early recognition and prompt intervention can help to avoid the long-term consequences of this often devastating complication. The essential components of management are controlling the disease activity and providing adequate calories to allow for growth.

REFERENCES

1. McCaffrey TD, Khosrow N, Lawrence AM, et al: Severe growth retardation in children with inflammatory bowel disease. *Pediatrics* 1970; 45:386–393.
2. Burbige EJ, Huang S, Bayless TM: Clinical manifestations of Crohn's disease in children and adolescents. *Pediatrics* 1975; 55:866–871.
3. Kelts DC, Grand RJ, Shev G, et al: Nutritional basis of growth failure in children and adolescents with Crohn's disease. *Gastroenterology* 1979; 76:720–727.
4. Solomons NW, Rosenfield RL, Jacob RA, et al: Growth retardation and zinc nutrition. *Pediatr Res* 1976; 10:923–927.
5. Kirschner BS, DeFararo MV, Jensen W: Lactose malabsorption in children and adolescents with inflammatory bowel disease. *Gastroenterology* 1981; 81:829–832.
6. Barot LR, Rombeau JL, Steinberg JJ, et al: Energy expenditure in patients with inflammatory bowel disease. *Arch Surg* 1981; 116:460–462.
7. Chan ATH, Fleming CR, O'Fallon WM, et al: Estimated versus measured basal energy requirements in patients with Crohn's disease. *Gastroenterology* 1986; 91:75–78.
8. Driscoll RH Jr, Rosenberg IH: Total parenteral nutrition in inflammatory bowel disease. *Med Clin North Am* 1978; 62:185–201.
9. Beeken WL, Busch HL, Sylvester DL: Intestinal protein loss in Crohn's disease. *Gastroenterology* 1972; 62:207–215.
10. Dunne WT, Cooke WT, Allan RN: Enzymatic and morphometric evidence for Crohn's disease as a diffuse lesion of the gastrointestinal tract. *Gut* 1977; 18:290–294.
11. Grand RJ: Model for the treatment of growth failure in children with inflammatory bowel disease, in Suskind RM (ed): *Textbook of Pediatric Nutrition*. New York, Raven Press, 1981.
12. Andersson H, Dotevall G, Gillberg R, et al: Absorption studies in patients with Crohn's disease and in patients with ulcerative colitis. *Acta Med Scand* 1981; 190:407–410.
13. Franklin JL, Rosenberg IH: Impaired folic acid absorption in inflammatory bowel disease: Effects of salicylazosulfapyridine. *Gastroenterology* 1973; 64:517–525.
14. Kirschner BS, Sutton MM: Somatomedin-C levels in growth-impaired children and adolescents with chronic inflammatory bowel disease. *Gastroenterology* 1986; 91:830–836.
15. Rosenthal SR, Snyder JD, Hendricks KM, et al: Growth failure and inflammatory bowel disease: Approach to treatment of a complicated adolescent problem. *Pediatrics* 1983; 72:481–490.
16. Preece MA: Anthropometry and growth: Patterns of growth in disease starting at different ages, in Davideon M (ed): *Growth Retardation Among Children and Adolescents with Inflammatory Bowel Disease*. New York, National Foundation for Ileitis and Colitis, 1983.
17. Hyams JS, Carey DE, Leichtner AH, et al: Type I procollegen as a biochemical marker of growth in children with inflammatory bowel disease. *J Pediatr* 1986; 109:619–624.

18. Whittington PF, Barnes HV, Bayless TM: Medical management of Crohn's disease in adolescence. *Gastroenterology* 1977; 72:1338–1344.
19. Strobel CT, Byrne WJ, Ament ME: Home parenteral nutrition in children with Crohn's disease: An effective management alternative. *Gastroenterology* 1979; 77:272–279.
20. Seidman EG, Bouthillier L, Weber AM, et al: Elemental diet versus prednisone as primary treatment of Crohn's disease. *Gastroenterology* 1986; 90:1625.
21. Layden T, Rosenberg J, Nemchauaky B, et al: Reversal of growth arrest in adolescents with Crohn's disease after parenteral alimentation. *Gastroenterology* 1976; 70:1017–1026.
22. Morin CL, Rovlet M, Roy CC, et al: Continuous elemental enteral alimentation in children with Crohn's disease and growth failure. *Gastroenterology* 1980; 79:1205–1210.
23. Kirschner BS, Klich JR, Kalman SS, et al: Reversal of growth retardation in Crohn's disease with therapy emphasizing oral nutritional restitution. *Gastroenterology* 1981; 80:10–15.
24. Motil KJ, Altschuler SI, Grand RJ: Mineral balance during nutritional supplementation in adolescents with Crohn's disease and growth failure. *J Pediatr* 1985; 107:473–479.
25. O'Morain C, Segal AW, Levi AJ: Elemental diet in treatment of acute Crohn's disease. *Br Med J* 1980; 281:1173–1175.
26. Navarro J, Vargas J, Cegard JP, et al: Prolonged consistent rate elemental enteral nutrition in Crohn's disease. *J Pediatr Gastroenteral Nutr* 1982; 1:541–546.

11 Medical and Nutritional Management of Inflammatory Bowel Disease

Esther Jacobowitz Israel, M.D.

A 17-year-old girl was evaluated because of a 1-month history of right lower quadrant abdominal pain, vomiting, and a 10-lb (4.5-kg) weight loss. She had one formed, brown stool every third day without blood. Her appetite and energy level were poor. She had two febrile episodes over the month and had missed her menses though she denied sexual activity. The patient also denied arthritis, rashes, night sweats, apthous ulcers, or photophobia. Her past medical and family history was unremarkable.

Her physical examination showed an alert, cheerful girl in no obvious distress. Her weight was at the 15th percentile and her height at the 60th percentile. Positive findings were confined to the abdomen, which was remarkable for generalized guarding and a 10×10-cm tender mass in the right lower quadrant. Her liver and spleen were not enlarged. No mass was palpated on rectal examination, and the stool was negative for occult blood. She was at Tanner stage V.

Her laboratory studies included hematocrit 35%, normal white blood cell count, platelet count 488,000/mm^3; erythrocyte sedimentation rate 40 mm/hour; total protein level 7.1 gm/dl; and albumin level 3.6 gm/dl. The liver enzyme and amylase values were normal, and the stools showed no evidence of bacterial or parasitic organisms. An upper gastrointestinal (GI) series with small bowel follow-through showed a narrowed, thickened distal 15 cm of ileum (Fig 11–1). The duodenum also showed mild mucosal irregularity. A barium enema showed mucosal involvement in the transverse and descending colon but not in the ascending and sigmoid colon. A rigid sigmoidoscopy and biopsy were normal. An upper endoscopy showed increased duodenal nodularity with punctate ulcers. Although acute and chronic inflammation of the mucosa was seen microscopically, no granulomas were identified. A tuberculin skin test result was normal.

She initially did well on 40 mg/day of prednisone but developed severe mid-epigastric pain and fever when tapered to 15 mg/day. Her symptoms resolved on 50 mg/day of prednisone, and she was gradually tapered and then maintained on 20 mg every other day. She was also given sulfasalazine, 2 gm/day.

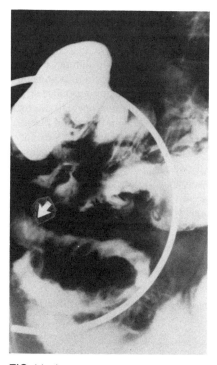

FIG 11-1.
Upper GI radiographic series
demonstrating thickened walls with
narrowing of the terminal ileum *(arrow).*

After 2 years of alternate-day prednisone and daily sulfasalazine therapy, abdominal pain, anorexia, weight loss, and a tender right lower quadrant mass developed. A barium enema showed irregularity of the cecum and the contiguous portion of the colon and a probable fistula between the ileum and the hepatic flexure. Prednisone at 40 mg/day quieted her symptoms, and she was eventually tapered to 30 mg every other day over the next 5 months. Because of her mass and probable fistula, metronidazole was started but was stopped when she experienced severe abdominal pain and headache. Alimentation with an elemental formula by mouth was switched to nighttime nasogastric infusions, and her symptoms improved dramatically.

After a taper of her steroids and a return to a regular diet, she developed an incomplete bowel obstruction, which improved with intravenous (IV) steroids and hydration. Elemental enteral feedings did not improve her symptoms of fatigue and pain, and she underwent resection of the terminal ileum, ileocecal valve, and two fistulas to the ascending colon. Since the surgery she has required cholestyramine for diarrhea and vitamin B_{12} injections. A subsequent flare of her disease required therapy with prednisone and total parenteral nutrition (TPN). Because her symptoms recurred when the TPN was stopped, azathioprine was started. She is now maintained on azathioprine and low-dose steroid therapy every other day.

DISCUSSION

Clinical Features

The patient's clinical presentation includes a number of commonly reported signs and symptoms of Crohn's disease, including the insidious onset of abdominal pain, anorexia, and weight loss. Other symptoms frequently seen, though more commonly in ulcerative colitis than in Crohn's disease, include diarrhea and rectal bleeding. The variations in the symptoms result from the site of disease.[1] Growth retardation, frequently seen in Crohn's disease (see Chapter 10) was not present in this patient, nor any of the extraintestinal manifestations of inflammatory bowel disease (IBD), including skin lesions (pyoderma gangrenosum or erythema nodosum), iritis, arthralgias and arthritis, photophobia, oral mucosal ulcerations, and liver disease.[2]

Inflammation of the bowel secondary to Crohn's disease can occur anywhere from the mouth to the anus with a preponderance of ileocolonic involvement (60% of Crohn's disease),[3] as was seen in this patient. The location of the disease plays a significant role in the clinical features and, hence, in the approach to management.

Treatment

The most commonly used therapeutic modalities for IBD are included in Table 11–1.

Corticosteroids.—The mainstay of medical therapy in IBD is oral prednisone, at a dose of 2 mg/kg/day up to a maximum of 40 to 60 mg/day. As the symptoms and signs of inflammation improve, the prednisone dose is tapered slowly

TABLE 11–1.
Medical and Nutritional Therapy in Inflammatory Bowel Disease

	Usefulness of Therapy	
	Crohn's Disease	Ulcerative Colitis
Medications		
Corticosteroids	Mainstay	Mainstay
Sulfasalazine	With colitis	Mainstay
Imuran and 6-mercaptopurine	Probably reduces steroid dependence	May reduce steroid dependence
Metronidazole	Effective especially with perirectal disease and fistulas	Less useful
Nutritional therapy		
TPN	Effective	Probably not effective
Enteral feeding	Effective	Probably not effective

since no evidence for a prophylactic benefit from ongoing steroid therapy exists.[4] The tapering is usually started about 1 month after treatment is started. Patients may have relapse of their symptoms while being tapered, requiring an abrupt return to maximal-dose prednisone therapy followed by a slower tapering process. The steroids may be tapered first to an alternate-day regimen, which has been shown to reduce the side effects of steroid therapy.[5] The side effects of steroid therapy are well recognized and include fluid retention, acne, increased subcutaneous tissue, striae, weight gain, cataracts, bone demineralization, and growth retardation. Steroid use is a factor in the poor growth seen in 20% to 30% of children and adolescents with Crohn's disease and in about 10% of patients with ulcerative colitis. The steroid effect is partially related to alteration of epiphyseal growth and maturation. Some patients are able to stop their steroid intake completely, whereas others clinically appear to require a low-dose regimen, 10 to 20 mg every other day.

Sulfasalazine.—If the patient has colonic disease, sulfasalazine is added to the medical regimen. The dose for sulfasalazine is 30 to 50 mg/kg/day (maximum dose of 4 gm), and it is generally started at 250 to 500 mg/day and then increased by 250- to 500-mg increments to help reduce the development of side effects. Side effects with sulfasalazine are usually dose related,[6] are relatively frequent but not severe, and appear to be related to the sulfapyridine component of the drug.[7] The most common side effects are nausea, vomiting, abdominal discomfort, and headache. Leukopenia and hemolysis can also occur and appear to be a dose-related phenomenon. Like other sulfonamides, sulfasalazine also produces idiosyncratic hypersensitivity reactions, including skin rashes, hemolytic and aplastic anemia, and agranulocytosis.[7] If signs of toxicity are noted, sulfasalazine is discontinued and may be restarted again once the symptoms remit.

The usefulness of sulfasalazine in prophylaxis against recurrence in Crohn's disease of the colon is unclear, but sulfasalazine has proved to help prevent recurrence of ulcerative colitis.[8] Once it is tolerated, however, many clinicians continue therapy even after remission has been achieved in Crohn's colitis. The therapeutic component of sulfasalazine is the 5-aminosalicylic acid (5-ASA) moiety,[9] and the achievement of therapeutic effects requires high concentrations of 5-ASA in the colon.[10] This has led to the development of oral 5-ASA agents and enemas containing 5-ASA, which are currently being tested in adults and children.[10, 11]

Immunosuppressants.—The use of immunosuppressive therapy for IBD has been controversial. The National Cooperative Crohn's Disease Study reported that azathioprine is no more effective than placebo in suppressing active Crohn's disease,[4] whereas other studies indicate that immunosuppressants are effective.[12] There appear to be some situations in which azathioprine or 6-mercaptopurine may be indicated. In patients who have failed to respond fully to adrenocorticosteroids, the combination of azathioprine and steroids can be superior to the continuation of steroids alone in obtaining a remission of symptoms.[12] The use of the immunosuppressive agent can help to maintain a remission and allow for tapering of the steroid without a flare of disease.[12] The efficacy of azathioprine is directly related to the dosage and the length of time it is used. The suggested dose of azathioprine is 1 to 2 mg/kg/day, though remissions have been obtained at lower doses, and it may take as long as 9 months to obtain results.[12] Because immunosuppressive drugs have not been effective in inducing remission in IBD when used alone, they do not appear to be an appropriate first-line drug for the management of acute Crohn's disease or ulcerative colitis. Immunosuppressive therapy has also been used to treat fistulas in Crohn's disease with some success.

Potential toxic reactions are a major consideration in the decision concerning ongoing prophylactic azathioprine or 6-mercaptopurine therapy. Reactions sufficiently severe to cause discontinuation of the drug occur in 15% of patients given 2.5 mg/kg/day without concomitant steroids.[13] Up to 25% of this toxicity is due to acute pancreatitis (self-limited with withdrawal of the drug).[14] The excess risk of cancer in patients given azathioprine for nontransplant, noncancer indications is a 1.6-fold increase.[15] The long-term toxicity of the drug as a prophylactic agent against flare-up or recurrence of Crohn's disease remains unknown.

The major role for immunosuppressives at this time is for patients with considerable disability who are unresponsive to sulfasalazine, whose disease relapses when steroids are withdrawn, and for whom other measures (e.g., surgery) are inappropriate. The optimal dose of treatment with immunosuppressants is still an unanswered question.

Metronidazole.—Numerous antibiotics have been used with little success in the management of IBD. One antibiotic, metronidazole, however, has been demonstrated to be effective in the management of one of the complications of IBD, rectal fistulas. The presence of perirectal disease leading to fistula and abscess formation has historically been a very difficult complication of Crohn's disease to treat. Antibiotics, local care, and steroids have all been attempted with little long-term success; however, the use of metronidazole has met with relatively good success.[16] The two most serious adverse reactions reported in patients treated with metronidazole have been seizures and peripheral neuropathy.[17] The most common reactions are referable to the GI tract, including nausea, anorexia, vomiting, diarrhea, epigastric distress, and abdominal cramping; headaches are also often seen.

Nutritional intervention.—Nutritional therapy has been used as an important modality in treatment of GI fistulas and in the control of the general disease activity in IBD. Gastrointestinal fistulas occur in at least one half of the patients with chronic Crohn's disease and lead to a variety of complications.[18] Fistulas frequently end in indolent abscess cavities, which are the source of palpable masses, persistent fevers, and pain. Enteroenteric fistulas between loops of small or large bowel may contribute to recirculation of intestinal contents, and the consequent stasis promotes bacterial overgrowth within the small bowel, leading to nutritional problems. Fistulas between bowel and urinary bladder (1%–2% of cases) lead to persistent urinary tract infection, and pneumaturia may be a manifestation of such fistulas. Total parenteral nutrition has considerably improved the prognosis of these fistulas.[19] Enteral nutrition with an elemental formulation has also been used, as with the patient described here, although its use in the closure of fistulas has not been studied rigorously.

The beneficial use of TPN and elemental diets as primary treatment for acute

Crohn's disease and as adjunctive treatment for complications such as subacute obstruction, bile salt–induced diarrhea, perianal fissures, and growth failure has been suggested in several reports.[20, 21] However, the exact mechanism by which these nutritional therapies induce remission of the disease is not clear. The alteration in the course of the disease may be related to the enhanced nutritional status of the patient, the nutritional therapy's hypoallergenicity (by minimizing the macromolecular antigenic load to the intestine), and possibly by an alteration in the bowel flora. Nutritional management (parenteral and enteral) has also been used as adjunctive therapy and has been associated with better surgical outcome.[22] Although quite effective in Crohn's disease, nutritional therapy has not been of much help in the management of chronic ulcerative colitis.[23]

The elemental enteral formulations available are relatively unpalatable, although some patients have been able to drink their required daily amount. Generally, a constant or nighttime nasogastric infusion allows the bypassing of the gustatory sensation as well as providing the slow provision of appropriate calories, avoiding the problems of bloating, nausea with vomiting, and anorexia in patients with severe Crohn's disease. The formulation is started slowly, first providing about 25% of the required calories and then advancing as tolerated to total calories. The major limitation with this nutritional management is the high relapse rate, with the general length of remission being about 4 to 6 months.

Elemental enteral feedings are often helpful as an adjunct in the management of strictures, particularly if the patient has difficulty with solid food. As in the case of this patient, enteral feedings were initially helpful, and although the remission was short lived (about 4 months), she was able to complete her school semester and was then better able to face the need for surgery.

Strictures secondary to chronic inflammation and fibrosis sometimes do not resolve entirely with a medical and nutritional management protocol. Surgery is usually the answer for these patients and sometimes can bring on a longer remission than the other modes of management, permitting complete tapering of the steroids. However, the relapse rate with surgery is high in Crohn's disease,[24] and repeated surgical intervention can lead to the complications of short bowel syndrome, which are very difficult to manage.

In addition to the effect on disease activity and its intestinal complications, there are numerous nutritional and metabolic imbalances in IBD that require attention. Many of these problems are related to the diseased ileum, which is particularly important in the digestive, absorptive, metabolic, and nutritional activities of the GI tract. Ileal disease or resection can be associated with diminished or absent absorption of vitamin B_{12} and bile acids, lactose intolerance, or protein-losing enteropathy. The decreased reabsorption of bile salts results in a lowered concentration of bile salts in the proximal intestine with decreased micelle formation and fat absorption. Bile salt concentrations in gallbladder bile are decreased, and alterations in lipid metabolism, defective absorption of vitamin D metabolites, and diminished absorption of trace metals such as zinc, calcium, and magnesium occur. The administration of cholectyramine to bind bile acids can minimize the diarrhea associated with this malabsorption.

SUMMARY

The management of IBD is a complex, ongoing process. The review of this patient's course has provided the opportunity to discuss the pharmacologic and nutritional interventions that may be used alone or in concert in patients with IBD (see Table 11–1). With a relatively limited number of pharmacologic agents available, much interest is now focused on the nutritional mode of therapy, which has a relatively low morbidity. Certainly, further work is necessary to identify the methods by which nutritional therapy is effective and how to best combine nutritional, medical, and surgical intervention.

REFERENCES

1. Farmer RG, Hawk WA, Turnbull RB: Clinical patterns in Crohn's disease. A statistical study of 615 patients. *Gastroenterology* 1975; 68:627–635.
2. Greenstein AJ, Janowitz HD, Saeher DB: The extraintestinal complications of Crohn's disease and ulcerative colitis: A study of 700 patients. *Medicine* (Baltimore) 1976; 55:401–402.
3. Gyboski JD, Spiro HW: Prognosis in children with Crohn's disease. *Gastroenterology* 1978; 74:807–817.
4. Summers RW, Swartz DM, Sessions JT, et al: National Cooperative Crohn's Disease Study: Results of drug treatment. *Gastroenterology* 1979; 77:847–869.
5. Sadeghy-Nejed A, Senior B: The treatment of ulcerative colitis in children with alternate-day corticosteroids. *Pediatrics* 1968; 43:840–845.
6. Taffet SL, Das KM: Sulfasalazine adverse effects and investigation. *Dig Dis Sci* 1983; 28:833–842.
7. Stenson WF: Pharmacology of sulfasalazine. *Viewpoint Dig Dis* 1984; 16:13–16.
8. Dissanayake AS, Truelove SC: A controlled therapeutic trial of long-term maintenance treatment of ulcerative colitis with sulfasalazine. *Gut* 1973; 14:818.
9. Kahn AKA, Piris J, Truelove SC: An experiment to determine the active therapeutic moiety of sulfasalazine. *Lancet* 1977; 2:892–895.
10. Rosmussen SN, Binder V, Maili R, et al: Treatment of Crohn's disease with peroral 5-aminosalicylic acid. *Gastroenterology* 1983; 85:1350–1355.
11. Campieri M, Lafranchi GA, Bazzocchi G, et al: Treatment of ulcerative colitis with high-dose 5-aminosalicylic acid enemas. *Lancet* 1981; 2:270–271.
12. Present DH, Kotelitz BI, Wisch N, et al: Treatment of Crohn's disease with 6-mercaptopurine. *N Engl J Med* 1980; 302:981–987.
13. Singleton JW, Law DH, Kelley ML, et al: National Cooperative Crohn's Disease Study: Adverse reactions to study drugs. *Gastroenterology* 1979; 77:870–882.
14. Studerant RAL, Singleton JW, Deren JJ: Azathioprine-related pancreatitis in patients with Crohn's disease. *Gastroenterology* 1977; 77:883–886.
15. Kinlen LJ, Sheril AGR, Peto J, Doll R: Collaborative United Kingdom-Australian study of cancer in patients treated with immunosuppressive drugs. *Br Med J* 1979; 2:1461–1466.
16. Bernstein LH, Frank MS, Braudt LJ, et al: Healing of perineal Crohn's disease with metronidazole. *Gastroenterology* 1980; 79:357–365.
17. Duffy LF, Daum F, Fisher SE, et al: Peripheral neuropathy in Crohn's disease patients treated with metronidazole. *Gastroenterology* 1985; 88:681–684.

18. Korelitz BI, Present DH: Favorable effect of 6-mercaptopurine on fistulae of Crohn's disease. *Dig Dis Sci* 1985; 30:58–64.
19. N-Fekete C, Ricour C, Duhamel JF, et al: Enterocutaneous fistulas of the small bowel in children (25 cases). *J Pediatr Surg* 1978; 13:1–4.
20. Strobel CT, Byrne WJ, Ament ME: Home parenteral nutrition in children with Crohn's disease: An effective management alternative. *Gastroenterology* 1979; 77:272–279.
21. O'Morain C, Segal AJ, Levi AJ: Elemental diet in treatment of acute Crohn's disease. *Br Med J* 1980; 281:1173–1175.
22. Lake AM, Kim S, Mathis RK, et al: Influence of preoperative parenteral alimentation on postoperative growth in adolescent Crohn's disease. *J Pediatr Gastroenterol Nutr* 1985; 4:182–186.
23. McIntyre PB, Powell-Tuck J, Wood SR, et al: Controlled trial of bowel rest in the treatment of severe acute colitis. *Gut* 1986; 27:481–485.
24. Lock MR, Farmer RG, Fazio VW, et al: Recurrence and reoperation for Crohn's disease. *N Engl J Med* 1981; 304:1585–1588.

12 Surgical Management of Ulcerative Colitis

Robert C. Shamberger, M.D.

A 16-year old girl presented with a 2-month history of intermittent bloody stools. One week before admission she developed diarrhea and intermittent fevers. Sigmoidoscopy revealed severe diffuse active colitis. Stool cultures, examination for ova and parasites, and a tuberculin skin test were obtained, and results were negative. Three days before admission she developed anorexia, nausea, and vomiting. At admission she was febrile (39.2°C) with a mildly distended, tender abdomen. The white blood cell count was 16,700/mm^3 with 23% polymorphonuclear lymphocytes and 44% band forms. The abdominal radiographs demonstrated absence of colonic haustra but no significant increase in bowel diameter. Intravenous (IV) antibiotics and high-dose steroids were instituted, as was bowel rest and parenteral nutrition. Despite these maneuvers and a trial of azathioprine, more than 1 L of bloody diarrhea per day persisted over the next 3 weeks, requiring multiple blood transfusions. Colonoscopy demonstrated diffuse ulceration of the entire colon. A barium upper gastrointestinal (GI) study was entirely normal. Because the patient did not improve on maximum medical management, an abdominal colectomy, Brooke ileostomy, and closure of the rectal stump were performed. Six months later she had an ileoanal pullthrough with a diverting ileostomy. The ileostomy was closed at 4 months, and excellent continence has been achieved.

DISCUSSION

Ulcerative colitis is a diffuse inflammatory process involving the mucosal layer of the colon. The etiology of this disease remains a mystery. Medical management of ulcerative colitis with steroids, azulfidine, azathioprine, and diet (discussed in Chapter 11) is usually successful in controlling acute exacerbations of inflammation and the resulting bloody diarrhea, tenesmus, and crampy abdominal pain. The goal of treatment is to achieve remission of acute inflammation, maintain normal growth and development, and limit the number and duration of symptomatic attacks. No medical treatment, however, has been successful in curing this illness. In severe cases, treatment often includes surgical removal of the colonic mucosa, which is the only cure for the disease.

The timing of surgery depends on the initial presentation of the disease and response to treatment. Three conditions lead to surgery in children: a surgical emergency, disease that is unresponsive to optimal medical management, and chronic debilitating disease that causes an unacceptable quality of life (Table 12–1). Of the conditions that are unresponsive to maximal medical management, toxic megacolon is the most acute and, fortunately, the least common.[1] Surgery may be required within 48 to 72 hours of initial symptoms. Signs of toxic megacolon include high fever, leukocytosis, a large fluid requirement, and thrombocytopenia. Delay in recognizing and treating this condition of fulminant systemic symptoms and high risk for colonic perforation may be truly life threatening. More frequently, surgical intervention is required for uncontrolled colonic hemorrhage or failure to achieve an initial remission despite high-dose steroids and bowel rest, as occurred in this patient.

The indications for surgery for the first two categories are fairly clear cut. However, the decision to go to surgery because of an unacceptable quality of life is made on much more subjective grounds. The overall well-being of the patient considering such factors as school attendance and participation in extracurricular and family activities is based primarily on the patient's tolerance of his or her symptoms. Other factors that can lead to surgery in the pediatric age group are growth failure and delayed development of sexual maturity, intractable extraintestinal manifestations, and morbidity from long-term steroids. The decision to undergo surgery for chronic debilitating disease is entered into only after lengthy discussions involving the patient and parents, the surgeon, and the gastroenterologist and must be balanced against the psychologic effect of major surgery in the tumultuous teenage years. When surgery is contemplated, we often ask the patient to discuss his/her concerns and questions with another young person with ulcerative colitis who has already undergone the surgery.

The risk of the development of cancer is a very real concern for patients with ulcerative colitis, but fortunately the risk is very low in the first 10 years of the disease. The risk is low (<3%) but not absent during the first decade of the illness but increases thereafter at an initially estimated rate of 20% per decade.[2] More recent

TABLE 12–1.
Indications for Surgery

I. Surgical emergency
A. Colonic perforation
B. Uncontrolled colonic hemorrhage
II. Severe disease unresponsive to medical management
A. Toxic megacolon
B. Continued severe symptoms after 2 weeks of maximum support and IV steroids
III. Unacceptable quality of life
A. Recurrent or intractable colitis
B. Growth failure
C. Intractable extraintestinal manifestations
D. Morbidity from long-term systemic steroids
E. Risk for developing colonic cancer

studies suggest a somewhat lower cumulative risk of cancer at 25 years of 33.7 ± 8.6%.[3] The occurrence of carcinoma is commoner among patients with universal colitis and an unremitting course both characteristic of ulcerative colitis in the pediatric group, so these patients must have close follow-up as they become adults. Mild or limited disease does not obviate the ultimate risk of neoplasia.

Surgical Management

A rapid evolution has occurred in the surgical management of ulcerative colitis, and currently several treatment alternatives are available to the patient and surgeon. Prior to 1950, colectomy was seldom performed for ulcerative colitis.[4] The usually moribund patient was previously subjected to some form of "venting" procedure, such as appendicostomy, cecostomy, or double-barrel ileostomy through which various irrigants could be administered. The standard ileostomy performed in that era often resulted in serositis of the exposed bowel wall, high stoma output, fluid and salt depletion, and severe and painful skin inflammation. Recognition of the need to perform a proctocolectomy to provide a disease-free outcome and improvements in the ileostomy by Brooke were the first great advances.[5] Since Brooke's operative breakthrough, recent efforts have focused on technical improvements and the achievement of fecal continence. All results regarding morbidity, mortality, and long-term satisfaction should be compared with his benchmark efforts.

The initial surgery performed is determined by the clinical condition of the patient. In the acute setting when colonic resection is required for toxic megacolon, fulminant colitis, hemorrhage, or perforation, the procedure should be limited to an abdominal colectomy, closure but not removal of the distal rectum, and Brooke ileostomy, as in this patient. When the acute episode is over or in the elective setting, several reconstructive procedures can be considered, including proctocolectomy and ileostomy, abdominal colectomy and ileorectal anastomosis, proctocolectomy and a continent ileostomy (Kock's pouch), and the ileoanal pull-through with anal preservation (Fig 12–1).

Surgery in the Acute Setting

Colectomy and Brooke's ileostomy are the operation of choice in the acute setting because it is associated with the lowest frequency of complications and can be accomplished most expeditiously in the acutely ill patient. It has as its major drawback the external stoma and a required appliance. It is technically the simplest procedure for ulcerative colitis and in a recent review revision was required in only 11% of patients.[6] More than 90% of adult patients in responding to a questionnaire stated they were satisfied with their diets, were employed, and had few problems with the management of their stomas.[6] Three fourths of the patients experienced no restrictions in their daily activities, and 95% expressed overall satisfaction with the surgery and ileostomy. The majority (72%) stated they would not consider a change in the type of ileostomy they had. On the negative side is the considerable cost of stoma supplies. In addition, 40% of patients had some peristomal skin irritation during their postoperative course, and persistent unhealed perineal wounds occurred in about one third of patients. The most telling of the figures is the fact that of

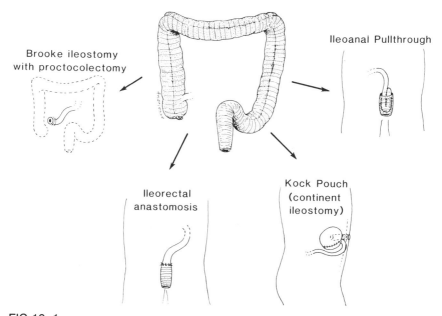

FIG 12–1.
The surgical alternatives for ulcerative colitis are depicted. They include removal of the entire colon and creation of an end ileostomy, removal of the intra-abdominal colon and anastomosis of the ileum to the rectum, removal of the entire colon and creation of a continent ileostomy, or removal of the abdominal colon and a mucosal proctectomy with an ileoanal anastomosis.

patients aware of alternative procedures, 40% desire or would consider a change. Adolescents are particularly reluctant to accept permanent ileostomy.

Surgery in the Elective Setting

The ileorectal anastomosis (see Fig 12–1) with preservation of the rectum has been a controversial alternative to proctocolectomy and the Brooke ileostomy and is not widely accepted. The major concerns raised about this procedure have centered around leaving the involved rectal mucosa intact with its capacity for malignant degeneration; colorectal cancer has been reported in patients who are left with the rectal stump.[7, 8] The use of this procedure is generally reserved for special situations where a stoma or fecal incontinence would be difficult to manage. If ileorectal anastomosis is selected, close follow-up and periodic endoscopy are essential.

The continent ileostomy or the Kock pouch was designed in an effort to free the patient of an ostomy device while still allowing drainage of a stoma on the abdominal wall.[9] A reservoir is created from the terminal portion of the ileum, and an intussusception nipple valve that allows eggress of pouch contents only when intubated by a specially constructed ileostomy catheter is constructed.

The major advantage of this method is avoidance of an external ostomy device. Its major disadvantages are threefold. First, it requires intubation by the patient on a regular schedule, a demand often hard to achieve in the teenage patient. Second, it requires manipulation of the stoma, which is often as disagreeable to the patient as is dealing with the ostomy device. Finally, even in the best of hands the procedure has been plagued by the need for surgical revision.[10–12] The Kock pouch has not been used significantly in the pediatric population.

The ileoanal pullthrough is the final surgical alternative, which has only recently gained wide favor since the technical details of the procedure have been established and favorable results have been reported.[13] Key technical factors for successful ileoanal pull-through include creation of some reservoir capacity and placement of the pouch within the pelvis below the peritoneal floor, which results in improved emptying. Submucosal dissection of the rectal mucosa in ulcerative colitis is difficult because the inflamed friable mucosa makes this a very lengthy, tedious, and often sanguine procedure. A rectal muscular cuff of 5 to 6 cm has proved adequate for continence (Fig 12–2).

The factors that will ultimately determine continence following ileoanal pull-through are multiple. First, without the colon to reabsorb water the effluent will be

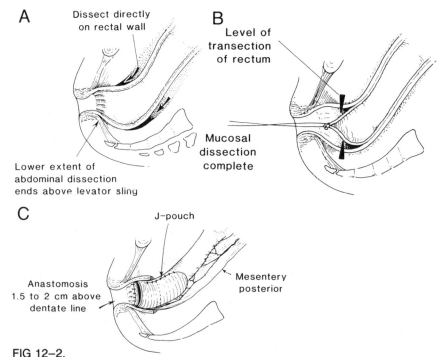

FIG 12–2.
The pelvic dissection for the ileoanal pullthrough is demonstrated. The rectum is dissected from the abdominal approach down to the levator sling with the dissection carried out directly on the rectal wall to avoid injury to the pelvic innervation **(A)**. The rectal mucosa is dissected from the perineal approach in the submucosal plane to a point above the levator sling. The rectal muscular wall is then divided above the levator sling and below the level of the mucosal dissection **(B)**. The J pouch is then brought down through the muscular tube of the rectum and joined to the remaining rectal mucosa **(C)**.

liquid in contrast with the normal consistency of stool. Second, some reservoir capacity must be achieved through either construction of a pouch or dilatation of the ileum because studies have shown that ileal capacity, compliance, and complete emptying correlate very well with good functional outcome.[14, 15] Distension of the ileum will result in propulsive peristalsis of the intact ileal wall as well as relaxation of the internal sphincter muscle. Third, the external and internal sphincters and the puborectalis muscle, the muscles involved with continence, must be preserved.

This procedure is not performed in the emergency setting or in patients nutritionally depleted or receiving high-dose steroids because of the increased frequency of complications. For these reasons, this patient underwent a staged sequence of surgeries beginning with an abdominal colectomy and a diverting Brooke ileostomy. By exclusion of patients with Crohn's colitis, elective operation on nutritionally intact patients, and creation of a diverting ileostomy, early complications of pelvic sepsis, fistula, and anastomotic breakdown have been uncommon.[16]

The most important postoperative concerns for patients center around the adequacy of fecal continence. Stool frequency is generally of secondary importance. The success of the procedure has varied, but several centers have reported good results. Telander and Dozois reported in a pediatric population no major difficulty with daytime leakage and a 3% to 13% occurrence of nocturnal leakage requiring use of a pad.[17] Only 3 of 65 patients required subsequent ileostomy and are considered poor results. Two patients have had persistent moderate nocturnal soiling lasting more than 6 months following their surgery. Coran et al. have utilized the straight ileoanal anastomosis without a pouch and preserved the distal 1 cm of mucosa.[18] In their experience, patients have been continent during the daytime and only rarely incontinent at night. Stool frequency in this series was from 2 to 20 per day early in their courses and have required psyllium hydrophilic mucilloid (Metamucil), diphenoxylate-atropine (Lomotil), and loperamide (Imodium) for symptomatic relief. This frequency has decreased with postoperative enlargement and accommodation of the ileum to an average of six movements per day at 1 year. Daytime incontinence in patients whose surgery was done at the Mayo Clinic was minor in 25% and major in 2.5%.[19] Some degree of nocturnal incontinence was found in almost one half of the patients. Five percent of the patients required conversion to a conventional ileostomy because of pelvic sepsis, Crohn's disease, or intractable diarrhea. Fonkalsrud reported 78% of patients completely continent during the day, 18% with minor "seepage," and 4% with occasional soiling.[20] Three of 77 patients were converted to ileostomy. All groups have had a significant rate of small bowel obstruction reported from 9% to 17% of patients. This has been attributed to the extensive mobilization of the small bowel and the creation of mesenteric defects that are required for the ileum to readily reach into the pelvis.

SUMMARY

There are three general indications for surgery in patients with ulcerative colitis: surgical emergency, disease unresponsive to medical management, and unacceptable quality of life (see Table 12–1). Currently several surgical alternatives are available to the patient with ulcerative colitis. Each procedure has limitations, and modification of the techniques will continue as additional experience is gained. Full discussion of each surgical possibility with the patient and family is essential to help them make the best choice and to prepare them for possible complications that may be encountered. If an emergency colectomy is required, the rectum should be retained to allow future ileoanal pull-through if this alternative is selected.

REFERENCES

1. Ehrenpreis T: Ulcerative colitis, in Mustard WT, Ravitch MM, Snyder WH Jr, et al (eds): *Pediatric Surgery*, ed 2. Chicago; Year Book Medical Publishers, 1969, pp 940–948.
2. Devroede GJ, Taylor WF, Sauer WG, et al: Cancer risk and life expectancy of children with ulcerative colitis. *N Engl J Med* 1971; 285:17–21.
3. Kewenter J, Ahlman H, Hulten L: Cancer risk in extensive ulcerative colitis. *Ann Surg* 1978; 188:824–828.
4. Gardner C, Miller GG: Total colectomy for ulcerative colitis. *Arch Surg* 1951; 63:370–372.
5. Brooke BN: The management of an ileostomy including its complications. *Lancet* 1952; 2:102–104.
6. Pemberton JH, Phillips SF, Dozois RR, et al: Current clinical results, in Dozois RR (ed): *Alternatives to Conventional Ileostomy*. Chicago, Year Book Medical Publisher, 1985, pp 40–50.
7. Baker WNW, Glass RE, Ritchie JK, et al: Cancer of the rectum following colectomy and ileorectal anastomosis for ulcerative colitis. *Br J Surg* 1978; 65:862–868.
8. Grundfest SF, Fazio V, Weiss RA, et al: The risk of cancer following colectomy and ileorectal anastomosis for extensive mucosal ulcerative colitis. *Ann Surg* 1981; 193:9–14.
9. Kock NG: Intraabdominal "reservoir" in patients with permanent ileostomy. Arch Surg 1969; 99:223–231.
10. Kock NG, Myrvold HE, Nilsson LO, et al: Continent ileostomy: The Swedish experience, in Dozois RR (ed): *Alternatives to Conventional Ileostomy*. Chicago, Year Book Medical Publisher, 1985, pp 163–175.
11. Dozois RR, Kelly KA, Beart RW, et al: Improved results with continent ileostomy. *Ann Surg* 1980; 192:319–324.
12. Dozois RR, Kelly KA, Beart RW Jr, et al: Continent ileostomy: The Mayo Clinic experience, in Dozois RR (ed): *Alternatives to Conventional Ileostomy*. Chicago, Year Book Medical Publisher, 1985, pp 180–191.
13. Martin LW, LeCoultre C, Schubert WK: Total colectomy and mucosal proctectomy with preservation of continence in ulcerative colitis. *Ann Surg* 1977; 186:477–480.
14. Stryker SJ, Phillips SF, Dozois RR, et al: Anal and neorectal function after ileal pouch-anal anastomosis. *Ann Surg* 1986; 203:55–61.
15. Taylor BM, Cranley B, Kelly KA, et al: A clinico-physiological comparison of ileal pouch-anal and straight ileoanal anastomoses. *Ann Surg* 1983; 198:462–468.
16. Beart RW Jr, Metcalf AM, Dozois RR, et al: The "J" ileal pouch-anal anastomosis: The Mayo Clinic experience, in Dozois RR (ed): *Alternatives to Conventional Ileostomy*. Chicago, Year Book Medical Publisher, 1985, pp 384–397.
17. Telander RL, Dozois RR: The endorectal ileoanal anastomosis in Farnell MB, McIlrath DC (eds): *Problems in General Surgery*. Philadelphia, JB Lippincott Co, 1984, p 39.
18. Coran AG, Sarahan TM, Dent TL, et al: The endorectal pull-through for the manage-

ment of ulcerative colitis in children and adults. *Ann Surg* 1983; 197:99–105.
19. Metcalf AM, Dozois RR, Kelly KA, et al: Ileal "J" pouch-anal anastomosis: Clinical outcome. *Ann Surg* 1985; 202:735–739.
20. Fonkalsrud EW: Endorectal ileal pullthrough with isoperistaltic ileal reservoir for colitis and polyposis. *Ann Surg* 1985; 202:145–152.

13　Acute Diarrhea

John D. Snyder, M.D.

A 13-month-old boy was in his usual state of excellent health until he developed the acute onset of diarrhea 5 days earlier without fever, rash, or vomiting. His mother noted that his stools had changed from one formed brown movement per day to five to eight watery movements per day associated with mild abdominal discomfort. He had no accompanying respiratory symptoms, change in his urinary habits, abdominal distention, or hematochezia. His appetite and energy levels were decreased. No other family members were ill, and the child had no antecedent history of frequent infections, recent travel, manipulations of his normal diet, exposure to well water or animals, or recent use of antibiotics or other medications. The child attended a day-care center regularly.

He was initially switched from his regular diet of full table foods and milk to clear liquids, especially apple juice, for 2 days without improvement. He was then given alternating days of a milk-free diet (including bananas, applesauce, crackers, toast, and juice) and clear liquids with no change in his stooling.

On examination the child was irritable but consolable, alert, and drank thirstily. His height and head circumference were at the 50th percentile, and his weight was at the 25th percentile. His skin turgor was slightly decreased, his mucous membranes were mildly dry, but his orbits were firm, and he had no postural changes in pulse or blood pressure. He was assessed to be 5% dehydrated. Results of his examination were otherwise normal and included a soft, nontender abdomen without masses. The stool examination results were negative for blood, reducing substances, fat staining, or polymorphonuclear leukocytes. A stool culture and a stool sample for ova and parasite analysis were taken. Examinations for viral particles and stool electrolytes were not done.

The child was initially given an oral glucose-electrolyte solution containing 139 mmole/L of glucose, 75 mmole/L of sodium, 20 mmole/L of potassium, 60 mmole/L of chloride, and 35 mmole/L of citrate. He drank avidly and then produced a urine sample with a specific gravity of 1.032. He took 800 ml of the fluid in 4 hours, and his weight increased from 21.4 lb (9.7 kg) on presentation to 22.5 lb (10.2 kg). He was discharged from the emergency room on the glucose-electrolyte solution with directions to begin eating again utilizing an initial diet of rice cereal, noodles, and half-strength milk. His hydration status remained good, and the volume of diarrhea began to diminish by the next day. His stool evaluation was negative for *Salmonella, Shigella, Campylobacter, Yersinia enterocolitica, Giardia lamblia, Cryptosporidium,* and *Entamoeba histolytica.*

DISCUSSION

Clinical Features

This case highlights several important points about the evaluation and therapy of a child with acute infectious diarrhea. The history should seek information about an associated illness or risk factors to help identify a causative agent. This child had no evidence of an upper respiratory tract, pulmonary, or urinary tract infection that can often be associated with diarrhea. No history of exposure to well water or animals was elicited that would have indicated an increased risk of infectious diarrhea from *Salmonella, Shigella, Campylobacter, Y. enterocolitica, Giardia,* and *Cryptosporidium.* Travel to lesser developed countries would have increased his risk for infection from many of these pathogens and from enteropathogenic and enterotoxigenic *Escherichia coli* and parasites, including *E. histolytica.* The dietary history is very important since children whose diets differ greatly from the usual proportion of fat (40%–50%), carbohydrate (40%–50%), and protein (10%–15%) can also develop diarrhea.[1] The child had no history of exposure to antibiotics that would have increased his risk for *Clostridium difficile* infection. He did attend a day-care center, which is a significant risk factor for enteric infections in young children.[2] Day-care center outbreaks of a variety of enteric pathogens have been reported, with *Salmonella, Shigella, Campylobacter,* and *Giardia* infections being especially common.[3] Many cases of *Cryptosporidium,* a newly recognized parasitic pathogen, have been reported from day-care settings.[4]

The physical examination in this child demonstrated 5% dehydration but no other diagnostic findings. The assessment of dehydration should include evaluation of the skin turgor, moisture of the mucous membranes, firmness of the orbits, alertness, and presence or absence of postural changes in the heart rate or blood pressure.

The laboratory examination of the acutely dehydrated child with a history and physical examination that point to a probable infectious etiology can usually be fairly limited. Infectious diarrheas are caused by pathogens from one of three classes of microorganisms: bacteria, viruses, or parasites, which often produce illness that is very similar. A more helpful classification is to group pathogens by their inflammatory or noninflammatory nature since most enteric pathogens act in one of these two ways (Table 13–1).[5] Most common bacterial pathogens in North America cause inflammatory lesions that often cause white blood cells (WBCs) or red blood cells (RBCs) in the stools.[5] The viruses and common parasites (*Giardia lamblia* and *Cryptospor-*

TABLE 13–1.
Mechanisms of Illness Caused by Common North American Enteric Pathogens

Inflammatory	Noninflammatory
Salmonella	Rotavirus
Shigella	Norwalk virus
Campylobacter	Enteric adenovirus
Y. enterocolitica	*G. lamblia*
C. difficile	*Cryptosporidium*

idium) are more likely not to show inflammatory changes. A microscopic examination of the stool using either a Wright's stain or Gram stain should be done to determine whether RBCs or WBCs are present in the stool. Without such evidence of inflammation, the yield of finding a bacterial enteric pathogen is exceedingly low. Guerrant et al. reported a greater than 10-fold increase in positive stool cultures when initial screening for fecal leukocytes was instituted.[6]

Therapy

Since most acute diarrheal episodes are self-limited and do not require antimicrobial therapy, the need to seek an enteric pathogen in a case like this can be questioned. The usual course to follow is to treat any dehydration and ongoing losses with oral rehydration therapy (ORT) using a glucose-electrolyte solution and then reintroduce feedings.

Oral rehydration therapy has been successfully used since the late 1960s to provide replacement and maintenance fluids for children with diarrhea.[7] Successful controlled clinical trials have been carried out in more than 60 developing and developed countries around the world usually using formulations similar to the World Health Organization (WHO) and UNICEF–approved formula of 111 mEq/L of glucose, 90 mEq/L of sodium, 20 mEq/L of potassium, 80 mEq/L of chloride, and 30 mEq/L of citrate.[7] Acceptance in the United States has lagged behind the rest of the world, and physicians and families here still often use inappropriate fluids such as fruit juices and carbonated beverages (Table 13–2).[8] Fruit juices have a high osmolarity because their high carbohydrate concentration and have been shown to be a cause of prolonged diarrhea in children.[9] The sodium concentration in juices is too low even for a maintenance solution. Carbonated beverages, likewise, have a high carbohydrate and low electrolyte concentration and should not be used for either maintenance or rehydration therapy. Use of glucose-electrolyte solutions is now increasing in the United States, and a number of new commercial products are available (see Table 13–2).

Two major concerns about the use of glucose-electrolyte solutions continue to be raised. The first is the concern for hypernatremia especially using the WHO-UNICEF solution. In practice, this solution has been used effectively to treat hypernatremia,[10] and if early feeding or free water consumption is initiated, this solution can even effectively provide maintenance fluid and electrolytes to patients without dehydration who have normal renal function.[11] The excess sodium is excreted in the urine.[11] In the United States, extensive use with the commercially available solutions that have sodium concentrations of between 45 to 90 mEq/L have shown them to be effective and safe.[12, 13]

The second major concern about the use of ORT solutions is their use in children with vomiting, which frequently accompanies diarrhea. Oral rehydration therapy can be used effectively in children with vomiting if given in small, frequent doses with net retention of fluid and electrolytes as the goal.[14] Retention is often increased by giving ORT 5 ml at a time.

The second component of oral therapy for diarrhea is the early reinstitution of feeding. Debate has continued for many years about the efficacy of withholding or

TABLE 13–2.
Composition of Commonly Used Hydration Solutions

		mEq/L			
	Glucose (gm/dl)	Sodium	Potassium	Base	Osmoles
Apple juice	550–850 (10–15)	3	20	0	700
Cola drinks	275–550 (5–10)	2	0.1	13 (HCO_3)	550
Infalyte	111 (2)	50	20	30 (HCO_3)	270
Lytren	111 (2)	50	25	30 (citrate)	270
Pedialyte	139 (2.5)	45	20	30 (citrate)	270
Reosol	111 (2)	50	20	23 (citrate)	270
Rehydrolyte	139 (2.5)	75	20	35 (citrate)	309
WHO-UNICEF ORS	111 (2)	90	20	30 (citrate)	310

giving food during diarrhea.[15] Until recently, little data have supported either position; however, several recent studies have indicated that earlier feeding may be the best method to quicken the recovery.[16–18] Use of simple foods such as rice powder to provide the carbohydrate source for rehydration solutions has resulted in decreased stool volume and duration when compared with a standard glucose-electrolyte solution.[16] Santosham et al. have shown increased weight gain and decreased stool output in children begun on formula feedings after 4 hours of ORT compared with children receiving only ORT and no food for 48 hours.[17] The current recommendation is to begin feedings when a child has been rehydrated using easily absorbed foods such as rice or wheat and emphasizing breast-feeding if possible.[15]

SUMMARY

This case has emphasized several important points about the evaluation and management of a child with acute diarrhea. From the history, risk factors including water supply, exposure to animals, travel history, and day-care attendance can be clues for enteric infection. Assessment of hydration status is the most important part of the physical examination. The laboratory evaluation should include a stool smear since the presence of WBCs and RBCs is more commonly seen with bacterial infections. Since most diarrheal episodes are self-limited, therapy should center on fluid and electrolyte replacement to treat or prevent dehydration. Oral rehydration therapy has proved to be the simplest, most effective, and least expensive method of therapy. Mounting evidence indicates that appropriate feeding of easily digested foods can help speed recovery from a diarrheal episode.

REFERENCES

1. Cohen SA, Hendricks KM, Mathis RK, et al: Chronic nonspecific diarrhea: Dietary relationships. *Pediatrics* 1979; 64:402–407.
2. Pickering LK, Bartlett AV, Woodward WE: Acute infectious diarrhea among children in day care: Epidemiology and control. *Rev Infect Dis* 1986; 4:539–547.
3. Pickering LK, Woodward WE: Diarrhea in day care centers. *Pediatr Infect Dis* 1982; 1:47–52.
4. Wolfson JS, Hopkins CC, Weber DJ, et al: An association between *Cryptosporidium* and *Giardia* in stool. *N Engl J Med* 1984; 310:788.
5. Guerrant RL: Gastrointestinal infections and food poisoning: Principles and definition of syndromes, in Mandell GL, Douglas RG, Bennett JE (eds): *Principles and Practice of Infectious Diseases,* ed 2. New York; John Wiley & Sons 1985, pp 635–646.
6. Guerrant RL, Shields DS, Thorson SM, et al: Evaluation and diagnosis of acute infectious diarrhea. *Am J Med* 1985; 78:91–96.
7. *Oral Rehydration Therapy: An Annotated Bibliography.* Washington, DC, Pan American Health Organization Scientific Publication no 445, 1983.
8. Snyder JD: From Pedialyte to popsicles: A look at oral rehydration therapy used in the United States and Canada. *Am J Clin Nutr* 1982; 35:157–161.

9. Hyams JS, Leichtner AM: Apple juice: An unappreciated cause of chronic diarrhea. *Am J Dis Child* 1985; 139:503–505.
10. Pizarro D, Posado G, Villavicencio N, et al: Oral rehydration in hypernatremic and hyponatremic diarrheal dehydration. *Am J Dis Child* 1983; 137:730–734.
11. Santosham M, Daum RS, Dillman L, et al: Oral rehydration therapy of infantile diarrhea: A controlled study of well nourished children hospitalized in the United States and Panama. *N Engl J Med* 1982; 306:1070–1076.
12. Santosham M, Burns B, Nadkarni V, et al: Oral rehydration therapy for acute diarrhea in ambulatory children in the United States: A double-blind comparison of four different solutions. *Pediatrics* 1985; 76:159–166.
13. Listernik R, Zieserl E, David AT: Outpatient oral rehydration in the United States. *Am J Dis Child* 1986; 140:211–215.
14. Finberg L: Oral rehydration: Finding the right solution. *Contemp Pediatr* 1987; 2:61–67.
15. Brown KH, MacLean WC: Nutritional management of acute diarrhea: An appraisal of the alternatives. *Pediatrics* 1984; 73:119–125.
16. Molla AM, Hossain M, Sarker SA, et al: Rice-powder electrolyte solution as oral therapy in diarrhea due to *Vibrio cholerae* and *Escherichia coli*. *Lancet* 1982; 1:1317–1319.
17. Santosham M, Foster S, Reid R, et al: Role of soy-based, lactose-free formula during treatment of acute diarrhea. *Pediatrics* 1985; 76:292–298.
18. Mehta MN, Subramanian S: Comparison of rice water, rice electrolyte solution, and glucose electrolyte solution in the management of infantile diarrhea. *Lancet* 1986; 1:843–845.

14 Bloody Diarrhea: *Salmonella*

Joaquin Cortiella, M.D.

A 2-month-old boy was admitted to the hospital because of bloody diarrhea and fever. The patient had been the 7.5 lb (3.4 kg) product of a term, uncomplicated pregnancy, labor, and delivery and had fed well on Similac with iron. The child grew well until 3 weeks of age, when he developed an upper respiratory tract infection. At 5 weeks of age he developed fever, irritability, and frequent watery, nonmucous stools for 1 day without melena or frank blood. The child had no exposure to well water, animals, or day care and had no travel history; no one else at home was ill. On examination he weighed 12.3 lb (5.58 kg), which was at the 90th percentile for age. He was febrile to 39°C, was irritable but consolable, and had no obvious source for his fever. On laboratory examination, the white blood cell (WBC) count was 5,800/mm³ with a normal differential cell count, the hematocrit was 24.3%, and the reticulocyte count was 1.8%. Cultures of his spinal fluid, urine, and stools were obtained. He was then admitted and treated for 3 days with ampicillin and gentamicin and was discharged when his cultures were negative. After discharge, the child fed well on formula, gained weight, and had normal stools. Two weeks after being discharged, the patient presented again with a 24-hour history of 12 mucousy, bloody stools. He had no vomiting, and no one else at home was sick. On examination he weighed 14.4 lb (6.55 kg), was afebrile, and was smiling and playful. His physical examination was unremarkable except for mild abdominal tenderness. The laboratory evaluation included a WBC count of 12,000/mm³ with a normal differential count, and the hematocrit was 26%. His stool Gram stain was positive for sheets of polymorphonuclear leukocytes. Stool and blood culture specimens were taken.

Because he looked well, the child was then sent home and continued to feed well on his formula. However, his stool culture grew *Salmonella blockley;* the blood culture was negative. He was then admitted to the hospital with a temperature of 38.3°C. He was irritable but consolable, and his physical examination was unchanged from the previous examination. Repeated blood and stool cultures were sent. During the hospitalization, the patient was treated with a 10-day course of IV ampicillin and 4 days of oral amoxacillin. While on ampicillin therapy, he was advanced to full-strength Pregestimil feedings. Seven days after stopping the ampicillin, the patient became irritable and had bloody stools again. A rigid sigmoidoscopy showed friable mucosa with punctate hemorrhages; the histology revealed mild focal infiltrates of neutrophils and eosinophils in the surface epithelium, consistent with mild acute proctitis secondary to infection. The bloody stools resolved without further treatment, and the patient has done well.

DISCUSSION

This case provides a forum for reviewing the differential diagnosis of bloody diarrhea and the special considerations for treatment of an infant with *Salmonella enteritidis*. A full discussion of the diagnostic considerations for a child with bloody stools is included in Chapter 21. This discussion will focus on the infectious and inflammatory etiologies in an infant.

Clinical Features

A careful history and physical examination are essential to the evaluation of the infant with bloody diarrhea. This child had no obvious risk factors, including travel history or exposure to well water or animals. Fever, rashes, such as those seen in Henoch-Schönlein purpura, petechiae, and purpura should always be sought. Several important findings in this child pointed to an infectious or inflammatory etiology for his diarrhea. He had a low-grade fever, abdominal pain, and inflammatory cells and blood in his stool. The presence of the inflammatory cells is perhaps the most important single finding. Several recent studies have shown that the rate of recovery of enteric pathogens is greatly increased when inflammatory cells are present in the stool.[1, 2] The routine evaluation of stool smears using a Wright or Gram stain has proved to be a very cost-effective method for determining which stool samples should be sent for culture.[2]

Diagnosis

The commonest invasive enteric bacterial pathogens found in this country are *Campylobacter jejuni*, salmonellae, *Shigella*, and *Yersinia enterocolitica* (Table 14–1).[3] *Escherichia coli* is rarely an invasive pathogen in this country but should also be sought if the patient and his or her family have traveled to lesser developed countries. Other colitis-producing pathogens include *Entamoeba histolytica* and *Aeromonas hydrophilia*. The pathogenicity of *Clostridium difficile* is uncertain in infants since the organism and its toxin can be found in normal healthy infants.[4] This child had no evidence of being immunocompromised, which would expand the diagnostic list to include a number of viral and fungal pathogens. Such common enteric pathogens as rotavirus, *Giardia*, and *Cryptosporidium* do not invade the mucosa and so should not cause bloody diarrhea (see Chapter 13).

   Salmonella **Gastroenteritis.**—The stool cultures from this child grew *S. blockley*, which is one of the more than 1,400 serotypes of the species *S. enteriditis*. The other two species of salmonellae, *Salmonella choleraesuis*, and *Salmonella typhi*, consist of only one serotype each.

   Salmonella continues to be one of the commonest bacterial enteric pathogens

TABLE 14–1.

Enteric Pathogens That Cause Colitis in Infants

Organism	Mechanism
Common	
Salmonella	Invasion
Shigella	Invasion
C. jejuni	Invasion
Y. enterocolitica	Invasion
Uncommon	
E. coli	Invasion
Entamoeba histolytica	Invasion
Aeromonas hydrophilia	? Toxin
? *Clostridium difficile*	Toxin

in infants and children.[5] Domestic animals are the reservoir of most salmonellae infections in humans, excluding *S. typhi*. Disease is caused by oral ingestion of contaminated food or fecal material.

Infants are especially at risk for *Salmonella* infections, with boys infected more than girls.[5] The onset of symptoms is usually between 12 and 72 hours after the ingestion of contaminated food.[6] The commonest clinical syndrome caused by salmonellae is acute gastroenteritis, but septicemia with or without localized infection, enteric fever, and an asymptomatic carrier state are also possible.[7] Most episodes of gastroenteritis are relatively mild and self-limited with nausea, vomiting, and diarrhea as the major complaints.[7] Severe abdominal cramps may also be reported. The diarrhea is often watery, but bloody stools are not uncommon.[7]

Of special concern in infants is the risk for developing bacteremia and attendant sepsis or focal metastatic complications (Table 14–2). The rate of bacteremia in salmonellac infections is highest in infants and especially in infants less than 3 months of age.[9–11] The bacteremia is often transient and usually does not alter the course of the infection.[9] However, the bacteremia can result in life-threatening complications such as septicemia, osteomyelitis, and meningitis, which are seen much more commonly in neonates than in older infants and children.[12] Unfortunately, no clinical signs and symptoms are available to serve as predictors for which child will develop

TABLE 14–2.

Salmonella Sepsis in Infants

Study	No. of Patients	Age (mo)	Bacteremia	Metastatic Foci
Hyams et al.[9]	18	<3	7/17	0
	42	3–12	7/31	0
Davis[10]	151	<3	5	2
	232	3–12	2	1
Nelson and Granoff[11]	16	<1	5/11	6
	21	1–2	2/14	3
	15	3	0/4	2

bacteremia and subsequent complications. For this reason, all infants with salmonellae infections should have a blood culture.[7, 9–11]

Treatment

The approach to the treatment of inflammatory diarrhea should be the same as the approach to treatment of diarrhea in general and should focus on supportive care emphasizing proper fluid and electrolyte management and early reinstitution of feeding (see Chapter 13). Inflammatory diarrheas are frequently self-limited, and the patient is often improved by the time the culture result returns.

In older infants (>3 months) and children, antimicrobial therapy is not recommended for salmonellae gastroenteritis because of the usually self-limited nature of the illness and because antimicrobial agents may worsen the clinical course.[11] Nelson et al. have elegantly shown that antibiotic therapy for salmonellae infections prolongs the carrier state and increases the risk for gastrointestinal relapse after therapy is discontinued.[13]

However, salmonellae infections in infants less than 3 months old represent a special situation because of the significantly increased risk for developing bacteremia and septic complications.[7, 10, 11] Current recommendations are to treat infected infants with 10 days to 2 weeks of antibiotics regardless of the results of the initial blood culture.[11] The antibiotic therapy may have little positive effect on the course of the diarrhea but is used to prevent hematogenous spread of the infection. Depending on the antibiotic susceptibility of the *Salmonella* isolated, ampicillin, trimethoprim-sulfamethoxazole, or chloramphenicol are the antimicrobials of choice.[10]

The child presented in this case was treated according to these guidelines and had prolonged diarrhea, including a relapse following the discontinuation of therapy. However, he remained free of evidence for bacteremia and did not develop sepsis. He eventually recovered completely and is doing well, as do almost all children who develop salmonellae infections.

SUMMARY

The differential diagnostic possibilities for infants presenting with bloody stools is lengthy (see Table 21–1). When a salmonellae infection is found in a child less than 3 months old, the usual guidelines of supportive care and no use of antibiotics must be changed because of the risk of hematogenous seeding of the infection. The child presented here was treated with antibiotics and eventually had a complete and uneventful recovery.

REFERENCES

1. Stoll BJ, Glass RI, Banu H, et al: Value of stool examination in patients with diarrhea. *Br Med J* 1983; 286:2037–2040.
2. Guerrant RL, Shields DS, Thorson SM, et al: Evaluation and diagnosis of acute infectious diarrhea. *Am J Med* 1985; 78:91–96.

3. Pai CH, Sorger S, Lackman L, et al: *Campylobacter* gastroenteritis in children. *J Pediatr* 1979; 94:589–591.

4. Stark PL, Lee A, Parsonage BD: Colonization of the large bowel by *Clostridium difficile* in healthy infants: Quantitative study. *Infect Immun* 1982; 35:895–899.

5. Ryder RW, Merson MH, Pollard RA, et al: Salmonellosis in the United States 1968–1974. *J Infect Dis* 1976; 133:483–486.

6. Blaser MJ: Bacterial gastrointestinal infections. *Gastroenterol Ann* 1986; 3:317–340.

7. Saphra I, Winter JW: Clinical manifestations of salmonellosis in man. *N Engl J Med* 1957; 256:1128–1134.

8. Bishop WP, Ulshen MH: Bacterial gastroenteritis. *Pediatr Clin North Am* 1988; 35:69–87.

9. Hyams JS, Durbin WA, Grand RJ, et al: *Salmonella* bacteremia in the first year of life. *J Pediatr* 1980; 96:57–59.

10. Davis RC: *Salmonella* sepsis in infancy. *Am J Dis Child* 1981; 135:1096–1099.

11. Nelson SJ, Granoff D: *Salmonella* gastroenteritis in the first three months of life. A review of management and complications. *Clin Pediatr* 1982; 21:709–712.

12. Cherubin CE, Nell HC, Imperato PJ, et al: Septicemia with non-typhoid salmonella. *Medicine* (Baltimore) 1974; 53:365–376.

13. Nelson JD, Kusmicsz H, Jackson LH, et al: Treatment of *Salmonella* gastroenteritis with ampicillin, amoxicillin, or placebo. *Pediatrics* 1980; 65:1125–1130.

15 Chronic Diarrhea

Clifford W. Lo, M.D., M.P.H., Sc.D.

A 12-month-old girl developed diarrhea 1 month prior to admission. She started having approximately 10 watery stools per day while on a trip to Mexico with her family. All other family members also developed diarrhea and vomiting during the trip; although they recovered, she did not. She was seen by the family physician, who suggested a rice, apples, and bread diet, without success. She was then admitted to a local hospital for intravenous (IV) fluid therapy, but the diarrhea continued for more than 1 week. She was then transferred to Children's Hospital, where she was noted to be very emaciated, with a temperature of 40.3°C. Her weight was 13.6 lb (6.16 kg) (<5th percentile, ideal body weight for age was 22.1 lb [10 kg]), height 74 cm (25th percentile, weight for height <5th percentile), and head circumference 42.5 cm (5th percentile). The complete blood cell (CBC) count showed a white blood cell count of 25,500/mm^3 with 20% segmented neutrophils, 23% bands, and 44% lymphocytes. She was hyponatremic with an initial serum sodium concentration of 121 mEq/L, hypochloremic with a chloride concentration of 87 mEq/L, and acidotic with a bicarbonate of 17.5 mEq/L. Her serum potassium concentration was 4.1 mg/dl, glucose level 106 mg/dl, creatinine level 0.4 mg/dl, and BUN value 3 mg/dl. Her total serum protein level was 4.0 g/dl, albumin level 1.9 g/dl, calcium level 7.3 mg/dl, phosphorus level 2.6 mg/dl, and magnesium level 1.4 mg/dl, all depressed. Liver function test results were slightly elevated, with an alanine aminotranferase (ALT) concentration of 28 mU/ml, an aspartate aminotranferase (AST) concentration of 21 mU/ml, and a total bilirubin concentration of 0.8 mg/dl. After initial IV rehydration, her serum electrolyte concentration improved to 132 mEq of sodium/dl, 94 mEq of chloride/dl, 2.4 mEq of potassium/dl, and 22.7 mEq of bicarbonate/dl. A central venous catheter was placed in her left jugular vein, and total parenteral nutrition was started, initially providing 80 to 100 kcal/kg/day. Within 1 week, the patient was able to tolerate a continuous enteral infusion of diluted elemental formula, and she improved steadily over the next month without further diarrhea or any other complications.

DISCUSSION

With estimates of 3 to 5 billion cases per year (an average of roughly 1/person/year),[1] diarrheal diseases continue to be the leading cause of morbidity and mortality in the world today. Young children in developing countries are especially at risk, with 5 to 18 million deaths/year occurring in this group.[2] Until 50 years ago, diarrheal diseases were the leading cause of infant mortality in the United States.[3] In many

TABLE 15–1.
Causes of Protracted Diarrhea*

Postinfectious diarrhea
  Shigella, Salmonella, Escherichia coli, Yersinia,
    Campylobacter
  Rotavirus, Norwalk agent, adenovirus,
    calcivirus, coronavirus, astrovirus, other
    enteroviruses
Celiac sprue
Allergic gastroenteropathy
  Cow's milk allergy
  Soy protein intolerance
Pancreatic insufficiency
  Cystic fibrosis
  Shwachman-Diamond syndrome
Congenital enzyme deficiencies
  Sucrose-isomaltase deficiency, enterokinase
    deficiency, glucose-galactose malabsorption,
    lactase deficiency, congenital chloridorrhea
Parasitic infection
  Giardiasis, strongyloidiasis, amebiasis,
    capillariasis, coccidiosis
Bacterial overgrowth, stasis syndromes
  Clostridium difficile
Short-bowel syndromes
Drugs
  Laxatives, phenolphthalein, antibiotics,
    antacids, sorbitol
Miscellaneous
  Intestinal lymphangiectasia,
    abetalipoproteinemia, Wolman's syndrome,
    Hirschsprung's disease, endocrine tumors,
    cholestasis, immunodeficiencies

*From Lo and Walker.[5] Used by permission.

industrialized countries, mortality of infants hospitalized for diarrhea still exceeds 1%.[4]

Etiology

A wide range of etiologic and pathophysiologic mechanisms may be involved in chronic diarrhea (Table 15–1).[5] Surprisingly, there is a lack of a precise definition of diarrhea, and neither stool frequency, weight, or consistency is a completely reliable guide to the dehydration, malabsorption, malnutrition, or failure to thrive that often accompanies it. A syndrome of "chronic nonspecific diarrhea" often occurs in children aged 6 to 30 months, with copious stools without any evidence of malabsorption or growth retardation.[6] Thus, information about the infant's weight and a few simple diagnostic tests on stool samples are crucial in determining the diagnosis, prognosis, and management of chronic diarrhea.

Postinfectious diarrhea is probably the most common cause of chronic protracted diarrhea, but much remains to be understood about the progression of disease and prolongation of diarrhea. The classic bacterial dysenteries caused by *Salmonella, Shigella,* and *E. coli* have been joined by a number of other pathogens such as *Yersinia enterocolitica* and *Campylobacter jejuni.* But the majority of epidemic infectious diarrheas are probably due to viruses, of which rotaviruses were among the first to be identified as pathogens.

Pathogenesis

Viral gastroenteritis and many other causes of chronic diarrhea (e.g., celiac disease, cow's milk allergy) result in similar structural changes of intestinal villous atrophy, crypt hypertrophy, and inflammatory infiltrates.[7, 8] A severe decrease in effective absorptive area is accompanied by diminished disaccharidase activity (located on the microvillous brush border). Lactose and other undigested carbohydrates pull water into the gut lumen, causing an osmotic diarrhea and encouraging proliferation of enteric microflora in the small intestine. In some bacterial, viral, and congenital diarrheas, paralysis of the sodium–cyclic adenosine monophosphate pump results in a secretory diarrhea that continues even if no food is ingested. In most cases, the intestine regenerates a new epithelial brush border within a few days, but if the insult is prolonged or malnutrition prevents adequate healing, a vicious cycle of infection, mucosal damage, malabsorption, malnutrition, and depressed immunity and healing may lead to chronic diarrhea and failure to thrive (Fig 15–1).

Diagnosis

The great majority of acute infectious diarrheas are self-limited, will resolve in a matter of days, and require treatment with only oral glucose-electrolyte solutions to replace fluid and electrolyte losses. Occasionally, however, the diarrhea fails to resolve despite many changes of formula. In this case, the value of a detailed dietary history is apparent. Sorting out the various formula changes and their effects on stool frequency can take some time and requires some familiarity with the composition of infant formulas. A careful history of travel, illnesses, medications, development, family history, and social situation can sometimes provide the only clue to the origin of the diarrhea. Much important information is gained by plotting the infant's growth curve with serial measurements of weight, height, and weight for height.

On physical examination, the general appearance of a child with chronic diarrhea may show signs of marasmus with lethargy, emaciation, muscle wasting, hypotonia, and sunken cheeks, but these signs may be much more subtle in mild or moderate malnutrition. Edema, dermatitis, or physical signs of specific nutrient deficiencies are usually not seen unless the malnutrition is long standing.

Laboratory examination of the stool is often overlooked but usually provides far more information than most biochemical serum tests in the diagnosis of chronic

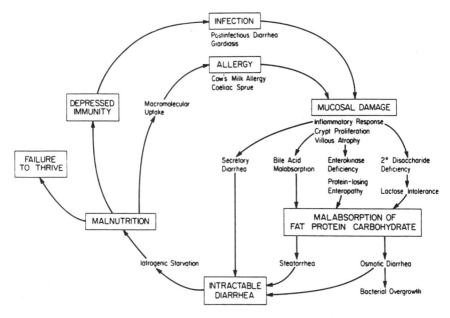

FIG 15–1.
Hypothetical pathogenesis for nutritional cause of intractable diarrhea of infancy. (From Lo CW, Walker WA: Chronic protracted diarrhea of infancy: A nutritional disease. *Pediatrics* 1983; 72:786. Reproduced by permission.)

diarrhea. The liquid portion of the stool sample can be quickly and easily tested for weight, acidity, sugars (reducing substances), occult blood, fat globules, leucocytes, ova, and parasites. Malabsorption of reducing sugars (glucose and lactose, but not sucrose) can be detected by a greater than 0.5% reading of a Clinitest tablet dropped in equal portions of liquid stool and water. If the infant is receiving sucrose (as in most soy formulas), the mixture must first be heated with 0.1N hydrochloric acid for a few minutes to hydrolyze the sugar. A positive stool guaiac test result suggests some source of gastrointestinal (GI) bleeding, perhaps colitis due to cow's milk allergy. Excessive fat globules can be seen easily under a low-power microscope, especially if highlighted with a Sudan red stain. A methylene blue stain may reveal fecal leukocytes, indicating a bacillary dysentary, or parasitic ova, trophozoites, or cysts.

Biochemical tests of nutritional status tend to be too expensive and limited for most situations, but a good initial screen might include a CBC count with differential and red blood cell morphology, serum electrolytes, total protein, and albumin. For further investigation, values of serum carotene, calcium, phosphorus, magnesium, iron, transferrin, zinc, copper, thyroxine, cholesterol, triglyceride, creatinine, BUN and liver function tests might considered. Stool cultures, multiple samples for ova and parasites, and a 72-hour collection for fecal fat (if the patient is ingesting at least 50 gm of fat/day) can be done. A D-xylose absorption test (measuring serum xylose after an oral test dose) or a lactose breath hydrogen test (measuring hydrogen produced by the action of colonic bacteria on malabsorbed carbohydrate) may be helpful in the assesment of chronic diarrhea after acute rehabilitation.

One of the most important tools for investigation of chronic diarrhea and failure to thrive is hospitalization for observation of stool pattern and weight gain. Daily weights, careful input and output records, and daily measurements of stool weight, pH, and reducing substances will quantitatively document the severity of the diarrhea and malabsorption. Occasionally, an upper GI contrast series with small bowel follow through, a barium enema, ultrasound studies, a small bowel biopsy and duodenal aspirate, sigmoidoscopy, or colonoscopy may be necessary to reveal the underlying cause (Fig 15–2).

Management

The basic principles of the treatment of chronic diarrhea are nutritional, replenishing not only salt and water losses but also protein, calorie, and other nutrient stores by enteral or parenteral means. Although fluid rehydration was known as a treatment for cholera as early as 150 years ago, high mortality continued until the use of IV sugar and salt solutions gained widespread acceptance 100 years later. However, if the diarrhea continued, infants were often subjected to a prolonged fast, or "bowel rest," without adequate attention paid to nutritional rehabilitation to promote gut healing. Indeed, recent evidence suggests that both gut villous morphology and disaccharidase activity improved faster when stimulated by early enteral feedings than with prolonged bowel rest and IV alimentation.[9]

Oral glucose-electrolyte solutions have been used increasingly as initial therapy in diarrhea and dehydration due to a wide variety of infectious agents. They contain simple monosaccharides and minerals that can usually be absorbed by active transport across damaged gut mucosal surfaces without normal villi.[10, 11] However, the caloric value of clear liquids is low, and they contain no protein source that can be used to heal damaged gut epithelium. Therefore, clear liquids alone should not be used for more than a few days without the provision of additional calorie or nitrogen sources.

Oral elemental diets containing simple monosaccharides, amino acids, and medium chain triglycerides (e.g., Pregestimil) are essentially completely predigested and are usually well tolerated by infants with even badly damaged gut epithelium.[12] These elemental formulas, claimed to be hypoallergenic, are also useful if the problem involves some form of dietary allergy. If bolus feedings cannot be tolerated, a slow continuous drip through a nasogastric tube may be tried. Patients with severe malnutrition often have severe electrolyte problems, which may become even worse on nutritional rehabilitation as rapid fluid and metabolic shifts occur. Very gradual increases in the caloric supplements over a period of weeks or even months may be necessary to minimize the risk of refeeding edema or sudden cardiac arrhythmias.

Although oral elemental formulas will be sufficient in most cases, occasionally total parenteral nutrition may be necessary if diarrhea and malabsorption continue. Peripheral IV administration of dextrose–amino acid solutions with fat emulsions have been used to provide maintenance calories for short periods of time, but this does not allow for the large amount of extra calories often needed to sustain growth in an infant with prolonged diarrhea and malabsorption. Therefore, surgical placement of a Silastic catheter in a central vein may become necessary for infusion of hypertonic dextrose–amino acid and fat solutions.

Drug treatment of chronic diarrhea in children is usually not warranted. No advantage has been found in giving antibiotics in diarrhea unless systemic signs (fever) are present or unless reduction of infectivity is the goal. Intestinal paralytic agents, such as diphenoxylate-atropine (Lomotil), may relieve symptoms by decreasing peristalsis, but without a reduction in secretion, the excess water will instead tend to pool in distended loops of bowel, masking dehydration and delaying the usual excretion of infectious organisms.[13] Adsorbents such as kaolin-pectin suspension (Kao-pectate) may actually cause increased sodium and potassium losses. Bismuth subsalicylate (Pepto-Bismol) has recently been shown to be of use in traveler's diarrhea, but the large quantities necessary to have a measurable effect may put young infants at risk for toxic salicylism. Other common antidiarrheal agents are probably useless and may actually prolong diarrhea and be hazardous in young children and infants.[14]

Rehabilitation from severe intractable diarrhea with malnutrition may require a long, expensive hospitalization with not inconsiderable mortality. If diarrhea does

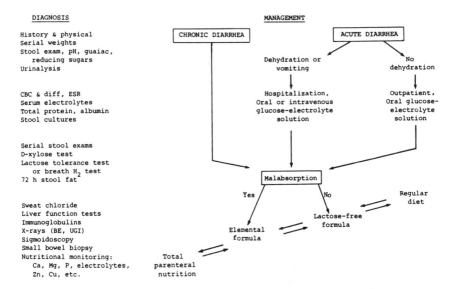

FIG 15–2.
Diagnostic tests and treatment alternatives in management of chronic diarrhea. Diagnostic tests are listed by groups in suggested order ranging from initial outpatient screening tests to more involved inpatient procedures. Not all tests need be or should be performed unless specifically indicated. Therapeutic changes of formulas should be selected according to persistence or resolution of carbohydrate malabsorption, progressing along a graded sequence from IV to elemental to lactose-free to regular diets as malabsorption resolves, or vice versa if it persists. BE = barium enema; UGI = upper GI series. (From Lo CW, Walker WA: Chronic protracted diarrhea of infancy: A nutritional disease. *Pediatrics* 1983; 72:786. Reproduced by permission.)

occur, proper attention to the infant's nutritional needs by the mother and the physician and avoidance of prolonged iatrogenic starvation on clear liquids or diluted formulas will prevent further deterioration into the vicious cycle of malnutrition, infection, and malabsorption.

SUMMARY

This patient exhibited a typical course of chronic diarrhea that started as an acute infectious gastroenteritis of unknown etiology. However, the insult to the small intestinal villous surface never healed, and the prolonged course was aggravated by malnutrition. Nutritional intervention with total parenteral nutrition and enteral elemental formulas interrupted this vicious cycle of infection, malnutrition, and malabsorption and resulted in steady rehabilitation over the next month.

REFERENCES

1. Walsh JA, Warren KS: Selective primary health care: An interim strategy for disease control in developing countries. *Soc Sci Med* 1980; 14:145–163.
2. Rhode JE, Northrup RS: Taking science where the diarrhea is. *Ciba Found Symp* 1975; 42:339.
3. Cone TE: *History of American Pediatrics.* Boston, Little, Brown & Co, 1979.
4. Tripp JH, Wilmers MJ, Wharton BA: Gastroenteritis: A continuing problem of child health in Britain. *Lancet* 1977; 2:233–236.
5. Lo CW, Walker WA: Chronic protracted diarrhea of infancy: A nutritional disease. *Pediatrics* 1983; 72:786–800.
6. Davidson M, Wasserman RL: The irritable colon of childhood (chronic nonspecific diarrhea syndrome). *J Pediatr* 1966; 69:1027–1038.
7. Rossi TM, Lebenthal E, Nord KS, et al: Extent and duration of small intestinal mucosal injury in intractable diarrhea of infancy. *Pediatrics* 1980; 66:730–735.
8. Brunser O: Effects of malnutrition on intestinal structure and function in children. *Clin Gastroenterol* 1977; 6:341–353.
9. Greene HL, McCabe DR, Merenstein GB: Protracted diarrhea and malnutrition in infancy: Changes in intestinal morphology and disaccharidase activities during treatment with total intravenous nutrition or oral elemental diets. *J Pediatr* 1975; 87:695–704.
10. Santosham M, Daum RS, Dillmann L, et al: Oral rehydration therapy of infantile diarrhea: A controlled study of well-nourished children hospitalized in the United States and Panama. *N Engl J Med* 1982; 306:1070–1076.
11. Sack RB, Pierce NF, Hirschhorn N: The current status of oral therapy in the treatment of acute diarrheal illness. *Am J Clin Nutr* 1978; 31:2252–2257.
12. MacLean WC Jr, Lopez de Romana G, Massa E, et al: Nutritional management of chronic diarrhea and malnutrition: Primary reliance on oral feeding. *J Pediatr* 1980; 97:316–323.
13. Dupont HL, Hornic RB: Adverse effects of Lomotil therapy in shigellosis. *JAMA* 1973; 226:1525–1528.
14. Portnoy BL, Dupont HL, Pruitt D, et al: Antidiarrheal agents in the treatment of acute diarrhea in children. *JAMA* 1976; 236:844–846.

16   Celiac Disease

Anne Munck, M.D.

A 12-month-old girl was admitted to the hospital for weight loss, diarrhea, and vomiting. She was born at 38 weeks' gestation after an uneventful pregnancy and had a birth weight of 7.3 lb (3.3 kg). The child was breast-fed for 3 months and then switched to cow's milk formula (Similac) without difficulty. At 6 months, other foods, including baby food cereals and fruit, were begun and were tolerated. However, at 9 months she developed constipation (one hard stool every other day), abdominal distention, decreasing activity, and emesis. Because of her distended abdomen, a barium enema was performed that showed a dilated cecum with a large amount of stool. The possibility of Hirschsprung's disease was considered, but results of a rectal biopsy were normal. Medical therapy, including a change of diet and mineral oil, improved the constipation, but her vomiting continued. Her subsequent weight gain was poor, and she had four loose, foul-smelling, greasy stools per day. The child became lethargic and irritable. There were no accompanying signs of acute illness such as fever, urinary tract symptoms, or allergies. The past medical history was otherwise unremarkable, and the family history was negative except for a maternal cousin who had milk protein intolerance. The child was referred to Children's Hospital.

On physical examination, the child was lethargic and pale. Her height and weight were substantially below the third percentile, and her head circumference was at the 10th percentile. Her examination was remarkable for a distended, tympanitic abdomen, a smooth, enlarged liver, and an absence of subcutaneous fat. Results of the remainder of the examination were normal, including no peripheral edema or lymph adenopathy. Laboratory studies included a normal white blood cell (WBC) count and differential, hemoglobin 11.0 mg/dl, total protein level 4.3 gm/dl, and albumin level 3.3 gm/dl. The urinalysis, stool evaluation for bacterial and protozoal pathogens, and sweat chloride test results were normal. Her stool was trace guaiac positive but negative for reducing substances. A 72-hour fecal fat determination revealed steatorrhea (25 gm of lipid in 125 gm of stool). The 1-hour serum D-xylose value was 8.9 (normal >25) and the serum folate level (1.4) and carotene level (4) were low. The patient's serum immunoglobulin levels were normal, and radioallergosorbent test (RAST) results for milk, soy, β-lactoglobulin, and casein were negative. Her bone age was 6 months.

A small bowel biopsy showed obvious atrophy of the jejunal villi accompanied by hyperplasia and irregularity of the crypts. The lamina propria was diffusely infiltrated by chronic inflammatory cells and eosinophils (Fig 16–1). Evaluation for bacterial and parasitic pathogens was normal. These findings were consistent with active celiac disease, and the child was discharged on a gluten-free, lactose-free diet. She improved rapidly on the diet, becoming a happy child with normal stools and no vomiting. Lactose was reintroduced gradually and was well tolerated.

The diagnosis of celiac disease was confirmed by two subsequent jejunal biopsies. The first biopsy, obtained after 1 year on the gluten-free diet, was normal (Fig 16–2). The child was then given a 4-week gluten challenge diet and developed decreased appetite. Her jejunal biopsy specimen after the 4-week gluten challenge showed regenerative surface epithelium and focal shortening of the villi. The surface epithelium was atrophic with an increased number of eosinophils and mononuclear cells and focal penetration of glands by eosinophils. These histologic findings of diffuse active enteritis after the gluten challenge confirmed the diagnosis of celiac disease.

DISCUSSION

Celiac disease, or gluten-sensitive enteropathy, is caused by intestinal intolerance to gliadin and results in severe mucosal lesions in susceptible individuals.[1] The disease

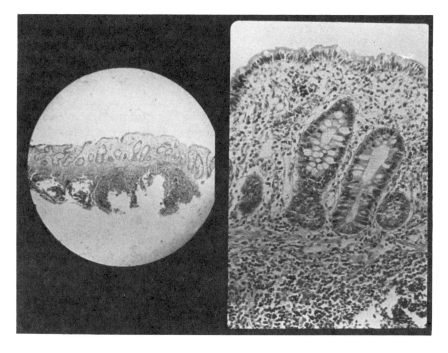

FIG 16–1.
A small intestinal mucosal biopsy showing subtotal villus atrophy (low power) and chronic inflammatory infiltrate of the lamina propria and infiltration of the epithelium by lymphocytes (high power).

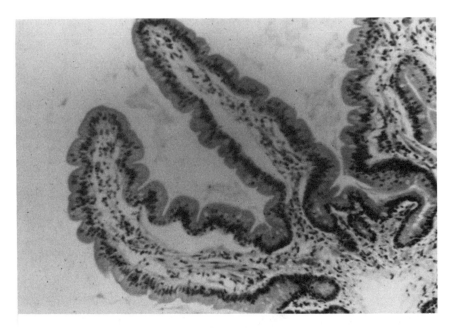

FIG 16–2.
Normal small intestinal biopsy specimen with villus/crypt ratio more than 2:1 (×200).

can be seen in all age groups, but most cases are identified in children less than 2 years old.[2] Girls are more often affected than boys.[2] The incidence is about 1:1,000 live births and appears to be higher in Europe than in the United States.[3]

Pathophysiology

The pathogenesis of celiac disease remains unknown. Several theories have been postulated to explain the mechanism of the gluten sensitivity.

The first hypothesis is that a deficiency of an intestinal peptidase allows the accumulation of a toxic metabolite of gliadin in the intestinal mucosa.[1] However, when the mucosa has healed after a gluten-free diet, no evidence of peptidase deficiency can be found. The second hypothesis is that a defect of the cell surface membrane allows gluten to act as a lectin by binding to intestinal cells and initiating a toxic reaction.[4]

The final theory, currently the most popular, is that celiac disease is an immunologic disorder with genetic and environmental components.[5] In this theory, gliadin is thought to play the role of an antigen that triggers an autoimmune response on the small bowel mucosa in genetically susceptible persons. Supporting this theory are family studies that demonstrate an increased incidence of celiac disease in first-degree relatives of patients.[6] In addition, several histocompatibility antigens (HLA-B8, HLA-Dw3, and HLA-DQw2) have been identified in many patients with celiac disease.[6, 7]

Clinical Features

The clinical picture usually includes many of the signs and symptoms demonstrated by this patient. She had onset of her symptoms at 12 months of age (the usual onset is between 8 and 24 months). Her symptoms included constipation, vomiting, lethargy, and irritability. She then developed diarrhea with bulky, greasy, foul-smelling stools and failure to thrive. Vomiting may dominate the clinical picture, and constipation can be seen in as many as 10% of patients.[8] However, the absence of gastrointestinal (GI) symptoms is not uncommon, and these patients often present with malnutrition, vitamin deficiencies, or growth failure.[9] Children with celiac disease may also present with peripheral edema, bleeding disorders, tetany, bone pain, fractures, iron deficiency anemia, rickets, or short stature.[8] Very rarely seen is the life-threatening celiac crisis characterized by dehydration, acidosis, and shock due to intractable diarrhea and vomiting.

This patient's laboratory evaluation was typical for a case of suspected celiac disease (Table 16–1). Infectious and allergic causes of diarrhea were sought but not found. The normal sweat test result ruled out cystic fibrosis, and the normal urine analysis and serum chemistries made a metabolic disorder unlikely. The abnormal D-xylose result gave evidence for small intestinal mucosal damage.

Malabsorption was assessed by measuring stool reducing substances (carbohydrate malabsorption) and by the 72-hour stool fat collection. In this case, there was no evidence of carbohydrate malabsorption, but 25 gm of fat were excreted in 72 hours. If a child is fed a standard diet containing at least 50 gm of fat per day, the presence of 3.5 gm (infant) or 4.5 gm (child) of fat in the stool is considered abnormal.[10] The low serum levels of carotene and folate gave further evidence of altered intestinal absorption. The child's hypoproteinemia and hypoalbuminemia could have been caused by decreased appetite or protein losing enteropathy. The bone age is usually delayed in these children with a chronic inflammatory process.

Diagnosis

Recent evidence indicates that testing for serum IgA antigliadin and reticulin antibodies (not done in this child) may also be helpful in diagnosing celiac disease.[11] Previous studies have shown the presence of circulating IgG antibodies to gluten, gliadin, and reticulin proteins in celiac disease, but the specificity was low.[11] Corresponding IgA antibodies are less sensitive but more specific. More recently, preliminary studies have indicated that IgA antiendomesial antibodies may be both highly sensitive and specific.[12]

Although these noninvasive tests hold promise for the future, the definitive diagnostic test remains the small bowel biopsy. This child's poor growth and evidence

TABLE 16–1.

Laboratory Evaluation of
Malabsorption

Blood Tests
  Complete blood cell count
  Iron
  Albumin, total protein
  Transferrin
  Prealbumin
  Immunoglobulins
  Calcium
  Phosphorus
  Zinc
  Magnesium
  Liver function tests
  Vitamin B_{12}
  Folate
  Prothrombin time
Stool tests
  WBC count
  Occult blood
  Sudan stain
  pH, reducing substances
  Culture
  Ova and parasites
Sweat test
Absorption tests
  D-Xylose
  72-hr fecal fat
  Lactose, sucrose breath test
Intestinal biopsy

---

for small intestinal dysfunction and malabsorption led to her biopsy. The histologic findings of villous atrophy, elongated crypts, loss of nuclear polarity, infiltration of lamina propria by inflammatory cells, and an increased mitotic index in the crypts were consistent with but not diagnostic of celiac disease (see Fig 16–1). If the diagnosis of celiac disease is to be established conclusively, a series of three small bowel biopsies after appropriate feeding challenges must be obtained. Following the initial biopsy with the child on a regular diet, a second biopsy is obtained 6 to 12 months after the child is placed on a strict gluten-free diet. The histologic findings of this biopsy should be normal in a child with celiac disease. A third biopsy is then obtained after gluten is reintroduced to the diet for 1 month. Results of this biopsy again show evidence of enteropathy. Children who do well initially after the gluten rechallenge should be followed closely because relapses of symptoms have occurred up to 10 months later.[13] This series of biopsies will eliminate other causes of malabsorption, including intestinal lymphangiectasia, eosinophilic gastroenteritis, immune disorders, lymphoma, cow's milk intolerance, and infestation with *Giardia lamblia.*

Treatment

Once the diagnosis is established, the child must be on a complete gluten-free diet excluding wheat, rye, barley, and oats. The disease is a lifelong condition, and mucosal damage or symptoms are likely to occur if the gluten-free diet is not followed.[7]

The initial treatment should also include a temporary restriction of lactose and sucrose because the disaccharidase activities are often depressed because of chronic inflammation.[7] Depending on the clinical status, the child will receive iron, vitamins, trace elements, or mineral supplements as required. Milk can usually be reintroduced after a few weeks. For children with severe malnutrition, a short period of peripheral or central parenteral alimentation may be helpful. The clinical improvement is usually striking, as was the case for this child, accompanied by marked improvement in behavior. Restoration of normal weight usually occurs within a few months, along with catch-up growth in height.

The gluten-free diet should be followed for life because symptoms may recur on rechallenge with gluten.[7] An increased risk of malignancy in patients with celiac disease has been reported, but the relation of malignancy to dietary therapy has not been clearly established.[14] The tumors have often been intestinal lymphomas, but adenocarcinoma and carcinoid tumors have also been described.[14, 15] There is no evidence that patients with continued symptoms on a gluten-free diet or persisting flat jejunal biopsy results are more prone to die of cancer than patients who respond well to the diet. Because of the increased risk of cancer, patients with celiac disease need to be followed and routinely evaluated for the remainder of their lives.[7]

SUMMARY

Celiac disease is an important cause of malabsorption, especially in young children. The pathogenesis is unknown, but immunologic factors probably play an important role. Children classically present with symptoms of diarrhea, poor growth, and irritability and evidence of malabsorption of carbohydrates, fats, and protein. The diagnosis is made by a series of small bowel biopsies timed with gluten challenges. Recent advances in noninvasive testing appear promising. Close surveillance of all patients is required because of the associated risk of malignancy.

REFERENCES

1. Cornell HJ, Rolles CJ: Further evidence of primary mucosal defect in coeliac disease. *Gut* 1978; 19:253–259.
2. Polanco I, Biemond I, van Leeuwen A, et al: Gluten sensitive enteropathy in Spain: Genetic and environmental factors, in McConnell RB: *Genetics of Coeliac Disease.* Liverpool, MTP Press, 1981, p 211.

3. Langman MJ: Can epidemiology help us to prevent coeliac disease? *Gastroenterology* 1986; 90:489–491.
4. Weiser MM, Douglas AP: An alternative mechanism for gluten toxicity in coeliac disease. *Lancet* 1976; 1:567–569.
5. Lebenthal E, Sagaro E, Jimenez N: Family studies of coeliac disease in Cuba. *Arch Dis Child* 1981; 56:132–133.
6. Carter C, Sheldon W, Walker C: The inheritance of coeliac disease. *Ann Hum Genet* 1959; 23:266–273.
7. Auricchio S, Greco L, Troncone R: Gluten-sensitive enteropathy in childhood. *Pediatr Clin* North Am. 1988; 35:157–187.
8. Young WF, Pringle EM: 110 children with coeliac disease. *Arch Dis Child* 1971; 46:421–436.
9. Cacciari E, Salardi S, Volta U, et al: Can antigliadin antibody detect symptomless coeliac disease in children with shoit stature? *Lancet* 1985; 1:1469–1471.
10. Schmerling DH, Forrer JCW, Prader A: Fecal fat and nitrogen in healthy children and in children with malabsorption or maldigestion. *Pediatrics* 1970; 46:690–695.
11. Unsworth DJ, Walker-Smith JA, Holborow EJ: Gliadin and reticulin antibodies in childhood coeliac disease. *Lancet* 1983; 1:874–875.
12. Kapuscinska A, Zalewskit, Chorzelski T, et al: Disease specificity and dynamics of changes in IgA class antiendomysial antibodies in celiac disease. *J Pediatr Gastroenterol Nutr* 1987; 6:529–534.
13. Kumar PJ, O'Donoghue DP, Stevenson K, et al: Reintroduction of gluten in adults and children with treated coeliac disease. *Gut* 1979; 20:743–749.
14. Holmes GKT, Stokes PL, Soraham TM, et al: Coeliac disease, gluten free diet and malignancy. *Gut* 1976; 17:612–619.
15. Hallert C, Norrby K: Malignant carcinoid tumor complicating coeliac disease. *Acta Med Scand* 1983; 213:313–316.

17 Short Bowel Syndrome

John D. Snyder, M.D.

The patient was an 8-lb (3.6 kg) product of an uncomplicated full-term pregnancy, labor, and delivery. He was initially fed a cow's milk formula, but because of frequent episodes of vomiting and an episode of aspiration, he was switched to soy and then an elemental formula. His symptoms persisted, and his growth was poor; at 2 months of age he underwent a fundoplication and insertion of a gastrostomy tube. He continued with poor weight gain and 3 months after the fundoplication developed fever, bilious vomiting, and abdominal distention. Surgical exploration revealed midgut volvulus with infarction and necrosis of most of the jejunum and ileum. His small bowel was resected from 20 cm distal to the ligament of Treitz to 30 cm proximal to the ileocecal valve. The next day further necrotic bowel was resected, leaving a total of 21 cm of small bowel and the ileocecal valve. A jeju-nostomy and an ileal mucous fistula were created, and a central total parenteral nutrition (TPN) line was placed. His postoperative course was a stormy one marked by several bouts of sepsis, and he was transferred to Children's Hospital. He was initially maintained on TPN but developed rising bilirubin and serum transaminase levels; an abdominal ultrasound revealed sludge in the biliary tree. Initial attempts at low-volume, dilute, continuous elemental formula feedings resulted in large volumes of diarrhea and mild dehydration. Eventually the continuous infusions of dilute elemental formula were tolerated with the aid of cholestyramine and then loperamide. Currently the patient receives 30% of his calories from the elemental formula and 70% from TPN. His cholestasis has resolved.

DISCUSSION

Short bowel syndrome has usually been defined in functional terms because more precise definitions based on a specific length or percentage of bowel resected are difficult to make.[1] The difficulties arise because the total length of bowel at birth varies, excised bowel is difficult to measure because it can be easily stretched, and measurement of nonexcised bowel can be only approximated.[1, 2] For the purpose of this discussion, short bowel syndrome will be defined as loss of enough small intestine to affect the normal absorption of nutrients.

The incidence of short bowel syndrome is unknown but arises mainly from a portion of the cases of midgut volvulus (as with the patient presented here) and necrotizing enterocolitis, its two most common causes.[1] Intestinal atresia, abdominal wall defects, and inflammatory bowel disease also contribute to the incidence.[3]

Pathophysiology

Short bowel syndrome arises from loss of intestinal tissue resulting in altered absorption of nutrients. Several factors directly affect the severity of the malabsorption, including the length of the bowel resected, the status of the ileocecal valve, the age of the child at the time of surgery, the location of the bowel resected, and the adaptive properties of the bowel remaining.[3] Children have survived greater than 90% resection of small intestine (leaving as little as 8–12 cm of small bowel) if the ileocecal valve is left intact.[4, 5] As a general rule, when more than 50% of the bowel is resected, impairment of absorption is likely to be prolonged or permanent.[6]

The presence of the ileocecal valve is critically important to the outcome because it helps to modulate intestinal transit time. The valve also helps to prevent small bowel colonization by bacteria that can deconjugate bile salts and alter fatty acids.[6, 7]

The age of the child is also of particular importance since small bowel length doubles between 19 and 36 weeks of gestation.[2] A preterm infant, therefore, may have a greater chance for bowel growth after resection than a term infant.[2]

The impact of the resection is also dependent on the specific level of bowel involved (Fig 17–1).[8] For example, resection of the terminal ileum removes the selective site for the active absorption of bile salts and vitamin B_{12}, and significant losses of these compounds can result.[7] The loss of bile salt absorption sites reduces the enterohepatic circulation of bile acids and can lead to severe steatorrhea. The ileum also plays a more important role than the jejunum in modulating intestinal transit time.[8] In contrast, the majority of nutrient absorption takes place in the jejunum.[9] The small intestine is also the site of reabsorption of the enormous quantities of saliva, bile, gastric, and pancreatic juice that are secreted each day. Eighty percent of these secretions, which can total 5 L in an adult, are absorbed in the small intestine.[6]

The adaptive properties of the bowel left after resection is the final factor influencing the outcome. The remaining bowel can undergo mucosal hyperplasia with increased villus height and number of absorptive cells[10] and thus show increased absorptive function. The adaptive changes are always greater after proximal than after distal resection and are maximal near the anastomotic site.[11, 12] The intensity of the hyperplastic response is directly proportional to the length of the intestine resected.[13]

Clinical Features

The clinical features of short bowel syndrome depend to a great extent on the pathophysiologic factors previously listed, especially the length and site of bowel resected, the presence or absence of the ileocecal valve, and the degree of injury to the remaining bowel.[14] However, the general course in patients following massive small bowel resection is similar. Initially, most patients have significant diarrhea that can cause marked fluid and electrolyte losses. Gastric hypersecretion is often

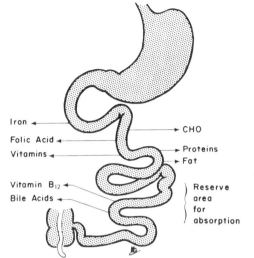

FIG 17–1.
The duodenum and jejunum are the sites of absorption of all substrates except vitamin B_{12} and bile acids, which are absorbed in the terminal ileum. (From Silverman A, Roy CC (eds): *Pediatric Clinical Gastroenterology*, ed 3. St Louis, CV Mosby, 1983, p 252. Used with permission.)

seen and can lead to peptic ulceration and an acidic intraluminal pH, which can impair pancreatic enzyme function.[7] Laboratory findings reflect the fluid losses and electrolyte derangements, especially depletion of potassium, sodium, calcium, and magnesium.

Treatment

The treatment of each patient should be individualized because of the variable interaction of the many pathophysiologic factors previously mentioned. However, because several difficulties commonly arise, some general guidelines to therapy can be given (Table 17–1). These interventions are directly related to the various pathophysiologic processes that usually operate in short bowel syndrome and are aimed mainly at slowing or stopping the diarrhea so that adequate absorption of nutrients and reabsorption of water and electrolytes can occur.

Almost all patients with short bowel syndrome will receive initial therapy via TPN because their fluid and electrolyte losses can be compounded by enteral feedings.[6] Total parenteral nutrition also provides nutritional support while initial gut adaptation is taking place. If gastric hypersecretion occurs, treatment with antacids and anticholinergic agents are indicated.

A gastrostomy tube is often placed at the time of surgical resection to aid in the initial enteral feedings, which begin with elemental formulas. The elemental formulas contain protein in the form of protein hydrolysates or amino acids, which can usually be assimilated even after significant loss of bowel surface area.[14] The carbohydrate component of these formulas is generally glucose polymers, which have a low osmotic activity and are hydrolyzed to glucose, which requires no enzyme for absorption. The formulas contain varying amounts of medium-chain triglycerides (MCT) as fat

TABLE 17–1.

Guidelines to Therapy for Diarrhea in Short
Bowel Syndrome

Medical
   Provide TPN to ensure nutritional stability
   Decrease gastric secretions
      H_2 blockers, anticholinergics
   Decrease osmotic load of feedings
      Elemental formulas, continuous feedings
   Decrease intestinal motility
      Opiods, loperamide
      Decrease bile acid pool
      Cholestyramine
      Treat small bowel overgrowth
      Antibiotics
Surgical
   Currently available techniques
      Segmental reversal of small intestine
      Colon interposition
      Sphincters and valves
      Intestinal loop lengthening
   Future possibilities
      Small intestinal transplantation
      Fetal intestinal transplantation

---

because MCTs are absorbed directly without the need for bile acids.

Continuous feedings are usually started because of increased nutrient absorption compared to bolus feedings.[15] Early initiation of feedings is attempted because enteral nutrients stimulate intestinal mucosal regeneration and are required for a complete return of bowel function.[11] Early initiation of enteral feedings can also help shorten the duration of hospitalization.[16] The risk of hepatobiliary complications from TPN is also reduced by starting enteral feedings (see Chapter 32).[17]

Drug therapy may also be of benefit. Antimotility agents such as loperamide can reduce bowel transit time and slow the diarrhea.[6] In patients with ileal resections, cholestyramine can bind unabsorbed bile acids and prevent their secretory action in the colon.[7] Bacterial colonization of the small bowel, especially if the ileocecal valve has been resected, can be an important cause of diarrhea.[6] Various antibiotics, including ampicillin and metronidazole, have been used to treat the resultant small bowel overgrowth.

A variety of surgical procedures have been attempted to maximize intestinal absorption, but most to date have not been widely used. Segmental reversal of the small intestine and colonic interposition have been used to try to slow the intestinal transit time, but experience with these techniques has been anecdotal.[14] Recirculating intestinal loops have been used to increase transit time and to reexpose luminal contents to the mucosal surface. However, stasis, bacterial overgrowth, and intestinal obstruction have all been reported with this procedure.[14] The creation of sphincters and valves has been tried in an attempt to replace the ileocecal valve. Although the technique has been described in the literature for more than 25 years, only anecdotal reports are available to assess their efficacy in humans.[14]

Intestinal loop lengthening procedures have perhaps the most potential usefulness of the current surgical procedures. The intestine is divided by use of a stapling device down the midline of the remaining bowel.[18] Two segments having equal length, but one half of the initial diameter are created and are anastomosed end to end. Because of the expected hypertrophy of the intestinal villi, this method can create twice as much usable bowel. Initial results with this procedure indicate that further trials are needed to evaluate its potential efficacy.[19]

Several surgical interventions, which are currently being experimentally evaluated, hold promise for the future. Small intestinal transplantation is the most logical and straightforward approach.[4, 14] The major problems of small intestinal transplantation at this time is the prevention of rejection. Even with the advent of cyclosporine, which has greatly increased the success of kidney, liver and heart transplants, the success rate in animal experiments is still discouraging.[14] Fetal intestinal transplantation and the use of small intestinal mucosal growth factors are also being studied.[14]

Outcome

The adaptation and hypertrophy of the intestine is a slow process, and progress to complete enteral feedings can take 1 year or more to occur.[11] Nutritional support from TPN has almost removed malnutrition as a cause of death in these patients. However, TPN toxicity can lead to hepatic cirrhosis, liver failure, and death. Hepatic failure and infection are now the commonest causes of death in patients with short bowel disease.[3] The patients who survive are often maintained on a number of medications and frequently may require elemental or easily digested diets.[15]

SUMMARY

Short bowel syndrome poses many management problems for the pediatrician. The specific abnormalities relate directly to the amount of bowel resected, the status of the ileocecal valve, the age of the child at the time of surgery, the level of the bowel resected, and the adaptive properties of the bowel remaining. The outcome has improved in recent years, especially with the use of TPN and improved elemental diets.

REFERENCES

1. Young WF, Swain VAJ, Pringle EM: Long-term prognosis after major resection of small bowel in early infancy. *Arch Dis Child* 1986; 44:465–470.
2. Tonloukian RJ, Walker-Smith JH: Normal intestinal length in preterm infants. *J Pediatr Surg* 1983; 18:720–723.
3. Cooper A, Floyd TJ, Ross AJ III, et al: Morbidity and mortality of short-bowel syndrome acquired in infancy: An update. *J Pediatr Surg* 1984; 19:711–718.

4. Holt D, Easa D, Shim W, et al: Survival after massive small intestinal resection in a neonate. *Am J Dis Child* 1982; 136:79–80.
5. Bell MJ, Martin LN, Schuburt WK, et al: Massive small-bowel resection in an infant: Long-term management and intestinal adaptation. *J Pediatr Surg* 1973; 8:197–204.
6. Jeejeebhoy KN: Therapy of the short gut syndrome. *Lancet* 1983; 1:1427–1430.
7. Weser E: The management of patients after small bowel resection. *Gastroenterology* 1976; 71:146–150.
8. Silverman A, Roy CC (eds): Malabsorption syndrome, in *Pediatric Clinical Gastroenterology,* ed 3. St Louis, CV Mosby Co, 1983, p 252.
9. Borgstion B, Dahlquist A, Lundh G, et al: Studies of intestinal digestion and absorption in the human. *J Clin Invest* 1957; 36:1521–1536.
10. Weser E, Hernandez MH: Studies of small bowel adaptation after intestinal resection in the rat. *Gastroenterology* 1971; 60:69–75.
11. Williamson RCN: Intestinal adaptation: Structural, functional and cytokinetic changes. *N Engl J Med* 1978; 298:1393–1402.
12. Dowling RH, Booth CC: Structural and functional changes following small intestinal resection in the rat. *Clin Sci* 1967; 32:139–149.
13. William RCN, Bauer FLR, Ross JS, et al: Proximal enterectomy stimulates distal hyperplasia more than bypass or pancreatic biliary diversion. *Gastroenterology* 1978; 74:16–23.
14. Schwatz MZ, Maeda K: Short bowel syndrome in infants and children. *Pediatr Clin N Am* 1985; 32:1265–1279.
15. Parker P, Stroop S, Greene H: A controlled trial of continuous versus intermittent feeding in the treatment of infants with intestinal disease. *J Pediatr* 1981; 99:360–364.
16. Christie DL, Ament ME: Dilute elemental diet and continuous infusion technique for management of small bowel syndrome. *J Pediatr* 1975; 87:705–708.
17. Beale EF, Nelson RM, Bucciarelli RT, et al: Intrahepatic cholestasis associated with parenteral nutrition in premature infants. *Pediatrics* 1979; 64:342–347.
18. Bianchi A: Intestinal loop lengthening—a technique for increasing small intestinal length. *J Pediatr Surg* 1980; 15:145–151.
19. Boeckman CR, Traylor R: Bowel lengthening for short gut syndrome. *J Pediatr Surg* 1981; 16:996–997.

18 Intestinal Malrotation

Craig W. Lillehei, M.D.

An 18-year-old boy presented with vomiting and dehydration. Since infancy he had experienced recurrent episodes of crampy abdominal pain associated with non-bilious vomiting and diarrhea. These episodes occurred nearly every month and lasted almost 1 week. At age 5 years, following an EEG showing left temporal lobe β-wave activity, the diagnosis of "abdominal migraines" was made, and he was started on primidone (Mysoline) and diphenylhydantoin without relief. The current episode began with epigastric pain 7 days prior to admission, followed by 5 days of nonbloody, nonbilious vomiting. Two days before admission, he developed watery diarrhea.

On physical examination the patient was dehydrated, but his blood pressure was 140/88 mm Hg. The abdomen was soft and slightly distended, and bowel sounds were present. He was mildly tender to deep palpation but had no guarding. The stool was guaiac negative.

Laboratory data included a hematocrit of 51%, BUN of 129 mg/dl, creatinine level of 6.4 mg/dl and an anion gap of 31. An upper gastrointestinal (GI) tract x-ray series showed malrotation. He was intravenously hydrated with rapid fall of his BUN and creatinine values to normal.

At laparotomy, malrotation with a midgut volvulus was found, but the entire bowel was viable. A Bill modification of the Ladd procedure was performed. He was discharged on postoperative day 6 and has had no further episodes of vomiting or abdominal pain.

DISCUSSION

Malrotation, or incomplete rotation of the bowel, is estimated to occur in about 1 in every 6,000 live births.[1] It is almost universally found in infants with large omphaloceles, gastroschisis, or congenital diaphragmatic hernias.[2][3] Patients with this abnormality may be entirely asymptomatic, or they may present with acute life-threatening volvulus, which demands immediate treatment. Chronic intermittent obstruction as described in this case can also be seen.

Pathophysiology

The key to understanding malrotation is an appreciation of the relevant midgut embryology. The midgut extends from the duodenojejunal junction to the middle of the transverse colon and is supplied by the superior mesenteric artery.[4] Usually there is rapid elongation of the midgut during the first few months of fetal life. As the bowel grows, it undergoes a process of rotation. The analogy of a loop fixed above at the stomach and below at the rectum is useful for visualizing this process (Fig 18–1).[4] The loop rotates about the axis of the superior mesenteric artery in a counterclockwise direction (as viewed anteriorly) over an arc of 270 degrees. As the midgut settles into the abdominal cavity at 12 weeks of fetal life, the duodenum lies behind the superior mesenteric artery, whereas the transverse colon crosses anteriorly so that the cecum is positioned in the right lower quadrant. There is broad mesenteric fixation from the ligament of Treitz to the cecum. Anomalies of this sequence of rotation and subsequent mesenteric fixation account for the pathologic findings of malrotation.

Malrotation actually represents a spectrum of anatomical abnormalities since the process of rotation may arrest at any point.[3] In nonrotation, or incomplete rotation, the midgut elongates on the superior mesenteric vessels. There is no ligament of Treitz, and the mesenteric attachment is quite narrow. The entire midgut hangs on the superior mesenteric vascular pedicle and is therefore prone to volvulus. In incomplete rotation either the duodenum, colon, or both fail to completely rotate into normal position.[4] In these conditions the mesenteric fixation is still narrow, and this deficient fixation predisposes to the risk for midgut volvulus. Abnormal mesenteric fixation often develops from the malpositioned viscera. Such mesenteric attachments may produce duodenal obstruction (so-called Ladd's bands) or sites for internal herniation.[4] Rarely, reverse rotation is seen in which the colon rotates behind the superior mesenteric artery with obstruction of the transverse colon by the overlying vessels and mesentery.[4]

Clinical Features

The clinical problems caused by malrotation are due to either defective mesenteric fixation, abnormal placement of fixation, or both. Although malrotation can certainly occur at any age, it is primarily a disease of childhood. Most patients present within the first year of life, and the majority are seen before they reach 1 month of age.[5, 6] Symptoms are typically those of duodenal obstruction with forceful, bilious vomiting. Abdominal distention is an unreliable sign since the site of obstruction is high and the stomach may be decompressed by emesis. Jaundice, usually unconjugated hyperbilirubinemia, can also be seen as in other causes of intestinal obstruction.[7] Hematochezia is seen in 10% of patients, raising concern for bowel viability.[5] The incidence of volvulus at surgery is approximately 50%.[5]

Malrotation may also present in older children or adults.[3, 8] Typically such cases develop chronic intermittent bowel obstruction, as described in this case. Recurrent abdominal pain, vomiting, and even malabsorption can be seen.[9] Although the incidence of midgut volvulus with infarction is certainly much lower in adults, the

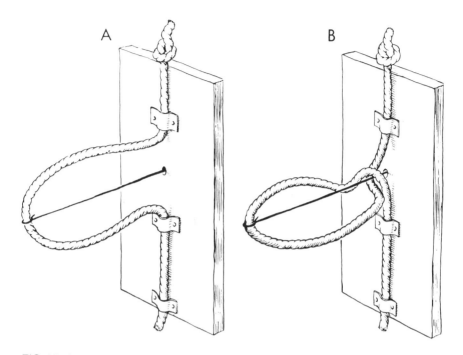

FIG 18–1.
Mechanics of intestinal rotation using a rope fixed to both ends and a wire representing the superior mesenteric artery fixed to the midportion. **A,** top limb corresponds to the duodenojejunal loop and the bottom limb to the cecocolic segment. **B,** rope is rotated through 270 degrees around the wire in a counterclockwise direction, resulting in the top limb becoming the bottom and the bottom segment becoming the top. (From Snyder WH, Chaffin L: Embryology and pathology of the intestinal tract: Presentation of 40 cases of malrotation. *Ann Surg* 1954; 140:368 380. Used with permission.)

possibility of malrotation needs to be considered in the differential diagnosis of bowel obstruction at any age.

Internal hernias may also develop from the abnormal mesenteric fixation. These hernias can cause recurrent entrapment of bowel, obstruction, and even strangulation.[10]

Finally, malrotation may be entirely asymptomatic. Occasionally the diagnosis is discovered incidentally from radiographic studies, at surgery, or at autopsy.[11] Given the potential for acute lethal complications, even asymptomatic patients with malrotation should be considered for surgical therapy.

Diagnosis

The first step to accurate diagnosis is to include malrotation and midgut volvulus in the differential diagnosis of all bowel obstructions. The index of suspicion must be particularly high in infants where the problem is common and the incidence of volvulus is highest. Other causes for bilious vomiting from bowel obstruction in the pediatric population are found in Table 18–1.

The key to diagnosis is a carefully performed upper GI x-ray series to identify the position of the ligament of Treitz. Although plain films, ultrasound, or computed tomographic (CT) scanning of the abdomen have occasionally been useful, these studies cannot reliably exclude the diagnosis.[12, 13] A contrast enema may be diagnostic, but a normally positioned cecum does not rule out the possibility of malrotation or even midgut volvulus.[12]

Treatment

The standard treatment for malrotation was outlined by Ladd more than 50 years ago.[14] Through an abdominal incision, the intestines are carefully inspected. Identification of the position of the duodenum and cecum is required to determine whether malrotation exists. If volvulus is present, the intestines are derotated, usually in a counterclockwise direction.[12] Division of the mesenteric bands overlying the duodenum is not only useful to relieve extrinsic obstruction but also permits correct identification of the anatomy. An intraluminal cathether should be passed to exclude the frequently associated intrinsic obstruction of a duodenal atresia or stenosis.[2] As the dissection proceeds, care must be taken to avoid injury to the mesenteric vascular pedicle. In Ladd's procedure, the jejunum is laid on the right side of the abdomen, and the cecum is placed next to the descending colon.[14] Most surgeons remove the appendix to avoid the possibility of future confusion about appendicitis. A modification advocated by Bill and Grauman involves stabilization of the mesentery by anchoring the bowel with suture fixation.[15]

Although resection of a gangrenous segment may be required, every effort is taken to maximize the amount of remaining bowel. A second-look operation in 24 hours can be used to assess bowel of borderline viability.

TABLE 18–1.
Important Mechanical Causes of Bowel Obstruction in Children

Neonates (<1 mo)	Older Children
Atresia/stenosis	Adhesions
Necrotizing enterocolitis	Intussusception
Meconium ileus	Appendicitis
Volvulus	Hernia
Hernia	Hirschsprung's disease
Hirschsprung's disease	Volvulus
Duplication	Malignancy

Outcome

With early recognition and prompt surgical treatment, the morbidity of malrotation has been substantially reduced. In a large review of patients from Children's Hospital of Los Angeles, the previously reported mortality of 23% had been lowered to 4%.[6] Death usually occurs when extrinsic bowel necrosis is present.[5, 6]

Stauffer and Herrmann have reported that the incidence of late reoperations for obstruction is high (10%–16%).[16] Unfortunately, this complication does not appear to be improved by intestinal fixation as described by Bill and Grauman.[15] Approximately 20% to 25% of the patients have mild to moderate abdominal complaints subsequently.

SUMMARY

Malrotation is a developmental anomaly resulting in abnormal mesenteric fixation. Although symptoms typically arise in infancy, they may present at any age. Since the consequences of malrotation may be devastating with midgut volvulus and necrosis of the entire small bowel, a high index of suspicion must be maintained in all cases of bowel obstruction. Early diagnosis and treatment are critical to minimize morbidity and mortality.

REFERENCES

1. Malrotation with or without volvulus of the midgut, in Silverman A, Roy, CC (eds): *Pediatric Clinical Gastroenterology,* ed 3. St Louis, C V Mosby Co, 1983, p 61.
2. Smith EI: Malrotation of the intestine, in Welch KJ, Randolph JG, Ravitch MM, et al (eds): *Pediatric Surgery* ed 4: Chicago, Year Book Medical Publishers, 1986, pp 892-893.
3. Wang CA, Welch CE: Anomalies of intestinal rotation in adolescents and adults. *Surgery* 1963; 54:839–855.
4. Snyder WH, Chaffin L: Embryology and pathology of the intestinal tract: Presentation of 40 cases of malrotation. *Ann Surg* 1954; 140:368–380.
5. Stewart DR, Colodny AL, Daggett WC: Malrotation of the bowel in infants and children: A 15 year review. *Surgery* 1976; 79:716–720.
6. Andrassy RJ, Mahour GH: Malrotation of the midgut in infants and children. *Arch Surg* 1981; 116:158–160.
7. Porto SO: Jaundice in congenital malrotation of the intestine. *Am J Dis Child* 1969; 117:684–688.
8. Yanez R, Spitz L: Intestinal malrotation presenting outside the neonatal period. *Arch Dis Child* 1986; 61:682–685.
9. Howell CG, Vozza F, Shaw S, et al: Malrotation, malnutrition and ischemic bowel disease. *J Pediatr Surg* 1982; 17:469–473.
10. Willwerth BM, Zollinger RM, Izant RJ: Congenital mesocolic (paraduodenal) hernia: Embryologic basis of repair. *Am J Surg* 1974; 128:358–361.
11. Houston CS, Wittenborg MH: Roentgen evaluation of anomalies of rotation and fixation of the bowel in children. *Radiology* 1965; 84:1–18.

12. Berdon, Baker DH, Bull S, et al: Midgut malrotation and volvulus: Which films are most helpful? *Radiology* 1970; 96:375–384.
13. Fisher JK: Computed tomographic diagnosis of volvulus in intestinal malrotation. *Radiology* 1981; 140:145–146.
14. Ladd WE: Congenital obstruction of the duodenum in children. *N Engl J Med* 1982; 206:277–283.
15. Bill AH, Grauman D: Rationale and technique for stabilization of the mesentery in cases of nonrotation of the midgut. *J Pediatr Surg* 1966; 1:127–136.
16. Stauffer UG, Herrmann P: Comparison of late results in patients with corrected intestinal malrotation with and without fixation of the mesentery. *J Pediatr Surg* 1980; 15:9–12.

19 Intussusception

Craig W. Lillehei, M.D.

A previously healthy 7-month-old girl, the product of a full-term pregnancy, had been feeding and growing well on a standard infant formula. Five days earlier she developed a mild upper respiratory tract infection. The evening prior to admission she was described by her parents as "restless" and subsequently vomited her feedings. A small amount of bright red blood was noted in her diaper. Her vital signs were stable and the skin; head, ear, eye, nose, and throat; pulmonary; and cardiac examination results were normal. The abdomen was nondistended; she exhibted moderate tenderness to abdominal palpation. No discrete mass was identified. Her stool was frankly bloody. An abdominal radiograph demonstrated several dilated small bowel loops. A barium enema identified an intussusception at the hepatic flexure (Fig 19–1). It was irreducible, so the patient was taken directly to the operating room where a laparotomy was performed. At operation an ileocolic intussusception that could be reduced to the proximal transverse colon but no further was found (Fig 19–2). The remaining intussusception was resected and bowel continuity restored with an end-to-end anatomosis. No specific lead point in the ileum was found. The infant had a benign postoperative course and was discharged home after 5 days.

Discussion

Intussusception is a common problem in infants and young children in which the proximal bowel (intussusceptum) invaginates into the distal bowel (intussuscipiens), producing obstruction and vascular compromise.[1] In its most frequent form the terminal ileum intussuscepts into the cecum as an ileocolic intussusception. The entity typically occurs within the first 2 years of life, with a peak incidence at 8 months of age. However, intussusception may occur at any age and has been identified in the fetus causing bowel atresia[2] and has also been seen in premature infants simulating necrotizing enterocolitis.[3] Epidemiologic studies indicate that the incidence is about 2 to 4 per 1,000 live births in England but appears to be less in the United States.[4] A male preponderance (3:2) is usually seen; there does not appear to be a major difference in incidence among racial groups.[5]

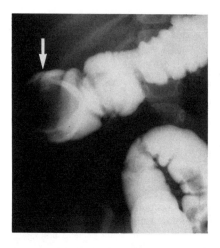

FIG 19–1.
Barium enema revealing the coiled spring appearance of the intussuscepted mass *(arrow).*

Pathophysiology

In most cases the etiology is unknown. It has been observed that intussusceptions often follow viral infections, especially adenoviruses.[6] This has led to speculation that hypertrophy of Peyer's patches or ileocolic lymphadenopathy may be involved. If this hypothesis is correct, the greatly increased amount of intestinal lymphoid tissue in infants compared with older children may predispose them to intussusception. Since almost 75% of intussusceptions occur at or near the ileocecal valve, abnormalities in this region have been vigorously sought. One current hypothesis is that the disproportion between the size of the ileum and the ileocecal valve in infants compared to older children predisposes infants to intussusception.[5]

Others have blamed local anatomic features.[7] In about 5% of cases a specific lead point can be identified. Examples include polyps, Meckel's diverticulum, enteric duplication, small bowel tumor, and inverted appendix. Children with an anatomic lead point tend to present at an older age, and surgical resection is usually required. Certain diseases may also increase the risk for intussusception. Henoch-Schönlein purpura can produce small bowel intussusceptions.[8] Children with cystic fibrosis have a higher incidence of intussusceptions, often colocolic, presumably secondary to inspissated feces acting as the lead point.[9] Postoperatively, bowel obstruction may be produced by intussusception even following operations in which there has been no bowel manipulation whatsoever.[10] Most often these intussusceptions are ileoileal and do not respond to nonoperative treatment. The clue to diagnosis is that the obstruction develops after resolution of the usual postoperative ileus.

Whatever the cause of the intussusception, the injury to the bowel is caused by compression of the invaginated bowel with acute angulation and restriction of the blood supply. Venous stasis and edema occur, and intraluminal mucus and blood seeping from the engorged bowel mix to form the typical currant jelly stools.[5] If the stasis and engorgement are not relieved, gangrene and necrosis occur.

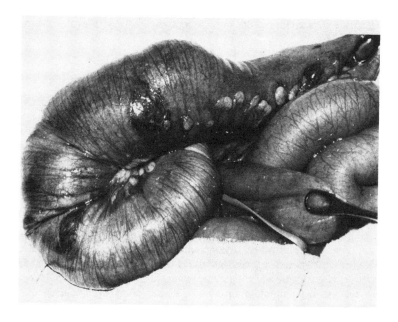

FIG 19–2.
Ileocolic intussusception with the intussuscepted mass seen at surgery.

Clinical Features

The classic symptoms of intussusception are the triad of abdominal colic, emesis, and hematochezia.[1] The frequency of the signs and symptoms of intussusception in infants and children is found in Table 19–1. Intussusception is usually seen in a previously healthy infant who suddenly develops intense abdominal pain. The child is inconsolable, crying in pain with his or her legs drawn up. Often, within minutes, the pain subsides and the child returns to his or her premorbid state, only to have the entire episode repeated. It is this history of severe abdominal cramping that must alert the physician to the possibility of intussusception. Emesis in association with the pain is common. As the duration of symptoms lengthens, the child becomes progressively lethargic. Occasionally infants may present with altered consciousness as the initial manifestation.[11] The passage of a bloody stool is often the symptom that initiates medical consultation.

The initial physical examination may reveal an infant who is asymptomatic, agonizing in pain, or somnolent. The skin should be carefully examined for mucosal pigmentation of Peutz-Jeghers syndrome or vasculitic lesions of Henoch-Schönlein purpura. Careful abdominal examination may reveal the sausage-shaped mass of the intussusception. It is often tethered by its mesentery into a crescent. The stools are classically described as ''currant jelly'' produced by a mixture of mucus and blood from the congested mucosa within the intussusception. However, they may be entirely normal at the outset. Rarely the intussusception will present as a mass prolapsing through the anus.

Management

Diagnosis and therapy must overlap. The key to diagnosis is a high index of suspicion based on the history and physical examination.before the barium enema, which is the single essential diagnostic test, the patient is stabilized with fluid and electrolytic replacement while arrangements are made for the radiologic study. If significant vomiting has occurred, nasogastric decompression is advisable. Preparations are made should operative reduction be required. The child is then transported to the radiology suite. Although a soft tissue mass may be identified on a plain film of the abdomen, its absence cannot be used to exclude the diagnosis.[12] Intussusceptions can also be recognized by ultrasound or computed tomography,[13][14] but these techniques do not offer the added benefit of therapy. The only absolute contraindication to the use of a barium enema is clinical or radiographic evidence of bowel perforation. Small bowel obstruction is not regarded as a contraindication to hydrostatic reduction.[15] Since the disease may present without the typical findings, a low threshold for utilizing barium enemas in young children must be employed. There is evidence that early diagnosis increases the likelihood of successful nonoperative hydrostatic reduction.[16]

The child is usually sedated prior to the barium enema examination. Our approach is to have a surgeon in attendance. The height of the barium column is limited to 90 cm above the patient to avoid excessive hydrostatic pressure. The temptation to use manual manipulation is resisted for the same reason. With these safeguards, the risk of perforation is small and appears to be associated with younger age (<6 months) and longer illness (>36 hours).[17] Although statistics vary, approximately 65% of ileocolic intussusceptions are reduced hydrostatically.[16] To ensure complete reduction, one must see free reflux of barium into the ileum. Although the swollen folds of the ileocecal valve may be misleading, a discrete filling defect or failure to achieve complete reduction are indications for surgery. The Chinese have reported considerable success with air pressure reduction, but experience in other centers with this technique has been limited.[18]

If the intussusception cannot be hydrostatically reduced, the child is taken directly

TABLE 19–1.
Signs and Symptoms of Intussusception*

	Infants	Older Children
Pain	+ + +	+ + +
Vomiting	+ + +	+ +
Bleeding	+ + +	+
Association with anatomic lead point	Rare	Almost all cases

*Plus signs indicate relative severity or frequency.

to the operating room. The intussusception is surgically exposed, and manual reduction is attempted. The bowel is gently compressed to milk the intussusceptum proximally. If the bowel mesentery has been intussuscepted too long, the bowel wall becomes edematous due to obstruction of venous outflow or ultimately gangrenous due to occlusion of arterial perfusion. In either case, it is no longer possible to achieve complete manual reduction, and a local bowel resection is required. Bowel continuity is restored by a primary end-to-end anastomosis. Resection is also required if a discrete lead point is identified. Curiously, the recurrence rate for intussusception is approximately 5% whether hydrostatic reduction, manual reduction, or resection is utilized.[5]

SUMMARY

Intussusception is a common cause of small bowel obstruction in infants and young children. The causes of intussusception are still largely unknown, but anatomic lead points and diseases such as Henoch-Schönlein purpura and cystic fibrosis can be seen especially in older children. The clinical signs of intermittent abdominal colic, vomiting, and hematochezia are the classical triad associated with intussusception. Since the etiology of most ileocolic intussusceptions is unknown and there is no preventive therapy, efforts must be directed toward early identification and treatment to minimize morbidity. The clinician should maintain a high level of suspicion and be ready to order a barium enema, which is the essential diagnostic study and can be the therapeutic intervention in about 65% of cases. If hydrostatic reduction of the intussusception is not possible, surgical intervention is required immediately.

REFERENCES

1. Gross RE, Ware PF: Intussusception in childhood: Experiences from 610 cases. *N Engl J Med* 1975; 259:645.
2. Parkkulainen KV: Intrauterine intussusception as a cause of intestinal atresia. *Surgery* 1958; 44:1106–1111.
3. Carman J, Grunebaum M, Gorenstein A, et al: Intussusception in a premature infant simulating necrotizing enterocolitis. *Z Kindenchir* 1987; 42:44-51.
4. Court D, Knox G: Incidence of intussusception in Newcastle children. *Br Med J* 1959; 2:408–409.
5. Ravitch MM: Intussusception, in Welch KJ, Randolph JG, Ravitch MM, et al (eds): *Pediatric Surgery*, ed 4. Year Book Medical Publishers, Chicago, 1986; pp 868–882.
6. Nichols JC, Ingrand D, Fortier B, et al: A one-year virological survey of acute intussusception in childhood. *J Med Virol* 1982; 9:267–271.
7. Schere T, Dechelotte P, Vanneuville G: Etiopathogenic theory of ileocecocolic intussusception. *Anat Clin* 1985; 7:103–106.
8. Martinez-Frontanilla LA, Haase GM, Ernster JA, et al: Surgical complications in Henoch-Schonlein purpura. *J. Pediatr Surg*, 1984; 19:434–436.
9. Holsclaw DS, Rocmens C, Shwachman H: Intussusception in patients with cystic fibrosis. *Pediatrics* 1971; 48:51–58.

10. Ein SH, Ferguson JM: Intussusception — the forgotten postoperative obstruction. *Arch Dis Child* 1984; 57:788–790.
11. Heidrich FJ: Lethargy as a presenting symptom in patients with intussusception. *Clin Pediatric* (Phila) 1986; 25:363–365.
12. White SJ, Blanc CE: Intussusception: Additional observations on the plain radiograph. *AJR* 1982; 139:511–513.
13. Swischuk LE, Hayden CK, Boulden J: Intussusception: Indications for ultrasonography and explanation of the doughnut and pseudokidney signs. *Pediatr Radiol* 1985; 15:388–391.
14. Merine D, Fishman EK, Jones B, et al: Enteroenteric intussusception: CT findings in nine patients. *AJR* 1987; 148:1129–1132.
15. Leonides JC: Treatment of intussusception with small bowel obstruction; application of decision analysis. *AJR* 1985; 145:665–669.
16. Liu KW, MacCarthy J. Guiney EJ, et al: Intussusception: Current trends in management. *Arch Dis Child* 1986; 61:75–77.
17. Humphry A, Ein SH, Mok PM: Perforation of the intussuscepted colon. *AJR* 1981; 137:1135–1138.
18. Gus JZ, Ma XX, Zhow QH: Results of air pressure enema reduction on intussusception: 6,396 cases in 13 years. *J. Pediatr Surg* 1986; 21:1201–1203.

20 Acute Appendicitis

Craig W. Lillehei, M.D.
John D. Snyder, M.D.

A 7-year-old boy had been in excellent health until the day before admission when he developed vague midabdominal pain. He was afebrile but complained of indigestion and anorexia without vomiting or diarrhea. His older brother had recently had the "flu" with symptoms including nausea, vomiting, diarrhea, and persistent abdominal pain. Over the night the pain worsened, and he had two episodes of nonbilious, nonbloody vomiting. The pain shifted to the right lower quadrant. When seen in the emergency room, he was a pale, ill-appearing child with stable vital signs. His positive physical findings were confined to the abdomen, which was mildly tender with hypoactive bowel sounds. Tenderness was greatest in the right lower quadrant, where involuntary guarding was noted. The rectal examination was unremarkable and included heme-negative soft brown stool, with no polymorphonuclear (PMN) cells on Gram stain. The laboratory evaluation revealed a normal hemoglobin and urinalysis. The white blood cell (WBC) count was elevated at 22,000/mm³ with a predominance of PMN cells and band forms; an erythrocyte sedimentation rate was also elevated at 35 mm/hour. The patient was taken to the operating room, where an inflamed appendix with a fecalith was removed (Figure 20–1).

DISCUSSION

Acute appendicitis is the most common abdominal surgical emergency in children and adolescents;[1] approximately 80,000 cases occur each year.[2] Appendicitis continues to carry a high rate of misdiagnosis (up to one third of all cases) and also has one of the highest rates of delayed diagnosis and perforation (up to 30% of cases).[3] The delay in diagnosis is often attributed to the fact that appendicitis is considered the great imitator and may frequently have an atypical presentation (Table 20–1). The mean age of presentation is 10 years, but cases have been reported in all ages, including newborn infants.[4]

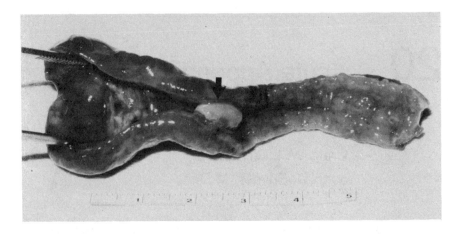

FIG 20–1.
Inflamed appendix with fecalith in lumen *(arrow)*.

Pathophysiology

The initial step in the development of appendicitis appears to be obstruction of the appendiceal lumen often by fecal material or local lymph node enlargement.[5] Secretions from mucosal glands, the volume of which may be increased by bacterial infection, produce progressive distention of the obstructed lumen. This distention of stretch receptors in the small blood vessels of the appendix is transmitted along visceral nerve fibers to the 10th thoracic ganglion, which supplies the dermatome of the umbilicus.[4, 6] Thus, periumbilical pain is often the first symptom of appendicitis.

As the obstruction continues and intraluminal pressure rises, there is compromise of lymphatic and venous drainage producing bowel wall edema and increased secretions.[4] When the pressure rises sufficiently to occlude arterial flow, gangrene and perforation are imminent.

TABLE 20–1.
Differential Diagnosis of Acute Abdomen Related to Age*

Infants	Older Children	All Ages
Intussusception	Pelvic inflammatory disease	Mesenteric adenitis
Volvulus	Mettelschmerz	Pneumonia
Hirschsprung's	Peptic ulcer disease	Urinary tract infection
enterocolitis	Cholecystitis	Trauma
Strangulated hernia	Ectopic pregnancy	Pancreatitis
	Crohn's disease	Meckel's diverticulum
		Renal stones
		Hepatitis

*Adapted from Hatch[4] and Cope.[6]

With increased pressure, small quantities of inflammatory fluid escape into the peritoneum, causing local irritation and shifting of the pain with increasing intensity to the right lower quadrant.[6] Without peritoneal irritation, pain will not be felt in the right lower quadrant. For example, retrocecal appendicitis even with perforation will cause only persistent periumbilical pain because of its retroperitoneal location.[4] When the appendix hangs over the brim of the true pelvis, pain is usually felt in both right and left iliac fossae and is felt on deep pressure at the brim of the pelvis; epigastric pain may be the predominant complaint.[6]

The evolution from appendiceal obstruction to perforation typically requires 24 to 48 hours. However, in the presence of an appendicolith, the evolution may accelerate to less than 12 hours. Acute appendicitis will usually progress to perforation if left untreated. By 48 hours after the onset of symptoms, 80% of untreated cases of appendicitis will have perforated.[7]

Clinical Features

The clinical history is the single most important tool in diagnosing acute appendicitis and should focus on three aspects: (1) the history immediately prior to the onset of pain, (2) symptoms and local signs of the attack, and (3) the order of occurrence of symptoms (Table 20–2).[4, 6] Before the onset of pain, the patient often complains for a few days of indigestion or flatulence and irregular bowel movements (constipation or diarrhea). A careful history of respiratory and urinary tract disease should always be sought because pneumonia, pyelonephritis, and renal stones can mimic the clinical picture of acute appendicitis. In pubescent girls, a detailed gynecologic history must be obtained and a pelvic examination performed, with special attention to the possible presence of pelvic inflammatory disease, mettelschmerz, and ectopic pregnancy.

The signs and symptoms of the attack are very helpful in making the diagnosis of appendicitis. The first symptom is almost always vague, poorly localized periumbilical discomfort that usually migrates to the right iliac region some hours later.[4, 6] Reflex vomiting, if present, follows periumbilical pain in contrast to gastroenteritis where vomiting is more likely to precede abdominal pain.[4] In the absence of vomiting, loss of appetite and nausea can also be important clues to the diagnosis.[6] The diarrhea seen with appendicitis is usually mucoid, infrequent, of small volume, and follows the onset of pain.[4]

Careful, complete, and gentle abdominal examinations, often repeated over time, are essential to help make the diagnosis. Abdominal muscular rigidity caused by inflammation of the parietal peritoneum is often absent early in the course of appendicitis and can be absent even after perforation of a pelvic appendix.[6] Local distention, when present, is caused by gaseous distention of the cecum. Hyperesthesia is usually seen on the right side of the abdomen in cases of inflamed unperforated appendicitis and is related to distention of the appendix.[6] Deep tenderness at McBurney's point (two thirds of the distance between the umbilicus and the anterior superior iliac spine) develops as time passes. The rectal examination becomes very important in localizing pain from an appendix located in the pelvis (see previous discussion).[6] In evaluation of the pain it is helpful to remember that the peritoneal cavity is analogous to a cube with six sides. Depending on the location of the inflamed appendix, anterior

TABLE 20–2.

Diagnostic Clues of Acute Appendicitis*

History prior to onset of pain
  Indigestion or flatulence for a few days
  Irregular bowel movements
Symptoms and local signs of the attack
  Pain migrating from epigastrium and becoming
    deep pain in the right iliac fossa
  Nausea and vomiting
  Diarrhea
  Local rigidity (inconstant)
  Local distention (inconstant)
  Superficial hyperestheia (inconstant)
  Fever
Order of occurrence of symptoms
  Pain, usually epigastric or periumbilical
  Nausea or vomiting
  Local iliac tenderness
  Fever
  Leukocytosis

*Adapted from Hatch[4] and Cope.[6]

abdominal tenderness, flank pain, iliopsoas irritation, hiccups, or pelvic rectal tenderness may be present.[6]

Fever usually develops after the migration of the pain to the right iliac fossa and the onset of nausea or vomiting (see Table 20–2). Low-grade fever is the rule before perforation, and often no temperature elevation is seen.[6]

The order of the occurrence of the signs and symptoms is probably the most important diagnostic clue (see Table 20–2). The classic sequence is umbilical (or epigastric) pain and then nausa or vomiting, followed by migration of the pain to the right iliac fossa.[6] Fever and leukocytosis are the final signs to develop.

The routine laboratory evaluation, which should include a complete blood cell count and urinalysis, is not diagnostic but can be helpful. The WBC count is very variable in children with appendicitis so that a normal WBC count should not delay surgical exploration.[8] The urinalysis indicates whether a urinary tract infection, pyelonephritis, or a renal calculus may be causing the symptoms. A few red blood cells (RBCs) or WBCs can be seen in acute appendicitis when the inflamed appendix is near the ureter or bladder.[4] In addition, a stool culture should be considered if RBCs or WBCs are found in the stool since *Yersinia enterocolitica* infection can mimic acute appendicitis.[9]

Radiographic studies are often obtained but usually offer only suggestive evidence of the diagnosis but may be helpful to exclude other diagnoses. An abdominal flat plate radiogram may demonstrate nonspecific findings, including an abnormal right lower quadrant gas pattern, scoliosis, and obliteration of the psoas shadow.[10] The finding of a fecalith, seen in 10% to 20% of cases, indicates that appendiceal obstruction has occurred.[3] The efficacy of the barium enema in diagnosing acute appendicitis is still debated. If the entire appendiceal lumen is seen, appendicitis is very unlikely. However, false positive and false negative results have been reported leading to the recommendation that the results of the study should not be the basis for operating on the child.[11] Ultrasonography has been of little help in diagnosing acute appendicitis but can be very helpful in identifying a periappendiceal abcess after perforation.

Differential Diagnosis

The differential diagnosis of an acute abdomen is lengthy and differs by age (see Table 20–1).[4, 6] The most commonly confused diagnoses are gastroenteritis, urinary tract infection, and mesenteric adenitis (especially from *Y. enterocolitica*). In infants, intussusception, volvulus, and Hirschsprung's enterocolitis must be considered. In older children and adolescents, pelvic inflammatory disease, mittelschmerz, ectopic pregnancy, peptic disease, cholecystitis, and Crohn's disease are possibilities. Several disease entities should be considered in all age groups, including mesenteric adenitis, pneumonia, trauma, pancreatitis, Meckel's diverticulum, renal stones, and hepatitis.

The early diagnosis of acute appendicitis remains difficult, and a diagnostic accuracy of 75% remains a high standard.[12] The accuracy falls appreciably in young children, where perforation rates of 50% to 70% can be seen.[13] When the risks of negative appendectomy are weighed against the hazards of a perforated appendix, the 75% diagnostic accuracy level is considered a desirable standard.[12]

Treatment

Acute appendicitis is a surgical emergency, and once the clinical diagnosis is made, surgical intervention should swiftly follow to reduce the chance for perforation. By 24 hours after the onset of symptoms, 20% of children will have perforated their appendix and at 36 and 48 hours, 50% and 80% of patients, respectively, will have perforated.[7]

A small right lower quadrant incision is usually made with wide abdominal preparation in case extension of the incision is required. For cosmetic reasons, a transverse or curvilinear incision along skin lines is made. The appendix can usually be removed by dividing its mesentery, amputating at its base, and inverting the stump. Occasionally resection of the cecal wall or even local ileocecal resection is required. If a normal appendix is found, it is nonetheless removed to prevent future confusion. In such cases, a careful search must be made intraoperatively to avoid overlooking other pathology. Specifically, the terminal ileum should be examined for evidence of Crohn's disease or Meckel's diverticulitis. Inspection of pelvic viscera is essential in girls to rule out gynecologic pathology.

Use of preoperative antibiotics has been shown to reduce wound infections.[14] Multiple antibiotics are used if perforation is likely.

When the appendix has perforated, the most common postoperative complications are infectious,[3] with *Escherichia coli* and *Bacteroides fragilis* being the most common infecting organisms.[15] If an abscess forms and is completely walled off, the child may have no signs of peritonitis or sepsis. Medical management has been used successfully to treat children with walled-off appendiceal abcesses, but very close observation and monitoring must be done.[16]

SUMMARY

Early diagnosis is essential to reduce the chance for severe complications of acute appendicitis. The diagnosis relies most heavily on clinical assessment, with the most important clues being the onset of periumbilical pain often associated with nausea and vomiting that migrates to the right iliac fossa area. Low-grade fever and leukocytosis follow these signs and symptoms (see Table 20–2).

Surgery is the sole treatment, and a 75% rate of diagnostic accuracy is considered an acceptable standard. When compared with the morbidity and mortality of a perforated appendix, a 25% rate of relatively benign negative appendectomy is widely accepted.

REFERENCES

1. Peltokallio P, Tykka H: Evolution of the age distribution and mortality of acute appendicitis. *Arch Surg* 1981; 116:153–155.
2. Ballentine TVN: Appendicitis. *Surg Clin North Am* 1981; 6:1117–1124.
3. Jess P, Bjerregaard B, Brynitz S, et al: Acute appendicitis: Prospective trial of concerning diagnostic accuracy and complications. *Am J Surg* 1981; 141:232–234.
4. Hatch EI Jr: The acute abdomen in children. *Pediatr Clin North Am* 1985; 32:1151–1164.
5. Schisgall RM: Appendiceal colic in childhood. The role of inspisated casts of stool within the appendix. *Ann Surg* 1980; 192:687–693.
6. Cope Z: *Cope's Early Diagnosis of the Acute Abdomen,* ed 16. (Revised by W Silen.) New York, Oxford University Press, 1983.
7. Brender JD, Marcuse EK, Koepsell, TD, et al: Childhood appendicitis: Factors associated with perforation. *Pediatrics* 1985; 72:301–306.
8. Doraiswamy NV: Leukocyte counts in the diagnosis of acute appendicitis in children. *Br J Surg* 1979; 66:782.
9. Black RE, Craun GF, Blake PA: Epidemic *Yersinia enterocolitica* infection due to contaminated chocolate milk. *N Engl J Med* 1978; 298:76–79.
10. Grosfield JL, Weinberger M, Clatworthy JW Jr: Acute appendicitis in the first two years of life. *J Pediatr Surg* 1973; 8:285–293.
11. Hatch EI Jr, Naffis D, Chandler NW: Pitfalls in the use of barium enema in early appendicitis in children. *J Pediatr Surg* 1981; 16:309–312.
12. Jess P, Bjerregaard B, Brynitz S, et al: Acute appendicitis: Prospective trial concerning diagnostic accuracy and complications. *Am J Surg* 1981; 141:232–234.
13. Graham JM, Pokorny WJ, Harberg FJ: Acute appendicitis in preschool age children. *Am J Surg* 1980; 139:24–50.
14. Flannigan GM, Clifford RP, Carver RA, et al: Antibiotic prophylaxis in acute appendicitis. *Surg Gynecol Obstet* 1983; 156:209–211.
15. Stone HH, Kolb LD, et al: Incidence and significance of intraperitoneal anaerobic bacteria. *Ann Surg* 1975; 181:705–715.
16. Janik JS, Ein SH, Shandling B, et al: Nonsurgical management of appendiceal mass in late presenting children. *J Pediatr Surg* 1980; 15:574–576.

21   Meckel's Diverticulum

Richard A. Schreiber, M.D.C.M., F.R.C.P.(C)

A 9-month-old boy was referred to Children's Hospital for gastrointestinal (GI) bleeding. He had been well until 4 days prior to admission when he passed a black tarry stool; he was otherwise asymptomatic. He then had one melanotic stool each day until the evening of admission, when he passed a large currant-jelly stool followed by rectal bleeding. Two episodes of nonbilious vomiting occurred during the day prior to admission, and a low-grade fever was noted. His appetite had not changed, and there was no history of crampy abdominal pain, diarrhea, constipation, medication use or abuse, or bleeding disorders. A 9-year-old sister had *Salmonella* gastroenteritis 1 month previously. The past history was significant for melena of 3 days' duration at the age of 9 months. There was no family history of intestinal disease. He was seen in the emergency room at another hospital where he was noted to be pale and tachycardic, but his blood pressure was stable. The hematocrit was 24%. A large-bore intravenous (IV) catheter was inserted. A nasogastric tube was passed, and the gastric lavage was clear. He was transfused and transferred to Children's Hospital. On physical examination there was no postural change in blood pressure or heart rate. No cutaneous lesions were noted. Examination of the head, eyes, ears, nose, throat, chest, and cardiovascular systems were unremarkable. The abdomen was nontender and without organomegaly, but a slight fullness was present in the right lower quadrant. The rectal examination revealed grossly bloody stools; no fissures were seen.

The hemoglobin value was 9.2 gm%, with a normal mean corpuscular volume. The white blood cell count, platelet count, prothrombin time, partial thromboplastin time, urinalysis, serum electrolyte levels, blood urea nitrogen value, and creatinine and glucose values were normal. A stool smear for leucocytes was negative. A barium enema did not show evidence of obstruction or colitis. The patient was observed for the next few hours, during which time he remained hemodynamically stable. He continued to pass blood rectally. Stool cultures were negative. A rigid sigmoidoscopy up to 20 cm revealed normal mucosa with evidence of blood coming from above. A Meckel's scan was done, but the results were inconclusive. The patient was taken to the operating room, where a Meckel's diverticulum was found and resected.

DISCUSSION

Rectal bleeding is not an uncommon event in the pediatric population, and the diagnosis can vary according to the child's age (Table 21–1). For example, milk allergy colitis is a possible cause of rectal bleeding in the newborn period, whereas this diagnosis would be rare in the school-age child. Volvulus is usually found in neonates, whereas polyps are generally found in older children. Underlying conditions such as sepsis or a bleeding diathesis should always be considered.

Clinical Features

The initial evaluation for the infant who presents with rectal bleeding includes a complete history and thorough physical examination looking for subtle clues to the etiology of the intestinal bleeding.[1] For example, a cutaneous strawberry hemangioma may indicate that intestinal hemangiomata are present. Hyperpigmented spots of the lips or buccal mucosa suggest the Peutz-Jaeger syndrome of intestinal polyps. Signs of ataxia may point to intestinal telangiectasia. Isolated splenomegaly may reflect portal hypertension, and clubbing can be a manifestation of inflammatory bowel disease.

Two points deserve special emphasis in the initial evaluation of the infant who presents with a history of significant blood loss. First, blood pressure measurements, although not routinely obtained in this age group, are essential in the assessment of

TABLE 21–1.
Differential Diagnosis of Lower Gastrointestinal
Bleeding by Age

Age	Condition
Neonates	Necrotizing enterocolitis
	Volvulus
	Duplication
Infants	Intussusception
	Meckel's diverticulum
	Allergic colitis
Children	Polyps
	Meckel's diverticulum
All ages	Anal fissure and excoriations
	Swallowed blood
	Colitis
	Infectious
	Idiopathic (IBD, HUS, HSP)*
	Hemangioma
	Arteriovenous malformations
	Foreign body

*IBD = inflammatory bowel disease; HUS = hemolytic uremic syndrome; HSP = Henoch-Schönlein purpura.

hemodynamic stability in a bleeding child. Second, insertion of a large bore IV catheter in anticipation of the need for rapid volume expansion in a compromised infant may prove to be lifesaving. This is an important early step, particularly in the pediatric patient in whom frequently only a limited-size (23- or 25-gauge) IV butterfly is placed. At the same time, blood can be drawn for a number of laboratory studies, including a cross-match, complete blood cell count, clotting times, electrolyte levels, glucose level, blood urea nitrogen value, and creatinine value.

Differential Diagnosis

Because the child presented here was 9 months old, the differential diagnosis of lower GI bleeding discussed will be confined to infancy. (see Table 21–1 for conditions found in neonates and children). A general approach to the evaluation of children with lower GI bleeding is included in Figure 21–1.

The clinician must remember that some cases of upper GI tract hemorrhage in infants may present with rectal bleeding. This is because blood in the intestinal tract can act as a cathartic and serves to shorten the intestinal transit time. Therefore, to help determine the site of the intestinal bleed, the stomach should be lavaged. In this case, the lavage was negative for blood, suggesting a lower site of GI hemorrhage. Stools should then be examined for leukocytes, and stool cultures should be obtained. As seen in Figure 21–1, the next step in the management will depend on the clinical setting.

The most common cause of rectal bleeding in infancy is an anal fissure.[2] Fissures can be found with careful inspection of the anus. Commonly they cause only a small amount of blood, which is usually seen streaked on the outside of the stool or on the diaper itself. Significant rectal bleeding should not be attributed to anal fissures without searching for other etiologies.

Infectious agents should always be considered as a cause for lower GI bleeding in infancy. Patients usually have fever and diarrhea as predominant symptoms, and there may be a history of infectious contact. Stools should be tested for the presence of polymorphonuclear leukocytes, a finding that suggests an active colitis. Stools from these patients should be screened for such invasive enteric pathogens as *Salmonella, Shigella, Yersinia enterocolitica, Campylobacter*, and the toxin-producing *Clostridium difficile*. Other causes of colitis such as allergic gastroenteritis, inflammatory bowel disease, Henoch-Schönlein purpura, and hemolytic uremic syndrome should also be considered.

Infants with intussusception usually present between the ages of 3 months and 3 years of age (see Chapter 19). Rectal bleeding, which is typically a red currant jelly stool, reflects impending bowel ischemia and infarction.[3] As soon as the diagnosis is suspected and the infant is stabilized, a barium enema should be obtained for both diagnostic and therapeutic purposes.

Lower GI hemorrhage resulting from intestinal polyps usually occurs in children older than 1 year and is often episodic and usually painless (see Chapter 22).[4] Other signs such as the hyperpigmented lesions of the lips as seen in patients with Peutz-Jaeger disease may be found on physical examination.[5] The majority of polyps are located in the descending colon, so a flexible sigmoidoscopy is usually the initial diagnostic procedure.

Additional causes of lower GI bleeding that should be considered include intestinal duplication, hemangioma, arteriovenous malformation, and foreign bodies.

Meckel's Diverticulum

Meckel's diverticulum represents the most common developmental malformation of the GI tract and is found in approximately 2% of the population.[6] The diverticulum develops as a vestigial remnant of the omphalomesenteric duct and is located about 60 to 90 cm from the ileocecal valve on the antimesenteric side. About 50% of Meckel's diverticula contain ectopic gastric mucosa.

Meckel's diverticulum is a common cause of GI bleeding in otherwise healthy infants. In a retrospective study of 148 pediatric patients with Meckel's diverticulum, more than 50% presented with rectal bleeding, and 40% had a previous history of hematochezia.[7] Of the remaining patients in this study, the majority had symptoms of abdominal pain and vomiting. Intestinal obstruction, resulting from volvulus around a vitello-umbilical cord, and intussusception with the diverticulum serving as a lead

RECTAL BLEEDING IN INFANCY

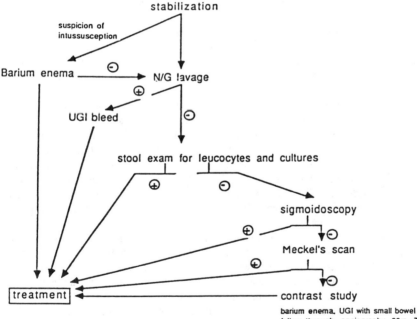

FIG 21–1.
Sequence of evaluating rectal bleeding in infancy.

point were among the operative findings in these patients. Meckel's diverticulum can also present with symptoms mimicking those of appendicitis, although this is usually seen in the older patient.

Pertechnetate scintigraphy is currently the best nonoperative method for definitive diagnosis.[8] Pertechnetate is actively taken up by gastric mucosal cells. Tagging this substance with a radioactive marker permits detection of gastric cells by nuclear scanning. Abdominal scintigraphy does not detect the diverticulum directly; rather, it will reveal the uptake of radiopertechnetate by the functioning ectopic gastric mucosa within the diverticulum. The test is easy to perform and is quite accurate. After injection of technetium 99m as sodium pertechnetate in a dose of 100 μCi/kg, the patient is kept supine, and serial images of the abdomen are taken with a gamma camera.[8] Normally, there is a gradual increase of tracer taken up in the wall of the stomach. The intestinal lumen then shows enhanced activity as the tracer is secreted into the gastric cavity and transits the GI tract. In addition, the kidneys, ureters, and bladder light up as the tracer is excreted in the urine. In patients with Meckel's diverticulum, tracer activity is detected in the distal small bowel early in the study, at a time when the gastric mucosa of the stomach wall is showing enhanced activity.

The first successful use of ^{99m}Tc pertechnetate scanning for ectopic gastric mucosa was reported in 1970.[9] Sfakianakis and Conway reviewed 10 years of clinical experience with pertechnetate scanning for the diagnosis of Meckel's diverticulum.[10] Of the surgically proved cases, they estimated that the scan has a sensitivity of 85% and a specificity of 95%, with an accuracy of 90%. The use of pentagastrin (6 μg/kg subcutaneously) to enhance the uptake of tracer into the gastric mucosa cells or the addition of cimetidine (40 mg/kg/day for 48 hours prior to the study) to concentrate the tracer within the cells has been shown to improve sensitivity in some studies.[11] Reasons for false negative scans include insufficient ectopic gastric mucosa, impaired vascular supply to the ectopic tissue, or improper technique. The presence of residual barium in the intestinal tract may obscure detection of tracer material, leading to a false negative result.[12]

Additional radiologic investigations used to locate an intestinal bleeding site include the tagged red blood cell scan and arteriography. These studies are usually reserved for the rare pediatric patient who is acutely bleeding and the site of hemorrhage cannot be determined by endoscopy or other conventional means, including intestinal contrast studies. Most often in pediatrics, arteriography is used to diagnose and define intestinal vascular malformations.

This patient presented with signs and symptoms suggestive of intussusception, and a barium enema was the initial study. Once this diagnosis was ruled out, a sigmoidoscopy was performed. This study helped to establish that the site of bleeding was more proximal than 8 in. (20 cm) and that there were no polyps or obvious colitis. A Meckel's scan with pentagastrin stimulation was the next step. The results of the study were inconclusive, and the radiologists could not agree as to whether increased uptake of tracer was present. Because the bleeding was severe, results of the other investigations were normal, and the scan suggested the possibility of an intestinal lesion, the infant was taken for exploratory laparotomy.

At operation, a Meckel's diverticulum was found and excised. Histologically, there was an abundance of ectopic gastric mucosa and part of the wall of the diverticulum was severely ulcerated. This severe ulceration and attendant poor vascular supply were thought to be possible reasons for the equivocal Meckel's scan result.

SUMMARY

Rectal bleeding in infancy may be life threatening, and the differential diagnosis is quite extensive. A systematic approach to these patients and expectant management is essential for a successful outcome (see Figure 21–1). Meckel's diverticulum is a common cause of rectal bleeding in the infant population. Typically, these patients present without any symptoms other than the intestinal bleed. The best nonoperative test for the diagnosis of this condition is abdominal scintigraphy using ^{99m}Tc pertechnetate. The treatment is surgical, and the prognosis is excellent.

REFERENCES

1. Oldham KT, Lobe TE: Gastrointestinal hemorrhage in children: A pragmatic update. *Pediatr Clin North Am* 1985; 32:1247–1263.
2. Hillmeier C: Rectal bleeding in childhood. *Pediatr Rev* 1983; 5:35–41.
3. Newman J, Schuh S: Intussusception in babies under 4 months of age. *Can Med Assoc J* 1987; 136:266–269.
4. Mestre JR: The changing pattern of juvenile polyps. *Am J Gastroenterol* 1986; 81:312–314.
5. Haggitt RC, Reid BJ: Hereditary gastrointestinal polyposis syndromes. *Am J Surg Pathol* 1986; 10:871–887.
6. Berquiot TH, Nolan NG, Adson MA, et al: Diagnosis of Meckel's diverticulum by radioisotope scanning. *Mayo Clin Proc* 1973; 48:98–102.
7. Rutherford R, Akers DR: Meckel's diverticulum: A review of 148 patients with special reference to the pattern of bleeding and mesodiverticular vascular bands. *Surgery* 1966; 59:618–626.
8. Treves ST, Grand R: Meckel's diverticulum, in *Pediatric Nuclear Medicine*. New York, Springer-Verlag, New York 1985, pp 179–187.
9. Jewett TC Jr, Duszynski DO, Allen JE: The visualization of Meckel's diverticulum with Tc-99m-pertechnetate. *Surgery* 1970; 68:567–570.
10. Sfakianakis GN, Conway JJ: Detection of ectopic gastric mucosa in Meckel's diverticulum and in other aberrations by scintigraphy: II. Indications and methods. A 10 year experience. *J Nucl Med* 1981; 22:732–738.
11. Yeker D, Buyukunal C, Benli M, et al: Radionuclide imaging of Meckel's diverticulum: Cimetidine versus pentagastrin plus glucagon. *Eur J Nucl Med* 1984; 9:316–319.
12. Meguid MM, Wilkinson RH, Canty T, et al: Futility of barium sulfate in diagnosis of bleeding Meckel's diverticulum. *Arch Surg* 1974; 108:361–362.

22 Intestinal Polyps

Mounif El-Youssef, M.D.
John D. Snyder, M.D.

A boy 4-years and 7 months old presented with the chief complaint of hematochezia. Approximately 5 months earlier, he complained of seeing a few dark red blood "spots" in his stool without mucus or melena. These spots were not associated with constipation, diarrhea, abdominal pain, pruritus ani, cramps, vomiting, trauma, medication use, or foreign body ingestion. He was then well until 1 week prior to presentation, when 5 ml of blood was seen with his stool without accompanying pain or diarrhea. The past medical history was noncontributory, and the family history was negative for blood dyscrasias or gastrointestinal (GI) disease.

On physical examination his height, weight, and head circumference were at the 50th percentile. The skin was normal without petechiae, purpura, rash, jaundice, or pallor. Results of head, ear, eye, nose, and throat; pulmonary; and cardiac examinations were normal. The abdomen was soft, nontender, and without masses. His rectal examination revealed no tags, fissures, or masses; the stool was soft, brown, and Hematest positive. The remainder of his examination was unremarkable.

The patient underwent a flexible sigmoidoscopy, which revealed a pedunculated 1 × 2-cm polyp at a distance of 14 cm from the anal verge. The polyp was removed by loop electrocautery and was found on histologic examination to be of the benign inflammatory type (Fig 22–1).

DISCUSSION

Intestinal polyps are tumors that protrude into the lumen of the bowel and are one of the commonest causes of bleeding in children.[1] The great majority (>90%) of the polyps that occur in children are benign inflammatory or juvenile polyps. The remainder are distributed among the polyposis syndromes (Table 22–1). This chapter will focus on juvenile polyps, followed by a brief review of the polyposis syndromes.

Juvenile polyps have been reported in all age groups but occur most commonly in children 2 to 6 years old.[1] They are rarely seen in children less than 1 year old[2] and are slightly more common in boys than girls.[1, 3] The incidence is not known, but juvenile polyps may occur in as many as 1% of all children.[4]

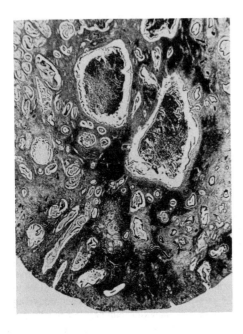

FIG 22–1.
Colonic juvenile polyp consisting of inflamed stroma containing numerous irregular glands, some of which are cystically dilated (×10).

Pathophysiology

The origin of juvenile polyps remains unknown, but they are believed to be most likely of either hamartomatous or inflammatory etiology.[5, 6] Juvenile polyps can be considered hamartomas (tumors that arise as malformations of normal tissue) because they contain no dysplastic or malignant components.[5] Juvenile polyps have a smooth surface overlying grossly dilated, mucus-filled spaces with a rich vascular supply. Histologically, the polyps are composed of irregularly branching mucus-filled glands set in an inflamed stroma and have also been called retention polyps because of these features (see Fig 22–1). The stalk is covered by normal colonic mucosa.

Support for an inflammatory origin of juvenile polyps comes from the identical histologic features of juvenile polyps and polyps formed from granulation tissue at the anastamotic line of previous surgery.[6] In both situations, granulation tissue is covered by regenerating epithelium from surrounding mucosa and forms the irregular, elongated cystic glands that are characteristic of juvenile polyps.[6]

The classic teaching is that juvenile polyps are always benign and have no risk of adenomatous or carcinomatous change.[4] Recent reports have questioned this teaching, especially since more than just solitary polyps are being found in children.[7–9] With an increased number of polyps, an increased risk of adenomatous change may be present.

In contrast to solitary or a limited number of juvenile polyps, all of the other categories of polyps (see Table 22–1) have the potential for either adenomatous or malignant changes.[10, 11] Even the syndromes of multiple juvenile polyps have been shown to have adenomatous potential.[12]

Clinical Features

The typical child with a juvenile polyp is a preschooler who develops painless, bright red rectal bleeding.[1] The bleeding is usually intermittent, of small amount, and often found streaked on the outside of the stool. Crampy abdominal pain is reported in about 15% of cases[1] and has been attributed to traction on the polyp during peristaltic activity. Prolapse of the polyp past the anus is seen in about 10% of cases. Rarely, diarrhea and tenesmus can also occur, and polyps can infrequently predispose to colonic intussusception or obstruction.[1] A detailed family history must be obtained because of the more serious nature of the polyposis syndromes.

A careful physical examination must be done to determine whether any signs of the polyposis syndromes are present. Pigmentation of the lips or buccal mucosa is an important clue for the Peutz-Jeghers syndrome.[10, 11] Soft tissue and bone tumors as well as dental anomalies are seen in Gardener's syndrome.[10] Alopecia, atrophic

TABLE 22–1.
Polyposis Syndromes*

	Location	Extraintestinal Lesions	Risk of Cancer
Familial			
Adenomatous			
Familial polyposis coli	Throughout but primarily colon	No	Marked
Gardener's syndrome	Throughout but primarily colon	Bone and soft tissue tumors, desmoid tumors after surgery	Marked
Turcot syndrome	Colon	Brain tumors	In brain
Hamartomatous			
Peutz-Jeghers syndrome	Throughout but especially small bowel	Melanin spots of lips, buccal mucosa, and digits	2%–3% risk of GI cancer
Juvenile polyposis	Throughout but especially colon	20% incidence of congenital abnormalities	Slight increase
Cowden syndrome	Throughout	Hamartomas of skin and mucous membranes, ganglioneuromas, lipomas, congenital abnormalities	No increased risk of GI cancer
Intestinal ganglio neuromatosis	Throughout	von Recklinghausen disease, multiple endocrine neoplasias	Low
Nonfamilial			
Cronkhite-Canada syndrome	Throughout	Alopecia, hyperpigmentation, onychatropia	Low

*Adapted from Erbe[10] and Haggitt and Reid.[11]

nails, and brown macular lesions of the skin are associated with the Cronkhite-Canada syndrome, whereas brain tumors can be seen with Turcot syndrome.[11]

There are no physical findings indicative of juvenile polyps, although palor may be seen if the bleeding has been heavy. The rectal examination is of critical importance since as many as 30% of juvenile polyps are located within 10 cm of the anal margin.[7, 13]

Diagnosis

The differential diagnosis of lower GI bleeding in children is included in Table 21–1, and a practical scheme to evaluate rectal bleeding is also found there. Infectious causes should always be considered; the stool should be examined for red and white blood cells, and cultures for enteric pathogens should be obtained. If these are negative, a flexible sigmoidoscopy is the next study undertaken. The flexible sigmoidoscopy is likely to identify the majority of juvenile polyps and evaluates enough bowel to indicate whether a polyposis syndrome is present.

The evidence that multiple polyps are often present and that they can be found in locations throughout the bowel argues for the use of colonoscopic examination.[8] However, if bright red blood per rectum is the presenting complaint, the likelihood of finding the offending polyp in the distal colon is great. Also, if the child has no evidence for a polyposis syndrome, the presence of asymptomatic juvenile polyps in the more proximal bowel is of little importance. If no lesion is found on flexible sigmoidoscopy or the bleeding recurs, a colonoscopy should be performed.[8, 13]

Barium contrast studies have also been used to diagnose polyps, but direct visualization with the endoscope is the procedure of choice.[13] Air contrast barium enemas are more helpful than conventional enema studies.

Treatment

Polyps seen on flexible sigmoidoscopy or colonoscopy should be excised for biopsy because of their tendency to bleed and cause mechanical obstruction.[7, 8] The polypectomy is routinely done with an electrocautery snare, which has proved to be a safe procedure in the hands of a skilled endoscopist.[13]

If a single juvenile polyp is found, no follow-up study is recommended because the risk of recurrence is low.[7] However, if multiple juvenile or adenomatous polyps are found, routine surveillance is indicated.

Polyposis Syndromes

The polyposis syndromes are generally classified into familial and nonfamilial categories (see Table 22–1).[10, 11] All of the familial polyposis syndromes are autosomal dominant diseases except the Turcot syndrome, which may be autosomal recessive.[10] They are usually subdivided into adenomatous and hamartomatous types.[11]

The prototype of the adenomatous familial polyposis syndromes is familial polyposis coli. Patients with this condition have at least 100 and often more than

1,000 small adenomas (<1 cm) confined primarily to the colon.[10, 11] These adenomas typically develop after puberty and are often associated with hematochezia and diarrhea. If they are left untreated, the observed rate of neoplasm is 80%.[10] Adenomas may also be found in other parts of the intestinal tract, but the rate of carcinoma in the small bowel appears to be low.[11]

Gardener's syndrome, which is characterized by the triad of intestinal polyps and soft tissue and bone abnormalities, is similar to familial polyposis coli in terms of the number of polyps, their distribution, and the mean age of onset.[10] Desmoid tumors (fibromas), which occur after trauma, are characteristic of the syndrome.[11] Osteomas of the mandible are seen in about one fourth of the patients.[11]

Turcot syndrome is distinguished from the two other forms of adenomatous familial polyposis in its probable autosomal recessive inheritance and its association with brain tumors.[10, 11] Fewer than 100 polyps have been reported in some of the affected patients.

There are four primary hamartomatous familial polyposis syndromes. Peutz-Jegher syndrome is associated with melanin spots on the lips and buccal mucosa, and the polyps can be found throughout the intestinal tract. Endocrine cells are present in the polyps of all sites.[10] Bowel carcinoma occurs in Peutz-Jegher syndrome but appears to be an infrequent complication.[11] Female patients have an increased risk of developing breast cancer.[11]

The polyps in familial juvenile polyposis have the characteristic appearance of juvenile polyps. Adenomas, high-grade dysplasia, and carcinoma have been reported in these patients.[12]

Gastrointestinal polyps, which are distinct from those of the other polyposis syndromes, are found in about one third of patients with Cowden's syndrome. The primary lesions are multiple hamartomas that affect the skin and mucous membranes.[11] There appears to be no increased risk of GI cancer, but cancer of the breast and thyroid have been reported.[11]

Intestinal ganglioneuromatosis, usually in the form of Von Recklinghausen's syndrome, may also involve the intestine. The risk of associated cancer is low.

The Cronkhite-Canada syndrome is the principal example nonfamilial polyposis. Patients typically have diffuse intestinal polyposis, alopecia, hyperpigmentation, and clubbing of the fingers and toes.[14] Presenting complaints include diarrhea and protein-losing enteropathy. The risk of cancer appears to be lower than for most of the familial polyposis syndromes.

SUMMARY

Juvenile polyps are by far the most common type of intestinal tumor in children and are a common cause of bleeding. The typical presentation is of painless, bright red rectal bleeding. Diagnosis and treatment is usually accomplished by flexible sigmoidoscopy and electrocautery snare removal. Individual or small numbers of juvenile polyps are benign and rarely recur. However, if one of the polyposis syndromes is identified, the risk of cancer rises, and close surveillance is mandatory.

142   *The Gastrointestinal Tract*

REFERENCES

1. Toccalino H, Gaustavind E, DePinni F, et al: Juvenile polyps of the colon and rectum. *Acta Paediatr Scand* 1973; 62:337–340.
2. Phillips DM: Case report: Juvenile polyp in a 10-month old infant. *Postgrad Med* 1978; 64:188–189.
3. Dajain YE, Kamal MF: Colorectal juvenile polyps, an epidemiological and histopathological study of 144 cases in Jordanians. *Histopathology* 1984; 8:765–779.
4. Anderson CM, Burke V: *Paediatric Gastroenterology.* Boston, Blackwell Scientific Publications, 1975; p 482.
5. Morson BC: Some peculiarities in the histology of intestinal polyps. *Dis Colon Rectum* 1962; 5:337–344.
6. Franzin G, Zamboni G, Dina R, et al: Juvenile and inflammatory polyps of the colon — a histological and histochemical study. *Histopathology* 1983; 7:719–728.
7. Mazier WP, MacKeigen JM, Billingham RP, et al: Juvenile polyps of the colon and rectum. *Surg Gynecol Obstet* 1982; 154: 829–832.
8. Mestre J: The changing pattern of juvenile polyps. *Am J Gastroenterol* 1986; 81:312–314.
9. Gryboski J: All juvenile polyps are not benign. *Am J Gastroenterol* 1986; 81:397.
10. Erbe WR: Inherited gastrointestinal polyposis syndromes. *N Engl J Med* 1976; 294:1101–1104.
11. Haggitt RC, Reid BJ: Hereditary gastrointestinal polyposis syndromes. *Am J Surg Pathol* 1986; 10:871–887.
12. Mills SE, Fechner RE: Unusual adenomatous polyps in juvenile polyposis coli. *Am J Surg Pathol* 1982; 6:177–183.
13. Euler AR, Seibert JJ: The role of sigmoidoscopy, radiography, and colonoscopy in the diagnosis and evaluation of pediatric patients with suspected juvenile polyps. *J Pediatr Surg* 1981; 16:500–504.
14. Scharf GM, Becker JHR, Laage NJ: Juvenile gastrointestinal polyposis or the infantile Cronkhite-Canada syndrome. *J Pediatr Surg* 1986; 21:953–954.

23   Pseudomembranous Colitis

Samuel Nurko, M.D.

A 17-year-old boy had a history of myelomeningocele and attendant bladder dysfunction that eventually led to chronic renal failure. He received a cadaveric renal transplant and underwent splenectomy when he was 10 years old, and due to rejection, he required a new renal transplant 5 years later. At age 15 years he developed rejection of his second transplant and since then has required multiple hospitalizations and, eventually, hemodialysis. His medications have included prednisone, azathioprine (Imuran), cyclosporine, hydralazine, propranolol, and prophylactic penicillin. When he was 15.5 years old, he developed a right otitis media, for which he was given 250 mg of amoxicillin every 8 hours. Three days later he developed left lower quadrant tenderness, anorexia, and profuse, watery diarrhea. He lost 7.1 lb (3.2 kg) and eventually developed a low-grade fever. When seen in the emergency room, he was lethargic, had a temperature of 38°C, and was 10% dehydrated. His abdomen was diffusely tender to palpation, but no rebound tenderness was present. His rectal examination revealed guaiac-positive stools. He was hospitalized for treatment. His initial laboratory results included hemoglobin value 15.7 gm/dl; white blood cell count 25,400/mm³; with 79 polymorphonuclear leukocytes, 15 bands, 1 lymphocyte, and 5 monocytes; BUN level 97 mg/dl, and creatinine level 4.6 mg/dl. The abdominal radiograph was normal. Stool cultures were negative, but an assay for *Clostridium difficile* toxin was positive at 1:1,000. He was treated with vancomycin for 2 weeks, and his amoxicillin was switched to trimetoprim-sulfamethoxazole. His diarrhea improved remarkably after 24 hours of vancomycin treatment, and he was completely asymptomatic at discharge.

Seven days after completing his antibiotic course, he became febrile to 39°C and again developed profuse watery diarrhea, which became grossly bloody. He was rehospitalized, and results of his physical examination were similar to those during previous admission, although his stool was now grossly bloody. A sigmoidoscopy was performed and revealed rectal mucosa that was red, edematous, and friable and had multiple raised yellow-white plaques (about 3 mm in diameter). The rectal biopsy specimens revealed a pseudomembrane consisting of polymorphonuclear leukocytes, fibrin, and necrotic cells (Figure 23–1). His stool cultures for bacterial pathogens were negative, but his *C. difficile* toxin was positive at 1:10,000, and he was again started on vancomycin therapy. He responded rapidly to the vancomycin and was sent home on a tapering dose. He has remained symptom free for the last 3 months. His prophylactic penicillin therapy has also been stopped.

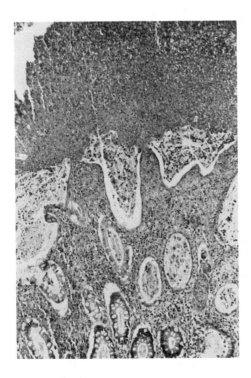

FIG 23–1.
Rectal biopsy showing a
pseudomembrane of
polymorphonuclear leukocytes,
fibrin, and necrotic cells *(arrow)*
(×150).

DISCUSSION

Antibiotic-associated diarrhea is now a well-described common side effect of the use of antibiotics.[1, 2] The diarrhea is usually self-limited and often stops after the antibiotic is discontinued.[1] Rarely this diarrhea can become worse than the initial disease for which the antibiotic was prescribed and can progress to dehydration, shock, and occasionally death.[1-3] This severe form of antibiotic-associated diarrhea is called pseudomembranous colitis (PMC), and the case of the patient described demonstrates many of the typical features.

Pathophysiology

Pseudomembranous colitis is caused by a toxin produced by *C. difficile*, a gram-positive obligate anaerobe, which was first isolated from the stools of newborn infants in 1935.[2] It was little more than a laboratory curiosity until the late 1970s, when it was first linked to the production of antibiotic-associated PMC in humans.[3] The pathogenic mechanism of *C. difficile*–associated colitis remains poorly understood, although it is now believed that a cytotoxin produced by the organism is responsible for the disease.[4] The *C. difficile* organism can be isolated in up to 2% of healthy adults and up to 50% of normal newborns.[5] The *C. difficile* toxin has been reported in up to 10% of normal infants and up to 55% of neonates in an intensive care unit.[6] Patients appear to become susceptible to colonization by this clostridial species as a consequence of antibiotic-induced suppression of the normal bacterial flora of the intestine.[3] Non-toxin-producing *C. difficile* has been isolated in more than 95% of these patients.[5, 7] In a study of 208 pediatric patients with diarrhea, the toxin was found in 8.6%.[8] It was identified more in younger patients (<11 months) and in those with hospital-associated illness and antibiotic-associated illness. The presence of *C. difficile* is not always associated with the full-blown picture of PMC, but PMC patients always have the toxin present in their stool.[9]

Pseudomembranous colitis has been associated with almost all antibiotics but is especially common with clindamycin, ampicillin, and the cephalosporins.[10, 11] In children, ampicillin is the most commonly implicated antibiotic.[1, 2] Not all cases of PMC are related to antibiotic therapy, as evidenced by the fact that PMC existed before the antibiotic era. Several other chemotherapeutic agents, including amphotericin B and methotrexate, have also been implicated.[1] Other predisposing risk factors include postoperative states, ischemic bowel, uremia, and intestinal obstruction.[3] These other causes should be carefully considered, especially in cases where relapses occur.

Clinical Features

The usual presentation of antibiotic-associated PMC in children is the acute onset of profuse, watery diarrhea, often associated with blood, which begins during the first 5 to 10 days of antibiotic therapy but may occur as early as the first or second day.[2, 3] About 25% of the patients develop the diarrhea from 2 to 10 weeks after the completion of the antimicrobial course.[3] Crampy hypogastric pain usually precedes or coincides with the onset of the diarrhea, and abdominal distention, nausea, and vomiting are frequent findings.[1–3] The patients usually have a low-grade fever but may have temperatures as high as 39.5°C.[3] Leukocytosis is frequent, and up to 20% of the patients have a picture suggestive of an acute abdomen. In uncomplicated cases the diarrhea and other symptoms resolve shortly after the antibiotic is stopped. However, the diarrhea may be severe enough to cause dehydration as well as the loss of a significant amount of serum protein, especially in young children and infants.[1, 2] Hypoalbuminemia with ascites, pleural effusion, and peripheral edema has been reported.[4]

Diagnosis

The diagnosis of PMC should be based on the demonstration of the *C. difficile* toxin and on the sigmoidoscopic findings of red, edematous, friable, colonic mucosa with multiple raised yellow-white pseudomembranous plaques, which usually measure between 2 to 5 mm.[2, 3, 12] Histologically, the biopsy shows a pseudomembrane consisting of polymorphonuclear leukocytes, fibrin, and necrotic cells (see Fig 23–1). The underlying mucosa is usually friable, but true ulcerations or abscesses are not found.[13] Plain films of the abdomen are nonspecific and can show air fluid levels and thumb printing.[4] If a barium enema is performed, the bowel appears edematous with mucosal ulcerations and scalloping.

Therapy

After the diagnosis has been established, the offending antibiotic should be discontinued and supportive care in the form of fluid and electrolyte replacement should be instituted (Table 23–1).[1–3] Antidiarrheal agents should be avoided. Appropriate methods of infection control should be instituted for hospitalized patients because *C. difficile* is a transferable enteric pathogen, and multiple outbreaks of PMC have been described within hospitals.[14]

The next decision to make is whether any specific therapy is required. Recent studies have demonstrated that most patients with *C. difficile* – induced enteric disease improve spontaneously as soon as the offending antibiotic is stopped.[3, 15] If the patient is severely ill or does not improve after discontinuation of the offending antimicrobial, a number of specific therapeutic modalities have been suggested based on current concepts regarding the pathophysiology.[15] The therapies may be divided into the following categories: (1) antimicrobial agents directed against *C. difficile*, (2) anion exchange resins that bind *C. difficile* toxin, and (3) replacement of fecal flora.

Three antimicrobial agents have been successfully used for the treatment of PMC: vancomycin, metronidazole, and bacitracin.[15, 16] Vancomycin has been most widely used because *C. difficile* is exquisitely sensitive to it, and randomized drug trials have shown vancomycin to be significantly more effective than placebo.[15, 16] When given orally, it is poorly absorbed, achieving very high fecal concentrations.[16] The recommended dose varies from 125 to 500 mg/daily in adults, and 500 mg/ 1.73 m^2 in children divided every 6 hours.[15] Because vancomycin is not absorbed, it can safely be used in patients with impaired renal function.[16] The usual clinical response is rapid, with improvement of the diarrhea, fever, and cramps by 3 or 4 days.[15] Side effects are rare, but relapses are reported in 15% to 25% of patients.[15] The major drawback to vancomycin is its great expense; a 10-day course costs about $500.

TABLE 23–1.
Therapy for Pseudomembranous Colitis

I. Discontinuation of previous antibiotic
II. Initial therapy
A. Severe disease
Vancomycin
B. Milder disease
Metronidazole
III. Treatment of relapse
A. First relapse:
Course of vancomycin
B. Second relapse:
Vancomycin and cholestyramine
Slow taper of vancomycin over 2 mo.

The other two antimicrobials, metronidazole and bacitracin, appear to be almost as effective as vancomycin. In one controlled study, metronidazole (250 mg every 6 hours for 10 days) was as effective as vancomycin (500 mg every 6 hours for 10 days) in the treatment of 101 patients with *C. difficile*–associated colitis in regard to cure rates, duration of diarrhea, or frequency of relapse.[17] The cost of a course of metronidazole was much lower ($12 vs. $520), and treatment was well tolerated by both groups. Metronidazole, however, has some potentially serious side effects, including convulsions, peripheral neuropathy, and neutropenia.[17] It also has the theoretical disadvantage of good absorption when given orally, potentially leading to suboptimal concentrations in the colon, and has been associated with the production of PMC.[15, 17] Metronidazole is also mutagenic, and when it is administered to animals, an increased incidence of mammary, lung, and lymphoreticular tumors has been reported.[17] However, in humans no evidence for cancer associated with metronidazole therapy has been uncovered.

Bacitracin offers the same theoretical advantage as vancomycin. The drug is absorbed poorly, and virtually all strains of *C. difficile* are sensitive to it. A recent randomized study comparing bacitracin with vancomycin in patients with PMC showed no difference in the response or relapse rates.[18] A potential problem has been that at the suggested dose of 20,000 units, the levels of bacitracin achieved in the stool are only 5 to 10 times the minimum inhibitory concentration for *C. difficile* compared with a 1,000 to 4,000 ratio for vancomycin at the low dose.[14]

The potential role of cholestyramine and other binding resins was originally reported even before the role of *C. difficile* in this disease was known.[17] The recent clinical experience has given conflicting results. Kreutzer and Milligan reported excellent results with cholestyramine in 12 patients[17]; however, Tadesco et al. found multiple treatment failures.[19] The complimentary modes of action of vancomycin and cholestyramine suggest that the combination of the two might prove superior. However, the resins can bind to the antibiotic, potentially decreasing the overall reponse.[14]

Finally, the normalization of the fecal flora with the use of fecal enemas has been tried with some success.[20] The major disadvantages of this approach are the possibility of transmitting an enteric pathogen and the lack of esthetic appeal.

As in this patient, relapses after successful treatment are common. Independent of the initial therapy, approximately 15% to 25% of the patients have a relapse, which can occur between 4 and 21 days after initial successful treatment.[20, 21] Usually there are no differences in the clinical risk factors for relapse, including initial dose, duration of therapy, or posttherapy toxin titer.[13, 21, 22] Unfortunately, *C. difficile* stool cultures or toxin assays do not consistently correlate with clinical recovery or likelihood of relapse and should not be used routinely to determine response to treatment.[13] Some individuals may have multiple relapses independent of the treatment used.[13] The presumed reason for the failure to eradicate the *C. difficile* in the presence of extremely high antibiotic levels is sporulation and the continued production of toxin. Another consideration is that an abnormal environment (diverticulosis, ischemia, etc.) may have a protective effect on the organism.[3]

Several approaches have been tried to reduce the chance for relapse. Bartlett et al. have advocated a 2-week course of vancomycin followed by cholestyramine, but subsequent relapses were demonstrated.[21] A first relapse is usually treated with a second course of antimicrobial therapy, often vancomycin.[23] If a subsequent relapse occurs, a combination of vancomycin and a binding resin is often employed. A long, slow tapering of vancomycin over 8 weeks has also been advocated.[24]

At this point vancomycin remains a highly attractive drug on the basis of bio-availability data, *in vitro* activity, and clinical experience. Most authorities continue to recommend vancomycin as the preferred drug for the seriously ill patient.[13, 17] For those who are less ill but still merit treatment, metronidazole is generally preferred as the best alternative on the basis of cost and efficacy.

SUMMARY

This patient's case is a reminder that PMC must be considered in the patient who develops diarrhea while on antibiotic therapy. Relapses after therapy is completed are not uncommon and often require prolonged therapy.

REFERENCES

1. Prince AS, Neu HC: Antibiotic associated pseudomembranous colitis in children. *Pediatr Clin North Am* 1979; 26:261–268.
2. Viscidi RP, Bartlett JG: Antibiotic associated pseudomembranous colitis in children. *Pediatrics* 1981; 67:381–386.
3. Tedesco FJ: Pseudomembranous colitis: Pathogenesis and therapy. *Med Clin North Am* 1982; 66:655–664.
4. Buts JP, Weber AM, Roy CC: Pseudomembranous enterocolitis in childhod. *Gastroenterology* 1977; 73:823–827.
5. Stark PL, Lee A: Clostridia isolated from the feces of infants during the first year of life. *J Pediatr* 1982; 100:362–365.
6. Donta ST, Meyers MG: *Clostridium difficile* toxin asymptomatic neonates. *J Pediatr* 1982; 100:431–434.
7. Viscidi R, Willeyv S, Bartlett JG: Isolation rates and toxigenic potential of *C. difficile* isolates from various patient populations. *Gastroenterology* 1981; 81:5–9.
8. Thompson CM, Gilligan PH, Fisher MC, et al: *Clostidium difficile* cytotoxin in a pediatric population. *Am J Dis Child* 1983; 137:271–274.
9. Lishman AH, Al-Jumaill IJ, Record GO: Spectrum of antibiotic associated diarrhea. *Gut* 1981; 22:34–37.
10. Silva J, Fecklety R, Werk C, et al: Inciting and etiologic agents of colitis. *Rev Infect Dis* 1984; S214–S221.
11. Gurwith MJ, Rabin HR, Love K: Diarrhea associated with clindamycin and ampicillin therapy: Preliminary results of a cooperative study. *J Infect Dis* 1977; 135(suppl): S104–110.
12. Randolph MF, Morris KE: Clindamycin-associated colitis in children: A prospective study and a negative report. *Clin Pediatr* 1977; 16:722–725.
13. Sumner HW, Tedesco FJ: Rectal biopsy in clindamycin associated colitis: An analysis of 23 cases. *Arch Pathol* 1975; 99:237–241.
14. Bartlett JG: Treatment of *Clostridium difficile* colitis [editorial]. *Gastroenterology* 1985; 89:1192–1195.

15. Bartlett JG: Treatment of antibiotic associated pseudomembranous colitis. *Rev Infect Dis* 1984; 16:S235–S241.
16. Teasley DG, Gerding DN, Olson MM, et al: Prospective randomized trial of metronidazole versus vancomycin for *Clostridium difficile*–associated diarrhea and colitis. *Lancet* 1983; 2:1043–1046.
17. Kreutzer EW, Milligan FD: Treatment of antibiotic-associated pseudomembranous colitis with cholestyramine resin. *Johns Hopkins Med J* 1978; 143:67–72.
18. Young GP, Ward PB, Bayley N, et al: Antibiotic associated colitis due to *Clostridium difficile*: Double-blind comparison of vancomycin with bacitracin. *Gastroenterology* 1985; 89:1038–1045.
19. Tedesco FJ, Napier J, Gamble W, et al: Cholestyramine therapy of antibiotic-associated pseudomembranous colitis. *Ann Gastroenterol* 1979; 1:51–54.
20. Bowden TA, Mansberger AR, Lykins LE: Pseudomembranous enterocolitis: Mechanism of restoring floral homeostasis. *Am Surg* 1981; 47:178–183.
21. Bartlett JG, Tedesco FJ, Shun S, et al: Symptomatic relapse after oral vancomycin therapy of antibiotic-associated pseudomembranous colitis. *Gastroenterology* 1980; 78:431–434.
22. Dink HT, Keinbaum S, Frottie, J: Treatment of antibiotic-induced colitis by metronidazole. *Lancet* 1979; 1:338–339.
23. Tedesco FJ: Treatment of recurrent antibiotic-associated pseudomembranous colitis. *Am J Gastroenterol* 1982; 77:110–111.
24. Tedesco FJ, Gordon D, Fortson WC: Approach to patients with multiple relapses of antibiotic-associated pseudomembranous colitis. *Am J Gastroenterol* 1985; 80:867–868.

24   Necrotizing Enterocolitis

Tracie L. Miller, M.D.
W. Allan Walker, M.D.

The patient was the 2.5-lb (1.15-kg) male product of a 31-week gestation com-plicated by intrauterine growth retardation. He was admitted to the neonatal intensive care unit because of prematurity. The delivery was induced because of fetal distress, but the child was vigorous at birth and had normal Apgar scores. He did well initially, never requiring ventilatory support or umbilical artery catheterization. He was fed sterile water on the second day of life and was advanced to full feedings of breast milk and supplemental infant formula by the fourth day. On day 7, the infant developed apnea, bradycardia, and metabolic acidosis (pH 7.25), passed guaiac-positive stools, and had large gastric residuals. The abdomen was firm, distended, and tender. There was no temperature instability, hypotension, thrombocytopenia, neutropenia, or coagulopathy. An abdominal radiograph revealed thickened, dilated loops of bowel, portal venous air, and pneumatosis intestinalis (intramural air) (Figure 24–1). Results of a full sepsis workup were normal. The diagnosis of necrotizing enterocolitis (NEC) was made on the basis of his clinical features and radiologic findings. All feedings were stopped, and he was started on ampicillin, gentamycin, and clindamycin therapy. The abdomen continued to be distended and tender. On day 12, free air was noted above the liver on a surveillance radiograph, without any other clinical changes. The child underwent exploratory laparotomy. Intraopera-tively, the distal 20 cm of ileum and cecum were noted to be necrotic with multiple walled-off perforations. The rest of the intestine was intact. An ileocecostomy was performed, and an ileostomy was created. Blood and peritoneal fluid cultures were positive for *Escherichia coli*. The child had an uneventful postoperative course and was discharged home 6 weeks after the resection; his bowel was reanastomosed at 1 year of age. He has done well since, except for mild symptoms of short bowel syndrome and slightly delayed growth.

DISCUSSION

Necrotizing enterocolitis is a gastrointestinal (GI) disease primarily of the premature infant, which is becoming more prevalent in the neonatal intensive care unit. Its broad clinical spectrum was described by Bell et al. as comprising three different

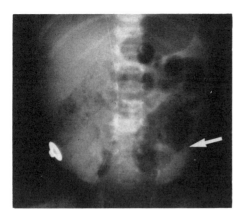

FIG 24–1.
Pneumatosis intestinalis. Abdominal radiograph showing intramural air *(arrow)*.

stages ranging from mild systemic and GI dysfunction to advanced symptoms of perforation and septic shock (Table 24–1).[1]

Epidemiology

The incidence of NEC, which was first described in the 19th century,[2] is increasing, most likely due to improved survival of premature infants. Necrotizing enterocolitis has been reported in 1% to 5% of the admissions to the neonatal intensive care unit[3] and may occur in up to 30% of infants who weigh less than 3.3 lb (1.5 kg).[4] These

TABLE 24–1.
Necrotizing Enterocolitis Staging System*

I. Stage I (suspect) A. Systemic symptoms—temperature instability, lethargy, apnea, and bradycardia B. Gastrointestinal symptoms—poor feeding, gastric residuals, emesis, mild abdominal distention, occult blood in stool C. Radiographic signs—distention with mild ileus
II. Stage II (definite) A. Stage I symptomatology plus persistent occult or gross GI bleeding and marked abdominal distention B. Radiographic signs—significant intestinal distention with ileus, bowel wall edema, persistently dilated bowel loops, pneumatosis intestinalis, and portal venous gas
III. Stage III (advanced) A. Stage I and II symptomatology plus unstable vital signs, shock or marked GI hemorrhage B. Radiographic signs—pneumoperitoneum plus other signs in stage II

*Adapted from Bell et al.[1]

statistics reflect that those at highest risk are the smaller, more premature infants. Maternal socioeconomic factors, sex, race, or seasonal variation do not affect the incidence of the illness.[2, 5]

The peak occurrence of NEC is in infants born between 32 to 34 weeks' gestation. Surprisingly, up to 10% of infants who develop NEC will be born full term.[3] These full-term infants usually have other medical problems, including cyanotic heart disease, polycythemia, enteritis, or birth asphyxia. Recently NEC has been reported in otherwise healthy full-term infants.[6]

Necrotizing enterocolitis usually occurs between day 3 and 10 of extrauterine life, but the diagnosis has been made from 1 to 90 days after birth.[3] It is thought to occur when the GI tract is least mature; therefore, full-term infants are at highest risk for only a brief postnatal period, and premature infants are susceptible at least until the postconceptual age of 35 to 36 weeks' gestation is reached.[7] Many potential risk factors for NEC, including fetal distress, low Apgar scores, premature rupture of membranes, hypotension, apnea, cyanosis, respiratory distress syndrome, umbilical artery catheterization, sepsis, polycythemia, hypertonic feedings, and exchange transfusions, have been studied. In large case control studies, none of these factors has been found more frequently in infants with NEC than in controls.[5] In fact, Kliegman et al. have failed to demonstrate any consistant risk factor other than prematurity.[8]

Pathophysiology

The pathogenesis of NEC is controversial. Three host factors have clearly been implicated in the development of NEC. These include (1) intestinal mucosal injury secondary to ischemia, (2) bacterial colonization, and (3) enteral feedings.[9]

Ischemic insult to the neonatal intestine may result from the dive reflex, which is a physiologic response by the vasculature to shunt blood from the splanchnic circulation such as the GI tract to more vital organs such as the brain and heart. This dive reflex is seen in infants with birth asphyxia, hypotension, umbilical artery catheters, polycythemia, patent ductus arteriosus, or any other circumstance that may predispose the infant to hypoxia. This ischemic insult may allow invasion of the intestinal wall by bacteria within the lumen.[10]

The link between NEC and an infectious etiology is weak because many cases of NEC are not associated with any organism, and infants may be colonized with potentially pathogenic organisms but do not develop the disease. Only 30% to 35% of patients with NEC have a positive blood culture.[1] Circumstantial evidence that NEC may be associated with distinct pathogens includes the facts that (1) NEC can occur in epidemics, (2) some outbreaks have been associated with specific bacterial pathogens, (3) epidemics have been interrupted by infection control measures, and (4) antibiotics may affect the course of NEC.[6]

Lending support to the bacterial colonization hypothesis is the fact that the intestinal transition from a germ-free *in utero* environment to normal colonization is a complex process. The organisms present in the neonatal intensive care unit are influenced by constant exposure to broad-spectrum antibiotics and may potentially interfere with normal intestinal colonization. Nosocomial pathogens may colonize

TABLE 24–2.
Signs and Symptoms of Necrotizing
Enterocolitis*

Finding	% of Patients
Abdominal distention	73%
Gastrointestinal bleeding	45%
Apnea, bradycardia	26%
Abdominal tenderness	21%
Gastric residuals	18%
Bilious emesis	11%
Abdominal cellultis	6%
Abdominal mass	2%

*Adapted from Walsh and Kliegman.[6]

the premature infant and become enteropathic in absence of microbial cross interference from normal flora.[11]

Feeding may also play a role in the development of NEC since most infants have been fed prior to the development of illness.[12] Fresh breast milk has been thought to be protective against NEC because it contains humoral antibodies, immunocompetent cells, and growth factors,[9] but cases have occurred in breast-fed infants.[12] Rapid advancement of feedings, hyperosmolar formula, which may contribute to bacterial colonization, and allergies to milk and soy protein have also been speculated to cause NEC.[9] In contrast, one study revealed an increased risk of NEC when feedings were delayed because delays may produce intestinal atrophy by nonuse.[4]

Clinical features

The clinical presentation of NEC is similar to that of sepsis, which must always be ruled out, but NEC has a predominance of GI findings. Necrotizing enterocolitis has been clinically divided into three stages, (see Table 24–1).[1] Stage I is classified as suspected NEC and includes nonspecific findings such as ileus, emesis, hematochezia, and feeding intolerance. Stage II is documented NEC reflected by all the signs of stage I plus abdominal tenderness and distention. There is radiographic evidence of pneumatosis intestinalis and possible intrahepatic venous air. Stage III is considered advanced disease because the patient may have unstable vital signs, respiratory failure, peritonitis, or intestinal perforation. Several other nonspecific signs of systemic disease may occur in NEC, including metabolic acidosis, apnea, and bradycardia. In addition, temperature instability, hypotension, thrombocytopenia, neutropenia, and coagulopathy can also occur (Table 24–2). This patient clearly had stage III disease because of bowel perforation and showed many of these other nonspecific signs.

The severity of NEC can be estimated from the history and presenting signs and symptoms. These include pH less than 7.3, bicarbonate less than 20 mEq/L, white blood cell differential count with greater than 13% immature forms, abdominal tenderness, and portal venous air.[12] This patient had all of these findings and would be expected to have severe disease. Interestingly, premature infants with minimal neonatal morbidity, such as this patient, may be at an increased risk to develop NEC because they may receive earlier feedings. Additional risk factors for infants who require surgery include asymptomatic patient ductus arteriosis, fewer days of antibiotics, fewer days of endotracheal tube intubation, and earlier diagnosis of the disease.[13]

Diagnosis

The differential diagnostic considerations in a neonate who presents with abdominal symptomatology is lengthy (Table 24–3). Sepsis as well as anatomic and inflammatory processes must first be ruled out.

The laboratory evaluation begins with a full sepsis workup consisting of blood, cerebral spinal fluid, and urine cultures, complete blood cell count with differential cell count, platelet count, electrolyte values, coagulation studies, and pH. Abdominal flat plate and cross-table lateral radiographic examinations are essential. Pneumatosis intestinalis is very suggestive of NEC, but it is not always present. Pneumatosis is often difficult to distinguish from air mixed with feces, and agreement between radiologists on the radiographic findings occurred in only 6% of cases in one study.[14]

Intrahepatic portal venous air has been reported in 5% to 25% of patients with NEC. Portal venous air always accompanies obvious pneumatosis, most likely due to intramural air tracking into the venous circulation. Abdominal ultrasound has recently been used to diagnose NEC because ultrasound is more sensitive than x-ray in detecting portal venous air.[14] Less specific radiographic findings suggestive of NEC include ileus, ascites, dilated fixed loop, and pneumoperitoneum.

A laboratory method to predict NEC has yet to be developed, but several tests are currently being evaluated. Elevated urinary thromboxane B_2 occurs with ischemic thrombosis and may be a nonspecific indicator of NEC.[10] A lysosomal acid hydrolase, hexosaminidase, also reflects intestinal ischemia and may be another potential marker for NEC.[14] Radionuclide scanning with technitium 99m diphosphate has been shown to detect intestinal necrosis.[14] The hydrogen breath test described by Kirchner demonstrates elevated levels of hydrogen gas in breath samples of patients with NEC.[6]

TABLE 24–3.
Differential Diagnosis for Necrotizing Enterocolitis

Sepsis
Gastroenteritis
Pyloric stenosis
Congenital intestinal atresia or stenosis
Midgut volvulus
Meconium ileus
Hirschsprung's disease
Milk protein intolerance
Neonatal appendicitis

Elevated breath hydrogen levels have been found in infants prior to the onset of NEC most likely due to bacterial fermentation.

Pathology

Necrotizing enterocolitis affects predominantly the ileum and the colon but may occur along any part of the small or large intestine. Microscopically, there is mucosal edema and hemorrhage. Patches of necrosis and abrasions of the superficial mucosal layer with an inflammatory cell reaction predominate initially. As the disease progresses, the necrosis extends below the muscular wall and may lead to perforation.[15] A pseudomembrane may form over the necrotic mucosa, which contains cellular debris, fibrinous exudate, and leukocytes.[2] Hydrogen gas cysts can be found in the submucosa. These are seen radiographically as pneumatosis intestinalis. In the healing process, the areas of active disease become fibrotic and may eventually form stenotic regions.

Therapy

The medical therapy of NEC centers on providing optimal supportive care, but surgical intervention is the only definitive treatment. Supportive management includes resuscitation, cardiotropic support, blood product replacement, nutritional support, and correction of metabolic problems such as acidosis. Specific management of NEC includes strict bowel rest, decompression of the bowel with a large bore nasogastric tube, frequent abdominal radiographs to detect possible perforation, and broad-spectrum antibiotics to treat sepsis, especially of gram-negative enteric flora. Enteral feedings are held and antibiotics are continued for 7 to 14 days, depending on the clinical stage. Improvement is seen in the majority of patients who are treated medically.[12]

When medical management fails, surgical intervention is required. Indications for surgical exploration include an abnormal paracentesis result, abdominal wall erythema, pneumoperitoneum, fixed palpable abdominal mass, and a persistently fixed dilated loop of bowel on x-ray film.[16] Other studies have also indicated that ascites and persistent acidosis in the clinical setting of NEC were also indications for surgery.[2]

At the time of surgery it is often difficult to differentiate necrotic bowel from hemorrhagic, viable bowel. Some centers plan second-look laparotomies if, at the time of the initial surgery, most of the intestine looks necrotic. The second laparotomy, which is performed 24 to 36 hours later, enables the surgeon to reassess questionable bowel, resect necrotic sections, irrigate purulent material, and search for further perforations.[17] If the area of necrosis is very small, end-to-end anastomosis is performed, but usually an enterostomy is placed. Mortality of patients requiring surgery is between 30% and 50%.[17]

Outcome

The overall mortality of NEC ranges from 15% to 40%.[2, 6, 12] Survival rates have improved because of earlier recognition and more aggressive therapy; deaths are usually reflective of immediate complications such as shock, sepsis, acute tubular necrosis, disseminated intravascular coagulation, perforations, and abdominal abscesses.[2]

Long-term complications, including intestinal stricture formation, occur in 10% to 22% of both medically and surgically treated survivors.[6] The colon is the site of 80% of all strictures, which is surprising since the terminal ileum is the most common site for NEC.[18] Obstipation, hematochezia, vomiting, and abdominal distention are symptoms that may be related to a stricture. Pathologically, there is cicatrical scarring at the site of the stricture. A radiographic contrast study may aid in defining the stricture in symptomatic patients.

The stricture is usually resected, although spontaneous resolution has been reported. Strictures that spontaneously resolve will usually do so within the first 2 months.

Infants requiring acute surgical bowel resection have a prolonged recovery phase. Intestinal adaptation takes months to years to occur. If more than 70% of the intestine is removed, malabsorption may be a chronic problem.[19] Often, these infants are dependent on total parenteral nutrition. Every effort is made to preserve the terminal ileum and ileocecal valve because these are important for fat, vitamin B_{12}, and bile salt absorption as well as regulation of intestinal emptying.[19]

The enterostomy can potentially be a source of sodium, water, and bicarbonate wasting, especially with minor GI illnesses.[6] Traditionally, reanastomosis of the bowel is delayed until the child's weight is approximately 11 lb (5 kg). However, recent studies suggest that early reanastomosis, even prior to discharge from the neonatal intensive care unit, may minimize nutritional and metabolic complications of enterostomies.[6]

The data on long-term growth and neurodevelopment are encouraging.[20] Except in patients with short bowel syndrome, the overall developmental morbidity is no higher than that due to prematurity, respiratory distress syndrome, or other problems prior to the onset of NEC.[6]

Prevention

Since the pathogenesis of NEC is unclear, effective preventive measures are not yet available. Ineffective measures have included the use of nonabsorbable antibiotics. Gammaglobulin, which has been beneficial in preventing rotaviral disease, may prove to be effective in NEC.[9] Pigbel, a NEC-like disease that occurs in Papua, New Guinea, has been effectively prevented by immunizing susceptible individuals with the active toxoid from *Clostridium* type B toxin.[9] In addition, prenatal steroids, by promoting intestinal maturity, may prove beneficial in the future.[21] Strict cohorting of affected patients and their care givers is the only proved preventive therapy to decrease the incidence of the disease.[22]

SUMMARY

Necrotizing enterocolitis is a disease of predominantly premature infants and is a significant cause of mortality in the neonatal intensive care unit. The pathogenesis is unknown but is thought to be multifactorial and may include intestinal injury secondary to ischemia, bacterial colonization, or response to the nature of enteral feedings. Patients present with a predominance of GI symptoms but may also appear systemically ill. Pneumatosis intestinalis is the radiologic hallmark, although it is not always present. The key therapeutic interventions include bowel rest, bowel decompression, and broad-spectrum antibiotics; surgical intervention is required when perforation occurs. Stricture formation is the most common long-term complication, but the overall long-term prognosis, once the patient is past the acute episode, is good.

REFERENCES

1. Bell MJ, Ternberg TJ, Feigin RD, et al: Neonatal necrotizing enterocolitis: Therapeutic decisions based upon clinical staging. *Ann Surg* 1978; 187:1–7.
2. Kliegman RM, Fanaroff AA: Necrotizing enterocolitis. *N Engl J Med* 1984; 310:1093–1103.
3. Kliegman RM, Fanaroff AA: Neonatal necrotizing enterocolitis: A nine year experience: I. Epidemiology and uncommon observations. *Am J Dis Child* 1981; 135:603–607.
4. LaGamma EF, Ostertag SG, Birenbaum H: Failure of delayed oral feedings to prevent necrotizing enterocolitis. *Am J Dis Child* 1985; 139:385–388.
5. Stoll BJ, Kanto WP Jr, Glass RI, et al: Epidemiology of necrotizing enterocolitis: A case control study. *J Pediatr* 1980; 96:447–451.
6. Walsh MC, Kliegman RM: Necrotizing enterocolitis: Treatment based on staging criteria. *Pediatr Clin North Am* 1986; 33:179–201.
7. Wilson R, Kanto WP Jr, McCarthy BJ, et al: Short communication. Age at onset of necrotizing enterocolitis: An epidemiologic analysis. *Pediatr Res* 1982; 16:82–84.
8. Kliegman RM, Hack M, Jones P, et al: Epidemiologic study of necrotizing enterocolitis among low birth weight infants. *J. Pediatr* 1982; 100:440–444.
9. Kosloske AM: Pathogenesis and prevention of necrotizing enterocolitis: A hypothesis based on personal observation and a review of the literature. *Pediatrics* 1984; 74:1086–1092.
10. Hyman PE, Abrams CE, Zipser RD: Enhanced urinary immunoreactive thromboxane in neonatal enterocolitis. *Am J Dis Child* 1987; 141:686–689.
11. Blakey JL, Lubitz L, Campbell NT, et al: Enteric colonization in sporadic neonatal necrotizing enterocolitis. *J Pediatr Gastroenterol Nutr* 1985; 4:591–595.
12. McCormack CJ, Emmens RW, Putnam TC: Evaluation of factors in high risk neonatal necrotizing enterocolitis. *J. Pediatr Surg* 1987; 22:488–491.
13. Barnard JA, Cotton RB, Lutin W: Necrotizing enterocolitis: Variables associated with the severity of the disease. *Am J Dis Child* 1985; 139:375–377.
14. Lindley S, Mollitt DL, Seibert JJ, et al: Portal vein ultrasonography in the early diagnosis of necrotizing enterocolitis. *J Pediatr Surg* 1986; 21:530–532.
15. Rousset S, Moscovici O, Lebon P, et al: Intestinal lesions containing coronalike particles in neonatal necrotizing enterocolitis: An ultrastructural analysis. *Pediatrics* 1984; 73:218–224.

16. Kosloske AM, Papile L, Burnstein J: Indications for operation in acute necrotizing enterocolitis of the neonate. *Surgery* 1980; 87:502–508.
17. Weber TR, Lewis JE: The role of second-look laparotomy in necrotizing enterocolitis. *J Pediatr Surg* 1986; 21:323–325.
18. Janik JS, Ein SH, Mancer K: Intestinal stricture after necrotizing enterocolitis. *J Pediatr Surg* 1981; 16:438–443.
19. Gertler JP, Seashore JH, Touloukian RJ: Early ileostomy closure in necrotizing enterocolitis. *J Pediatr Surg* 1987; 22:140–143.
20. Abbasi S, Pereira GB, Johnson L, et al: Long-term assessment of growth, nutritional status, and gastrointestinal function in survivors of necrotizing enterocolitis. *J Pediatr* 1984; 104:550–554.
21. Bauer CR, Morrison JC, Poole WK, et al: A decreased incidence of necrotizing enterocolitis after prenatal glucocorticoid therapy. *Pediatrics* 1984; 73:683–688.
22. Book LS, Overall JC, Herbst JJ, et al: Clustering of necrotizing enterocolitis: Interruption by infection-control measures. *N Engl J Med* 1977; 297:984–986.

25 Food Sensitivity: Cow's Milk Protein Intolerance

Anne Munck, M.D.,

Veronique Pelletier, M.D.

W. Allan Walker, M.D.

The patient was a 4-month-old boy who had been the 7.1-lb (3.2-kg) product of a full-term pregnancy terminated by an emergency cesarian section for unexplained fetal distress. His Apgar scores were normal, and he had an uneventful postnatal course. After discharge at 1 week with his mother, he fed well on breast milk and produced three to four loose stools per day.

He did well except for his loose stools until 3.5 weeks of age, when he was hospitalized for nonbloody diarrhea, vomiting, and a temperature of 39.5°C. He was treated for 3 days with intravenous (IV) ampicillin and gentamicin until the cultures were negative. He received a cow's milk infant formula for 1 day before breast-feeding was resumed. As he returned to his usual state of good health, several other family members developed similar symptoms of diarrhea, vomiting, and fever.

One week after hospital discharge, the child was noted to have specks of bright red blood in his loose stools. The diet continued to be solely breast milk except for the formula given in the hospital. His physical examination was normal, including growth at the 75th percentile and no evidence of rectal fissures. There was no evidence of rash or respiratory abnormalities. His mother had no mastitis or fissures of her nipples. Stool cultures were negative, and a complete blood cell (CBC) count included hematocrit 33%, white blood cell (WBC) count 13,000/mm³ with a normal differential count except for 5% eosinophils, and a normal platelet count. The prothrombin and partial thromboplastin times were normal.

The patient continued to enjoy general good health but had persistence of bloody stools. The CBC count was repeated and included: hematocrit 33%, WBC count 20,000/mm³ with 19% eosinophils, 27% neutrophils, 52% lymphocytes, and 2% monocytes. His mother was placed on a milk elimination diet, and the child's stools improved but continued to contain some blood.

The child's subsequent laboratory evaluation included a normal albumin level, negative radioallergosorbent assay test (RAST) results to milk and soy, and an elevated serum IgE level. A barium enema showed bowel wall thickening in the descending and transverse colon. A sigmoidoscopy revealed erythematous and friable mucosa, and biopsy specimens demonstrated increased eosinophilic infiltration of the lamina propria but no evidence of inflammation of the crypts, crypt abcesses, or granulomas (Fig 25–1). These findings were consistent with allergic colitis, and the child was placed on an elemental formula diet. The stools became guaiac negative within 2 days and have remained negative; his eosinophil count has returned to normal.

DISCUSSION

For the purposes of this discussion "food (milk) allergy" and "protein intolerance" will be used to refer to a reproducible reaction to a specific food and evidence of an immunologic reaction to it.[1] Allergic reactions to food antigens are relatively common in children and are usually grouped clinically into immediate and delayed types.[2] Cow's milk protein intolerance (CMPI) is the most common form of food allergy in children and usually presents as an immediate reaction.[3]

The prevalence of CMPI in the United States has been estimated from 0.3% to 7%.[4] The variation in prevalence rates can be explained by the lack of a single accepted set of diagnostic criteria.[1] Unfortunately, no reliable laboratory test on which to make the diagnosis exists.[4] Important risk factors for the development of CMPI appear to be a family history of atopy[4, 5] and early exposure to cow's milk feedings[6]; breast-feeding appears to be at least partially protective.[5, 7]

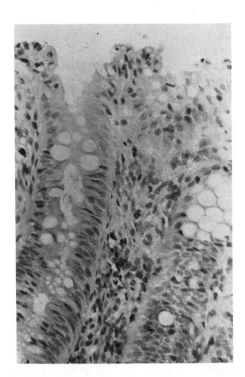

FIG 25–1.
High-power view of the rectal mucosal biopsy. The lamina propria contains clusters of eosinophils, and scattered eosinophils are present within the surface epithelium (×300).

Pathogenesis

The pathogenesis of food allergy can be divided into immediate and delayed reactions.[8] The immediate reactions are IgE mediated and cause an anaphylactic or immediate hypersensitivity response. The delayed reactions include cytotoxic, IgG–immune complex disease, or cell-mediated delayed hypersensitivity.[8] In most cases, the allergic reaction arises through a combination of these mechanisms.

Several systems appear to play a role in the immune reaction to food proteins. Macromolecular absorption of potential antigens across the mucosal barrier, intestinal antigen binding by secretory IgA, and local cell-mediated immune systems are important factors in developing an immune response.[9]

The secretory IgA response to ingested antigens is delayed in newborns and may affect protection against antigen uptake across the intestinal mucosal surface.[9] The components of gut-associated lymphoid tissues (GALT), including phagocytes, eosinophils, mast cells, and T and B lymphocytes, help provide an efficient local immune defense separate from the systemic immune system.[10] In addition, systemic tolerance usually occurs in response to orally ingested food proteins, but the failure of this tolerance to develop in infants appears to contribute to their increased incidence of gastrointestinal (GI) food allergy.[9]

Systemic allergic reactions can also play a role in food allergies. The finding of IgE antibodies to specific food antigens often correlates with the immediate onset of clinical symptoms of food allergy including anaphylaxis, vomiting, sneezing, and urticaria.[11] An elevated cord IgE level is an accurate predictor of atopic potential in young infants.[12] Failure to suppress IgE production by mucosal suppressor T cells may account for the response in allergy-prone infants. The specific mechanism of action is not known but appears to involve the release of histamine and prostaglandins that may serve as mediators of a local reaginic immune reaction.[4]

Evidence for immune complex hypersensitivity reactions has also been demonstrated in food allergy.[13] An immune reaction appears to be related to the development of enteropathy, but the trigger mechanism has not been identified.[4]

Whatever the mechanism, CMPI is primarily a disease of infancy. In contrast to most forms of allergy, children with CMPI usually have resolution of their symptoms by 1 to 3 years of age.[4]

Clinical Features

The clinical manifestations of CMPI are usually localized to the GI tract but may at times include systemic symptoms involving the respiratory tract and skin (Table 25–1).[4, 12, 13, 17] Intestinal CMPI can be divided into disease involving principally the colon and rectum or involving predominantly the upper portions and midportions of the intestine.[13]

Allergic proctitis is usually seen in infants and young children and is often caused by a single food allergen.[14] The commonest symptoms are rectal bleeding and diarrhea, which usually develop before 6 months of age and disappear by age 2 or 3 years.[4] When a child is rechallenged with milk, symptoms usually develop shortly after ingestion and may mimic an acute infectious gastroenteritis.[4] Less fre-

TABLE 25–1.

Clinical Manifestations of Cow's Milk Protein Intolerance*

Intestinal
    Rectal bleeding
    Diarrhea
    Abdominal pain
    Vomiting
    Growth failure
    Protein-losing enteropathy
Extraintestinal
    Rhinorrhea
    Sneezing
    Wheezing
    Perioral edema
    Urticaria
    Angioedema

*Adapted from Stern and Walker,[4] Proujansky,[12] Goldman and Proujansky,[13] and McCarty and Frick.[17]

quently symptoms may be delayed for more than 24 hours after ingestion and can rarely be seen days after the exposure.[4]

The colitis caused by CMPI is often associated with increased numbers of intraepithelial lymphocytes and eosinophils, elevated levels of serum IgE and IgE to specific food antibodies, and peripheral blood eosinophilia,[13, 14] as seen in this patient. This colitis usually improves when milk is removed from the diet and is not related to ulcerative colitis or Crohn's disease.

The case presented here is fairly typical of the colonic form of the transient CMPI of early infancy. The child had otherwise been healthy but was found to have blood in his stool. Stool cultures were negative, and there was no physical examination or laboratory evidence for a bleeding diathesis. The mechanism in this case was probably the presence of small amounts of cow's milk in the mother's breast milk since attempts at eliminating milk from the mother's diet led to improvement in symptoms. When the child was switched to an elemental formula, the bleeding stopped entirely.

The upper intestinal and midintestinal forms of CMPI differ from the lower colonic form.[13] Diarrhea has been found with similar frequency, but rectal blood loss is much less common; abdominal pain, vomiting, and growth failure were more frequently seen.[13] Multiple allergic manifestations and a family history of allergy have been more commonly reported in association with the upper intestinal form of allergy.[13] Intestinal allergy may also likely play a role in the rare disorder eosinophilic gastroenteritis, especially the mucosal form.[13]

In allergic gastroenteritis the esophagus, gastric antrum, and duodenum are particularly affected.[13] The findings include epithelial damage and infiltration with eosinophils. In milder cases, clusters of eosinophils are found in the lamina propria with only rare extension into the epithelial layer.

The relationship of other intestinal symptoms or symptom complexes often linked to intestinal allergy are more difficult to prove. The possibility that some cases of colic may be caused by CMPI has long been debated, but firm evidence is lacking. Irritable bowel syndrome and chronic constipation have also been mentioned as being caused by CMPI, but little evidence is available to support this relationship.[4] Cow's milk protein intolerance has also been speculated to be a cause of necrotizing enterocolitis, although epidemiologic studies have not identified milk ingestion as a risk factor.[15]

Extraintestinal manifestations of milk protein allergy may include rhinorrhea, sneezing, wheezing, lip swelling, urticaria and angioedema.[16, 17] Anaphylactic reactions have also rarely been reported.[4]

Diagnosis

The diagnosis of food allergy relies heavily on the clinical history and depends on the demonstration of symptoms in response to a specific food challenge. Classically the diagnosis has been made using the Goldman criteria, which require the development of symptoms within 48 hours of rechallenge with the antigen on three separate occasions.[18] These stringent criteria were suggested because the complex nature of food allergy can often make interpretation of food challenges confusing. However, most families will not accept the need for three rechallenges, and most clinicians currently use a single challenge.[17]

Detection of serum antibodies is also often done in suspected cases of milk protein allergy. Values of total serum IgE and IgE to milk protein are available through many clinical laboratories using the RAST. These tests will detect only IgE-mediated milk allergy and cannot determine other forms of food allergy. As a rule, children with the colonic form of CMPI are much less likely to have a marked increase in serum IgE levels, a positive RAST reponse to milk protein, or elevated eosinophil levels than are children with the small intestinal form.[13]

Skin testing has been touted by some to be an aid in the diagnosis but is unreliable in children less than 3 years of age and in delayed forms of allergy.[4] The importance of skin sensitivity as an indicator of an intestinal mucosal process is yet to be determined.

Intestinal biopsies can also be helpful in making the diagnosis of food allergy but are nonspecific and can only support the diagnosis. In the allergic proctitis form of food allergy, the proctitis is usually caused by a single food allergen and is probably mediated by a local IgE reaction. The overall mucosal architecture is normal, and no evidence of chronic colitis is found.[13] The main finding is an increased number of eosinophils in the lamina propria and clusters of eosinophils within the surface and crypt epithelium.[13] In the upper and midintestinal forms of food allergy, biopsies consistent with allergic enteritis (localized infiltrate of eosinophils) were found in 100% of antral biopsies compared to 79% of duodenal, 60% of esophageal, and 52% of gastric corpus biopsies.[13]

Treatment

The treatment of milk protein allergy is based on the elimination of milk from the diet. However, in contrast to celiac disease, this dietary restriction is usually transient since most children outgrow milk protein allergy.

In more general cases of food allergy, it is often difficult to identify the offending food.[19] In infants, a change is made to a hypoallergenic, elemental formula like Pregestamil or Nutramigen. In older children, milk products must be scrupulously avoided, which requires dietary counseling and careful reading of food labels. Drug therapy has not proved to have a primary role in the treatment of food allergy.[20]

SUMMARY

Fortunately, most children with CMPI do well when milk is removed from the diet and can tolerate an otherwise varied diet. In well-documented CMPI, milk products are usually withheld for 1 year and are then reintroduced under careful monitoring. The great majority of children with CMPI will eventually be able to tolerate milk products.

REFERENCES

1. Lessof MH: Food intolerance and allergy — a review. *Q J Med* 1983; 52:111–119.
2. Ford RPK, Hill DJ, Hosking CS: Cow's milk hypersensitivity: Immediate and delayed onset clinical patterns. *Arch Dis Child* 1983; 58:856–862.
3. Walker-Smith J: Cow's milk protein intolerance. Transient food intolerance of infancy. *Arch Dis Child* 1975; 50:347–350.
4. Stern M, Walker WA: Food allergy and intolerance. *Pediatr Clin North Am* 1985; 32:471–492.
5. Buisseret P: Common manifestations of cow's milk allergy in children. *Lancet* 1978; 1:304–305.
6. Lucas A, McLaughlan P, Coombs KRA: Latent anaphylactic sensitization of infants of low birth weight to cow's milk proteins. *Br Med J* 1984; 283:1254–1256.
7. Fallstrom SP, Ahlstedt S, Carlsson E, et al: Influence of breast feeding on the development of cow's milk protein antibodies and the IgE level. *Int Arch Allerg* 1984; 75:87–94.
8. Gallagher PJ, Goulding NJ, Gidney MJ, et al: Acute and chronic immunological response to dietary antigen. *Gut* 1983; 24:831–835.
9. Walker WA: Antigen handling by the small intestine. *Clin Gastroenterol* 1986; 15:1–20.
10. MacDermott MR, Bienenstock S: Evidence for a common mucosal immunologic system: I. Migration of B immunoblasts into intestinal, respiratory and genital tissues. *J Immunol* 1979; 122:1892–1898.
11. Burgin-Wolf A, Singer E, Friess HM, et al: The diagnostic significance of antibodies in various cow's milk proteins (fluorescent immunosorbent test). *Eur J Pediatr* 1980; 133:17–24.
12. Proujansky R, Winter HS, Walker WA: Gastrointestinal syndromes associated with food sensitivity. *Adv Pediatr* 1988; 35:219–238.

13. Goldman H, Proujansky R: Allergic proctitis and allergic gastroenteritis in children: Clinical and mucosal biopsy features in 53 cases. *Am J Surg Pathol* 1986; 10:75–86.
14. Jenkins HR, Pincott JR, Soothill JF, et al: Food allergy: The major cause of infantile colitis. *Arch Dis Child* 1984; 59:326–329.
15. Stoll BJ, Kanto WP Jr, Glass RI, et al: Epidemiology of necrotizing enterocolitis: A case control study. *J. Pediatr* 1980; 96:444–451.
16. Bock SA, Lee WY, Remigio L, et al: Studies of hypersensitivity reactions to food in infants and children. *J Allergy Clin Immunol* 1978; 62:327–334.
17. McCarty EP, Frick OL: Food sensitivity: Keys to diagnosis. *J Pediatr* 1983; 102:645–652.
18. Goldman AS, Anderson DW Jr, Sellers WA, et al: Milk allergy: 1. Oral challenge with milk and isolated milk proteins in allergic children. *Pediatrics* 1963; 32:425–443.
19. Zieger RS, Heller S, Mellon M, et al: Effectiveness of dietary manipulations in the prevention of food allergy. *J Allergy Clin Immunol* 1986; 78:224–237.
20. Sogan D: Medications and their use in the treatment of adverse reactions to foods. *J Allergy Clin Immunol* 1986; 78:238–243.

26 Recurrent Abdominal Pain

Barry Z. Hirsch, M.D.

A 14-year-old girl presented with recurrent abdominal pain, and an endoscopic retrograde cholangiopancreatogram (ERCP) was requested. Her problems began 1 year earlier and were associated with a month-long episode of recurrent vomiting, weakness, headaches, diarrhea, and weight loss, which caused her admission to a local hospital. A diagnosis of anorexia nervosa and bulimia was made, and she was placed on a high-caloric diet that featured frequent milkshakes. Over the ensuing year her vomiting resolved, but she developed a new complaint of subxiphoid pain that radiated subcostally to the back and was associated with nausea, diarrhea, and diaphoresis. The pain was stabbing, precipitated by meals, worse at night, and was partially relieved by sitting up and holding her stomach; she was never awakened at night by the pain. There was no associated abdominal distention, hematochezia, melena, hematemesis, or dysuria and no association with her menstrual cycle. The patient did, however, have problems with dysmenorrhea, for which she was treated with ibuprofen, a nonsteroidal anti-inflammatory agent. Six weeks prior to her clinic visit she was admitted to her local hospital for abdominal pain, where only blood tests were done, and the diagnosis of esophagitis was made. She was given a course of cimetidine and antacids without relief from her pain. Her past medical history was significant only for frequent hospitalizations as an infant for gastroenteritis. The family history was remarkable for her mother who had three operations for pancreatitis without relief of her pain. The mother's symptoms were remarkably similar to her daughter's. The mother did not know the etiology of her pancreatitis but stated that her amylase level had always been normal each time it was checked.

On physical examination the patient's height and weight were at the 10th percentile. She was healthy appearing and shy but cooperative. Examination results of the skin; head, ears, eyes, nose, and throat; lungs; and heart were normal. Examination of the thorax revealed costavertebral angle tenderness and mild tenderness over the anterior ribs. The abdominal examination findings were normal except for diffuse, mild tenderness to deep palpation. Her rectal, gynecologic, musculoskeletal, and neurologic examinations were unremarkable.

Results of the laboratory evaluation were negative including three stool examinations for ova and parasites and negative for stool guaiac. An abdominal ultrasound, upper gastrointestinal (GI) series with small bowel follow through, values for amylase, bilirubin, alanine aminotransferase (ALT), aspartate aminotransferase (AST), and erythrocyte sedimentation rate (ESR) were normal. Results of a lactose hydrogen breath test showed an abnormal rise to 109 ppm by 2 hours after ingestion associated with abdominal pain and diaphoresis, which was identical to her symptoms at home. She was diagnosed as having lactose intolerance and was placed on a lactose-free diet; when compliant with the diet, she has remained symptom free.

DISCUSSION

Recurrent abdominal pain is usually defined as three or more episodes of pain occurring over three months severe enough to affect routine activity.[1] This case illustrates the often long and frustrating attempt of families and physicians to identify the cause of recurrent abdominal pain. Although recurrent abdominal pain affects 10% to 18% of school-age children, diagnosible organic etiology can be found in fewer than 10% of cases.[1-3] Boys and girls are equally affected during the first 7 years of life, but girls greatly predominate in later childhood and adolescence.[2] A positive family history is likely to be found.[2] This chapter will provide guidelines for differentiating organic from nonorganic causes.

Pathophysiology

Recurrent abdominal pain can be caused by a long list of disorders and is usually divided into organic and psychogenic causes.[3] In the cases where organic causes are not found, environmental and psychosocial stresses are hypothesized to cause the pain.

Recently a more complex model has been proposed to explain nonorganic causes of pain based on multiple predisposing factors that converge to create the pain and modulate its severity.[3] These factors include somatic predisposition, effect of lifestyle, environment and temperament, and learned response patterns.

Clinical Features

The presenting complaints of patients with recurrent abdominal pain are often similar despite the wide variety of causes. However, some guidelines can be used to determine whether an organic or nonorganic cause is operative.

A careful history and physical examination can help to eliminate some of the many diagnostic possibilities and limit the cost and invasiveness of the evaluation. Important clues of possible organic disease include weight loss, sleep disruption, fever, arthritis, hematochezia or melena, and changes in the bowel or menstrual patterns. Description of the location, time course, and quality of the pain can help to sort out renal, gynecologic, and GI causes. For example, suprapubic pain may indicate cystitis, whereas excruciating flank and back pain can be associated with renal stones. Pain caused by pancreatitis or cholecystitis most often occurs after meals, whereas pain due to peptic disease may occur just prior to meals or 1 to 2 hours later.

In adolescent girls a menstrual history is crucial. Unlike dietary associations that are often nonspecific, linking the pain to events in the menstrual cycle can be very revealing. Dysmenorrhea, mittleschmerz, ovarian cysts, pregnancy, pelvic inflammatory disease, and endometriosis must all be considered. Consultation with either a gynecologist or an adolescent specialist is often required.

The source of drinking water is another important historic point because giardiasis is being increasingly identified as a cause of abdominal pain. Travel history to developing countries with its increased risk of enteric pathogens should also be sought.

The association between the pain and ingesting dairy products was quite helpful in this case and underscores the importance of asking a dietary history. However, the association of lactose ingestion and the occurrence of pain is often difficult to elicit since the symptoms can frequently occur hours later, or patients may be unaware of the lactose content of the foods they are eating.[4] Another important component of the diet history is determining the fiber content of the diet.

One of the most important results of the physical examination can be to reassure the physician that a significant medical problem is not being overlooked. Signs suggesting serious pathology include weight loss, guaiac positive stools, fevers, or poor growth. Documented weight loss, with no evidence for dieting, can indicate the presence of a serious medical or emotional problem. All patients with poor growth and abdominal pain should be evaluated for inflammatory bowel disease, especially Crohn's disease.

A full gynecologic examination is needed in all adolescent girls with recurrent abdominal pain. The examination should be done by an experienced physician who is most likely to detect subtle abnormalities.

Diagnosis

Although nonorganic causes are most commonly implicated in recurrent abdominal pain, these are diagnoses of exclusion. To help rule out the long list of possible organic causes (Table 26–1), a staged evaluation is recommended (Table 26–2). We generally screen all children with recurrent abdominal pain with a urinalysis, stool examination for parasites and blood, and a complete blood cell (CBC) count and ESR. These tests, along with the history and physical examination, help to rule out important causes such as infections, inflammatory bowel disease, and malignancy. Further investigations are obtained if indicated by the history, physical examination, or initial screening. In addition, a lactose hydrogen breath test is often obtained if another etiology has not been uncovered.

We also often employ one of three empiric trials for patients. A trial of a high-fiber diet is almost universally tried since children with irritable bowel syndrome are known to improve on such a regimen.[5] The diet is begun while the initial evaluation is undertaken. If history or physical findings consistent with constipation are found, a trial of stool softeners may also be given. Since antacid or H_2 blocker therapy is relatively safe and well tolerated, an empiric trial is often given if peptic disease, including esophagitis, seems likely.

Referral to a psychologist or psychiatrist can be done in conjunction with the evaluation for an organic cause. Parents and patients should be made aware of the

TABLE 26–1.

Organic Causes of Abdominal
Pain

Primary considerations
  Constipation
  Peptic ulcer
  Giardiasis
  Lactose intolerance
  Gastroesophageal reflux
  Urinary tract infection
  Mittelschmerz
  Dysmenorrhea
  Pregnancy
  Pelvic inflammatory disease
Secondary considerations
  Inflammatory bowel disease
  Intermittent volvulus
  Choledochal cyst
  Cholelithiasis
  Pancreatitis
  Renal calculous
  Pyelonephritis
  Ovarian cyst
  Endometriosis

TABLE 26–2.

Evaluation of Abdominal Pain

Initial screening
  Urinalysis
  Stools for ova and parasites
  Stool guaiac
  CBC and ESR
Additional tests*
  Lactose hydrogen breath test
  Liver profile
  Amylase and lipase
  Upper GI series
  Abdominal ultrasound
  Esophagogastroduodenoscopy
  Laparoscopy
  Urine porphyrins
  Intravenous pyelogram

*If indicated by specific history, physical examination, or laboratory findings.

relative infrequency of finding an organic etiology and the importance of evaluating sources of stress and the need to develop better coping mechanisms.[6, 7]

When the history and physical examination give clues to hepatic, biliary, pancreatic, or pelvic abnormality, an abdominal ultrasound can be an extremely useful tool (see Table 26–2). Without such indications, the sensitivity of the ultrasound in finding the cause of abdominal pain is extremely low.

Endoscopy should usually be reserved for patients with evidence for an organic process such as hematochezia, anemia, or weight loss. If peptic disease is considered likely, a therapeutic trial of antacids is usually given before endoscopy is performed. In those patients who do not respond to medication, a more aggressive approach may be taken. The goal of the evaluation should be to reassure the physician and the patient that serious medical causes have been ruled out.

The history and physical examinations in this patient did not identify an obvious organic cause for her pain. However, the use of a simple screening test implicated lactose intolerance. This case emphasizes the importance of considering an organic etiology in every patient with abdominal pain and also the importance of a practical, stepwise approach toward diagnosis.

Lactose Intolerance

Lactose malabsorption is the most frequently encountered form of carbohydrate intolerance and is usually manifested by a syndrome of abdominal pain, diarrhea, flatulence, and bloating.[8, 9] The intolerance may be congenital, secondary, or hereditary with delayed onset.[10]

The congenital form is extremely rare and is due to low or absent activity of brush border enzyme lactase at birth. The secondary form can be acquired at any age and results from an insult to the small bowel ranging from infectious and immunologic to malnutrition. Once the offending agent is removed or the environment changed, the intestinal villi should rapidly recover within a matter of days to weeks and again exhibit brush border lactase activity.

Hereditary lactose intolerance with delayed onset is the most common form seen in older children and adults such as this patient.[11] The defect is genetically inherited and is much more frequently found in Asian, Black, Native American, and Mexican populations. The highest incidence is in certain Nigerian tribes, where 99% of the adults are lactose intolerant.[11] The least affected groups are whites of North American and Northern European heritage; however, even among these groups up to 20% of adults are affected.[11, 12] Symptoms of lactose intolerance may start as early as 3 or 4 years of age, but typically they begin in adolescence or early adulthood.

Controversy exists as to what role lactose intolerance plays in recurrent abdominal pain. Although one recent study reported lactose intolerance in 40% of patients with recurrent abdominal pain, others have found it to be a very rare occurrence.[4, 9] Regardless of its incidence, the ease and safety of diagnosis and treatment make it an important diagnostic consideration in any patient with recurrent abdominal pain.

The diagnosis of lactose intolerance is usually made with a lactose hydrogen breath test. The theory behind this test is that malabsorbed lactose is fermented by the normal colonic flora, resulting in hydrogen gas detectable in the breath and in the production of symptoms.[13] The test can be performed on patients of any age who have fasted for 8 hours and who have not taken antibiotics for 2 weeks before the test.[13] A standard dose of lactose (2 gm/kg up to 50 gm) is dissolved in water and administered to the patient by mouth. The patient's breath is collected by a mask that is connected to a collection syringe. Breaths are obtained prior to the lactose load and every 30 minutes for 3 hours. The level of hydrogen is then analyzed by means of gas chromatography. A positive test result for lactose malabsorption is defined as a rise of greater than 10 ppm after 1 hour from a baseline less than 20 ppm.[13, 14] An abnormal test result is often accompanied by a symptomatic response, as seen in this patient.

Several conditions can make assessment of the lactose breath test difficult. An early rise of hydrogen gas or a high baseline can occur from either interaction with flora or rapid transit time through the small intestine.[13] Patients with small bowel overgrowth will have an early peak resulting from fermentation by small bowel flora, followed by a much larger colonic peak.[15] When rapid transit time is present, a single peak usually occurs in less than 30 minutes.

Once the diagnosis of lactose intolerance is made, the patient should be given a trial of a strict lactose-free diet.[16] Patients are often surprised at the number of commercial products that contain lactose, including many medications. After a strict trial off lactose and a pain-free period, small amounts of lactose-containing foods can be introduced into the diet. The fermentation process involved in the production of cheese and yogurt breaks down much of the lactose, making these products excellent initial trial foods.[17] Newly available lactase-treated milk, lactase drops, and lactase pills appear to be reasonably effective and can make the diet much more tolerable by permitting the intake of more dairy products.

SUMMARY

Although the cause of recurrent abdominal pain is most often not of organic origin, a practical approach to rule out the common organic causes should be undertaken (see Table 26–2). The evaluation often includes an empiric trial of a high-fiber diet, stool softeners, or antacid therapy. Referrral to a psychologist or psychiatrist can be done in conjunction with the initial evaluation.

REFERENCES

1. Apley J, Naish N: Recurrent abdominal pain: A field survey of 1000 school children. *Arch Dis Child* 1958; 33:165–170.
2. Apley J: *The Child with Abdominal Pains,* ed 2. Boston, Blackwell Scientific Publications, 1975.
3. Levine MD, Rappaport LA: Recurrent abdominal pain in school children: The loneliness of the long-distance physician. *Pediatr Clin North Am* 1984; 31:969–991.
4. Wald A, Chandra R, Fisher S, et al: Lactose malabsorption in recurrent abdominal pain of childhood. *J Pediatr* 1982; 100:65–68.

5. Feldman W, McGrath P, Hodgson C: The use of dietary fiber in the management of simple, childhood, idiopathic, recurrent, abdominal pain. *Am J Dis Child* 1985; 139:1216–1218.
6. Young ST, Alpers DH, Norland CC, et al: Psychiatric illness and the irritable bowel syndrome. *Gastroenterology* 1976; 70:162–166.
7. Hodges K, Kline J, Barbero G, et al: Depressive symptoms in children with recurrent abdominal pain and their families. *J Pediatr* 1985; 107:622–626.
8. AAP Committee on Nutrition: The practical significance of lactose intolerance in children. *Pediatrics* 1978; 62:240–245.
9. Barr R, Levine M, Watkins J: Recurrent abdominal pain in childhood due to a lactose intolerance. *N Engl J Med* 1979; 300:1449–1452.
10. Silverman A, Roy C: Carbohydrate intolerance, in *Pediatric Clinical Gastroenterology*, ed 3. St Louis, CV Mosby Co, 1983, pp 245–246.
11. Ferguson A, Maxwell JD: Genetic aetiology of lactose intolerance. *Lancet* 1967; 2:188–190.
12. Gray M: Intestinal disaccharidase deficiencies and glucose-galactose malabsorption, in Stanburg JB, Wyngaarden JB, Fredrickson DS, et al (eds): *The Metabolic Basis of Inherited Disease*, ed 5. New York, McGraw-Hill Book Co, 1983, pp 1729–1742.
13. Barr RG, Watkins JB, Perman JA, et al: Mucosal function and breath hydrogen excretion: Criteria for a normal response. *Pediatr Res* 1979; 13:395 [A].
14. Solomons N, Barillas C: The cut-off criterion for a positive hydrogen breath test in children: A reappraisal. *J Pediatr Gastroenterol Nutr* 1986; 5:920–925.
15. Rhodes JM, Middleton P, Jewell DP: The lactulose hydrogen breath test as a diagnostic test for small-bowel bacterial overgrowth. *Scand J Gastroenterol* 1979; 14:333–336.
16. Walker WA, Hendricks KM: *Manual of Pediatric Nutrition*, Philadelphia, WB Saunders Co, 1985, p 110.
17. Kolars JC, Levitt MD, Aouji M, et al: Yogurt—an autodigesting source of lactose. *N Engl J Med* 1984; 310:1–3.

27 Cystic Fibrosis

Richard A. Schreiber M.D.C.M., F.R.C.P.(C)

A 7-month-old girl presented to Children's Hospital because of generalized edema. She was born by cesarean section for transverse lie at 35 weeks' gestation with a birth weight of 6.2 lb (2.8 kg). She was breast-fed for 2 months and then switched to a cow's milk formula. Because of symptoms of colic, a soy-based formula was introduced. Three weeks prior to the current admission, an episode of bronchiolitis led to a 3-day hospitalization. She was then well until 6 days prior to admission when watery, nonbloody diarrhea developed. She was admitted for intravenous (IV) rehydration and 12 hours later was started back on oral feeds with a soy-based formula. Peripheral edema was noted, and the serum albumin level was 1.3 mg%. She was transferred to Children's Hospital for investigation. There was no family history for intestinal or renal disease.

On physical examination her weight was 15.7 lb (7.1 kg, 50th percentile) and her height was at the 10th percentile. She was afebrile, and her vital signs were stable. The head, ear, eye, nose, and throat; chest; and cardiovascular examinations were unremarkable. The abdomen was soft and nontender. The liver was 3 cm below the costal margin, and the spleen was not palpable. No shifting dullness or fluid wave could be elicited. There was marked pitting edema of the lower extremities up to the knees, and mild sacral edema was present.

The hemoglobin value was 10.6 mg/dl and the hematocrit 32.9%. The white blood cell count was 17,000/mm³ with 67% lymphocytes, 28% polymorphonuclear lymphocytes, and 4% monocytes. The platelets were normal. Multiple urine dipstick results for total protein were negative and the stools were Hemoccult negative. The serum protein level was 3.8 mg/dl (low), and the serum albumin level was 1.8 mg/dl (low). The serum electrolyte values, glucose level, prothrombin time, and partial thromboplastin time were normal. The aspartate aminotransferase (AST) level was 34 mU/ml (slightly elevated), the alanine aminotransferase (ALT) level was 32 mU/ml (slightly elevated), and the alkaline phosphatase and total bilirubin values were normal. Results of multiple stool examinations for bacteria, virus, and parasites were negative. An ultrasound of the abdomen showed a highly echogenic liver consistent with fatty infiltration. There was no ascites, and the biliary tract was normal.

The sweat chloride concentration was 114 mEq/L in a collection of 105 mg of sweat, consistent with a diagnosis of cystic fibrosis. She was given an elemental formula and pancreatic enzyme replacement. Within 4 days the edema had resolved; her weight dropped to 13.7 lb (6.2 kg), and the serum albumin level rose to 2.7 mg%. She continued to do well without diarrhea and was discharged home in stable condition.

DISCUSSION

Cystic fibrosis is the most frequent lethal genetic disease in whites.[1] Inherited in an autosomal recessive manner, the incidence in the white population is approximately 1:2,000 live births. Central to the pathogenesis of this disease is a generalized disturbance of exocrine gland function. Various excretory organs can be affected, including the pancreas and the gastrointestinal (GI), respiratory, hepatobiliary, and reproductive tracts. Thus, although chronic pulmonary disease contributes to much of the morbidity and practically all of the mortality in cystic fibrosis, the clinical spectrum of disease may be widespread. This discussion will focus on some of the GI complications of cystic fibrosis (Table 27–1). In addition, the unusual features of hypoproteinemia and edema as seen in this case will be reviewed.

Clinical Features

Cystic fibrosis is the leading cause of pancreatic insufficiency in North America.[1] Since pancreatic excretory enzymes are largely responsible for protein and fat digestion, a disturbance in pancreatic exocrine function can result in malabsorption of these major nutrients. This, in turn, gives rise to the clinical symptoms of poor growth and increased stool output characterized by steatorrhea and azotorrhea. In addition, fat-soluble vitamins and trace minerals may be lost in the stool, leading to deficiencies in vitamins A, D, E, and K as well as zinc and selenium.[2] Any child with chronic diarrhea, steatorrhea, or failure to thrive despite an adequate caloric intake should be screened for cystic fibrosis.

Pancreatic insufficiency is the most common of a variety of GI manifestations of cystic fibrosis and occurs in 80% to 85% of cases.[3] Pancreatic secretions are decreased in volume, viscid, and contain low concentrations of pancreatic enzymes and bicarbonate, leading to fat and protein malabsorption.[3] In addition to pancreatic insufficiency, patients with cystic fibrosis who do not have complete loss of pancreatic enzyme activity can develop recurrent acute pancreatitis. Thus, cystic fibrosis should also be considered in the patient with repeated episodes of pancreatitis.

Hepatobiliary complications have been reported in about 50% of cases of cystic fibrosis. In the neonatal period, cholestatic jaundice may be a presenting feature. Neonates with a conjugated hyperbilirubinemia should have a sweat test as part of their diagnostic evaluation. Hepatomegaly resulting from fatty infiltration of the liver is often found in patients with cystic fibrosis.[3] Other etiologies for an enlarged liver in these patients include viral or drug-induced hepatitis or cor pulmonale. Fulminant hepatocellular failure is quite unusual; although, about 5% of cases of cystic fibrosis with hepatic dysfunction will eventually develop cirrhosis. The significant consequence of liver disease is the potentially fatal complication of portal hypertension with resultant hypersplenism and esophageal varices.

The gallbladder and cystic duct can be functionally or anatomically abnormal in one third of cases.[3] Gallstones and their resultant complications have been well documented in these patients. Bile acid metabolism may be altered, but with appropriate use of pancreatic enzyme replacement, a normal bile acid pool is maintained.

TABLE 27–1.

The Gastrointestinal
Manifestations of Cystic Fibrosis

Pancreatic
  Pancreatic insufficiency
  Recurrent pancreatitis
Hepatobiliary
  Neonatal cholestatic jaundice
  Hepatomegaly
  Cirrhosis and portal hypertension
  Cholelithiasis
Intestinal
  Neonatal meconium ileus
  Neonatal small bowel atresia
  Intestinal mucosal dysfunction
  Meconium ileus equivalent
  Rectal prolapse

Intestinal mucosal function may also be impaired. Reduced oleic acid, phenylalanine, and glycine absorption have been demonstrated in these patients, suggesting the presence of small bowel mucosal defects.[4] Contrast studies of the upper small intestine may show multiple nonspecific abnormalities, including thickened folds, nodular filling defects, and redundancy. Histologically, there is normal villous architecture with an appropriate villous/crypt ratio; however, Brunner's glands appear to be enlarged, and there is an increased number of goblet cells.[4] Occasionally, increased mucoid material may be present in the intestinal lumen.

In the neonatal period, meconium ileus and small bowel atresia can occur. Cystic fibrosis must be considered in such cases of intestinal obstruction. Meconium ileus equivalent has been reported in 10% to 20% of adults with cystic fibrosis.[5] This bowel complication is seen in older patients, where the signs and symptoms of partial or complete intestinal obstruction mimic the picture of neonatal meconium ileus. In this condition, the stools are thick and viscid, precipitating a block to intestinal flow usually at the level of the terminal ileum and ascending colon. Patients can present with abdominal pain, distention, vomiting, and obstipation. Factors contributing to the development of meconium ileus equivalent include cessation of enzyme replacement, dehydration, or a change in diet. Most often, a precipitating cause will not be found. Interestingly, meconium ileus equivalent is not seen more frequently in patients who had meconium ileus in the neonatal period.[6] Acute episodes can be managed with IV rehydration, nasogastric suction for bowel decompression, and *N*-acetylcysteine enemas to relieve the obstructing stool.[7] In addition, pancreatic enzyme replacement should be continued.

Rectal prolapse can occur in about 20% of patients with cystic fibrosis and is usually seen in the younger age groups.[8] The cause of this condition is not known, although it may be related to poor muscular tone and malnutrition. The usual treatment is simple manual reduction of the prolapsed mucosa and surgery is rarely required. Prevention of constipation and improved respiratory condition by controlling infection and cough may be helpful.

This patient had an unusual presentation for cystic fibrosis. The features of hypoproteinemia and edema, which are probably related to an intestinal absorption defect, have been reported in less than 5% of all cases of cystic fibrosis. In one review of 229 cases of cystic fibrosis over an 18-year period, only 6 children presented with these features.[9] Most commonly, these infants are switched to a soy-based formula following a diarrheal illness and then develop the peripheral edema. However, hypoproteinemia and edema have also been reported in breast-fed and milk formula–fed infants with cystic fibrosis.[9] One study looked at the protein turnover in two patients with this syndrome and demonstrated that the hypoproteinemia was not secondary to a protein-losing enteropathy.[10] In another study, patients with cystic fibrosis fed a soy-based formula seemed to have a higher proportion of nitrogen excretion in their stools, suggesting that protein malabsorption rather than an enteropathy was responsible for the hypoproteinemia.[11] An antitrypsin effect has been demonstrated in soy formulas,[11] and this may be an important factor in the development of protein malabsorption and subsequent edema in patients with marginal pancreatic function. Certainly, further studies are required to clearly define the complex pathophysiology of this phenomenon. Nevertheless, soy-based formulas may be inappropriate for the infant with cystic fibrosis.

Diagnosis

The diagnosis of cystic fibrosis is confirmed by the sweat test. Using pilocarpine iontophoresis, the electrolyte composition of at least 100 mg of sweat is determined. A value of sweat chloride greater than 60 mEq/L is considered abnormal. False positive results may be seen in a variety of disorders, including adrenal insufficiency, glycogen storage disease type 1, hypothyroidism, and the mucopolysaccharidoses. A false negative result may occur in the presence of edema.[1]

Sometimes, particularly in the neonate, an adequate amount of sweat cannot be obtained and the sweat test is uninterpretable. To overcome this problem, a number of newer tests have been developed to diagnose cystic fibrosis in the neonatal period. Of these screening tests, the serum immunoreactive trypsinogen may be the most useful.[12] Trypsinogen, a proenzyme of trypsin that is synthesized by pancreatic acinar cells, is normally excreted via the pancreatic duct into the intestinal lumen. Younger patients with cystic fibrosis, who still maintain some pancreatic synthetic capability but have functional obstruction to excretory flow, will have excess "back leak" of acinar trypsinogen into the systemic circulation.[13] Thus, neonates with cystic fibrosis will have markedly elevated serum trypsinogen levels compared with normal newborns.

Pancreatic dysfunction or insufficiency can be determined by examination of duodenal fluid for reduced pancreatic enzyme secretion and abnormally low bicarbonate concentration following pancreatic stimulation.[14] Other indirect tests for pancreatic insufficiency include measurement of stool fat following a 72-hour collection or stool assays for trypsin and chymotrypsin. More recently, the para aminobenzoic acid (PABA) test has been used to screen for pancreatic dysfunction.[15] Bentiramide, which contains the PABA moiety, is ingested orally, and the PABA is cleaved by chymotrypsin. The PABA levels can be measured in the urine or serum.

Treatment

Cystic fibrosis is an inherited multisystem chronic disease. As such, optimal patient management necessitates a team approach with expertise drawn from various specialties. Respiratory, GI, nutritional, genetic, and psychosocial factors are among the numerous issues that concern these patients. To address each of these is beyond the scope of this discussion, but there are many excellent reviews.[16-18]

From the GI and nutritional standpoint, attention to caloric intake and assurance of adequate growth velocity are paramount to good patient care. Approximately 85% of cystic fibrosis patients will have pancreatic insufficiency and require enzyme replacement therapy and vitamin supplementation.[3] The dosage of synthetic enzyme should be titrated to the stool output. Overdoses of enzyme may be associated with perioral and perineal irritation. In addition, the high purine content of commercial enzyme preparations may lead to hyperuricosuria, but significant renal damage has not been documented.[19]

The use of pancreatic enzyme replacement therapy has allowed for a greater liberalization of the patient's diet and improved caloric intake, which ultimately has been shown to favorably affect prognosis.[20, 21] There is no longer any need for dietary restriction of fat in these patients. The patient described here, after being given an elemental formula and pancreatic enzyme supplementation, demonstrated rapid resolution of her edema. The serum protein levels normalized, and she continues to thrive.

SUMMARY

Cystic fibrosis is the leading cause of pancreatic insufficiency in the United States. Other GI manifestations include meconium ileus, cholestatic jaundice, rectal prolapse, and gallstones. A more unusual presentation for cystic fibrosis is hypoproteinemia and edema. One patient with this rare complication is discussed, and the possible causes of this particular constellation of symptoms are reviewed. The nutritional management for these patients includes pancreatic enzyme and vitamin supplementation and assurance of an adequate caloric diet aimed to maintain appropriate growth velocity.

REFERENCES

1. Wood RE, Boat TF, Doetshuk CF: State of the art: Cystic fibrosis. *Am Rev Respir Dis* 1976; 113:833–878.
2. Stead RJ, Redington AN, Hinks LJ, et al: Selenium deficiency and possible increased risk of carcinoma in adults with cystic fibrosis. *Lancet* 1985; 2:862–863.
3. Park RW, Grand RJ: Gastrointestinal manifestations of cystic fibrosis: A review. *Gastroenterology* 1981; 81:1143–1161.
4. Morin C, Roy C, Lasalle R, et al: Small bowel mucosal dysfunction in patients with cystic fibrosis. *J Pediatr* 1976; 88:213–216.
5. Rubinstein S, Moss R, Lewiston N: Constipation and meconium ileus equivalent in patients with cystic fibrosis. *Pediatrics* 1986; 78:473–479.

6. Rosenstein BJ, Langbaum TS: Incidence of distal intestinal obstruction syndrome in cystic fibrosis. *J Pediatr Gastroenterol Nutr* 1983; 2:299–301.
7. Weller PH: Clinical features, pathogenesis, and management of meconium ileus equivalent. *J R Soc Med* 1986; 79(suppl 12):36–37.
8. Stern RC, Izant RJ, Boat TF: Treatment and prognosis of rectal prolapse in cystic fibrosis. *Gastroenterology* 1982; 82:707–710.
9. Gunn T, Belmonte MM, Colle E, et al: Edema as the presenting symptom of cystic fibrosis: Difficulties in diagnosis. *Am J Dis Child* 1978; 132:317–318.
10. Nielsen OH, Larsen BF: The incidence of anemia, hypoproteinemia, and edema in infants presenting symptoms of cystic fibrosis: A retrospective study of the frequency of this symptom complex in 130 patients with cystic fibrosis. *J Pediatr Gastroenterol Nutr* 1982; 1:355–359.
11. Fleisher DS, DiGeorge A, Barness LA: Hypoproteinemia and edema in infants with cystic fibrosis of the pancreas. *J Pediatr* 1964; 64:341–348.
12. Ad hoc Committee Task Force on Neonatal Screening; Cystic Fibrosis Foundation: Neonatal screening for CF: Position paper. *Pediatrics* 1983; 72:741–745.
13. Crossley JR, Elliott RB, Smith PA: Dried blood spot screening for CF in the newborn. *Lancet* 1979; 1:472–474.
14. Zoppi G, Shmerling H, Gaburro D, et al: The electrolyte and protein contents and outputs in duodenal juice after pancreozymin and secretin stimulation in normal children and in patients with cystic fibrosis. *Acta Paediatr Scand* 1970; 59:692–696.
15. Nousia-Arvanitakis S, Arvanitakis C, Desai N, et al: Diagnosis of exocrine pancreatic insufficiency in cystic fibrosis by synthetic peptide N-benzoyl-L-tyrosyl-p-aminobenzoic acid. *J Pediatr* 1978; 92:734–737.
16. Matthews LW, Drotar D: Cystic fibrosis—a challenging long-term chronic disease. *Pediatr Clin North Am* 1984; 31:133–152.
17. Roy CC, Weber AM: Nutrition of the child with cystic fibrosis, in Walker WA, Watkins JB, (eds): *Nutrition in Pediatrics: Basic Science and Clinical Application.* Boston, Little, Brown & Co, 1985, pp 463–484.
18. Littlewood JM: An overview of the management of cystic fibrosis. *J R Soc Med* 1986; 79:55–63.
19. Davidson GP, Hassel FM, Crozier D, et al: Iatrogenic hyperuricemia in children with cystic fibrosis. *J Pediatr* 1978; 93:976–978.
20. Gaskin K, Gurwitz D, Durie P, et al: Improved respiratory prognosis in patients with cystic fibrosis and normal fat absorption. *J Pediatr* 1982; 100:857–862.
21. Neijens HJ, Duiverman EJ, Kerrebijn KF, et al: Influence of respiratory exacerbations on lung function and nutritional status in CF patients. *Acta Paediatr Scand* 1985; S317:39–41.

28 Constipation and Encopresis

Paul Harmatz, M.D.

A 5-year-old boy presented with a history of infrequent bowel movements, pain with bowel movements, intermittent rectal bleeding and soiling of underwear several times daily. At birth, following an uncomplicated pregnancy, labor, and delivery, the child passed meconium in the first 24 hours. He had several soft stools daily during the first 6 months of life while breast-feeding but subsequently developed constipation on a normal diet. By the age of 12 months, he was described as passing small hard lumps of stool every 1 to 3 days, associated with pain and straining. Small amounts of blood were intermittently seen on the outside of the stool. His stool frequency since starting kindergarten decreased to every 7 to 10 days, and soiling was noted for the first time. He had previously been treated with malt soup extract (Maltsupex), senna (Senokot), and mineral oil with only brief improvement.

Toilet training began in earnest at 3 years of age, and the child was toilet trained for both stool and urine by 3.5 years. His other medical history was unremarkable with the exception of three urinary tract infections. His development was age appropriate. The family history was positive for constipation in the father.

The child's family, including his 3-year-old sister, was supportive. The parents reported that he was very resistant to attending kindergarten and was often quite aggressive at home. The teacher described him as a quiet, withdrawn child at school. She did note several other students teasing him, saying that he smelled like ''poop.''

The child's physical examination included height and weight at the 50th percentile. The examination was unremarkable except for his abdominal examination, which revealed a palpable soft nontender mass in the left lower quadrant. Anorectal examination demonstrated a perianal fissure, normal position of the anus, normal anal wink and muscle tone, and a large mass of hard stool palpable just inside the rectum. Results of the neurologic examination in the lower extremities were normal.

A complete blood cell count and urinalysis were normal. An x-ray examination of the abdomen demonstrated a large amount of stool throughout the colon with no evidence of a spinal column defect. A rectal motility study demonstrated normal relaxation of the internal anal sphincter.

DISCUSSION

Constipation, with or without encopresis, is a very common, debilitating, and poorly managed problem among infants and children.[1, 2] Although most cases fall into the classification of "idiopathic" constipation, a careful evaluation is necessary to eliminate the possible organic causes.

A physician evaluating a child with the symptom of constipation must first determine precisely how the parent or child is defining the symptom. Much of our society considers a stool frequency of less than one stool per day as abnormal. In fact, the normal stool frequency in adults has been shown to range from three per day to three per week.[3] In pediatrics, obtaining such a standard definition based on frequency is more difficult because stool patterns change dramatically with age. Obviously, the association of pain, blood, decreased frequency, passage of very large-diameter stools, or soiling as was the case for this patient would all indicate a significant problem. It is important for the physician to differentiate normal variation in stool pattern from significant constipation to reassure parents in the first case and initiate appropriate evaluation and treatment in the second. The symptom, encopresis, can be defined as incontinence of stool after 4 years, an age when toilet training would normally be completed. By 5 years of age, the child presented here clearly fitted both quantitative and qualitative definitions of constipation and also developed evidence of encopresis.

Clinical Evaluation

The evaluation of constipation and encopresis should begin with a careful history and physical examination. This should be aimed at identifying possible medical conditions associated with constipation (Table 28–1). Attention should focus on bowel habits, including frequency, consistency, size, and difficulty of passage to determine if the patient truly has constipation. The time of onset can be helpful. For example, delayed passage of meconium (>24 hours) occurs in most patients with Hirschsprung's disease (aganglionic megacolon).[4] When the onset of constipation occurs within the first year of life and is resistant to medical intervention, there may be a 15% to 20% incidence of Hirschsprung's disease.[5]

A detailed behavioral history should be obtained, including school performance, socialization with peers, and behavioral problems at home or school. However, primary psychologic or behavioral problems leading to constipation account for only a small number of patients with "idiopathic" constipation. The majority of emotional or behavioral factors are generally secondary in this condition.

A complete physical examination should follow. Most patients with idiopathic constipation grow and gain weight normally. Deviations from the growth curves are unusual and require careful evaluation. The physical examination should emphasize the abdominal, rectal, and neurologic examinations. The abdominal examination is generally unremarkable, although one can often obtain some impression of the degree of stool retention. Anterior displacement of the anus and presence of a posterior "shelf" should be noted and have been suggested to play an etiologic role in certain cases of constipation.[6, 7] A rectum full of stool is usually found in "idiopathic" constipation. In contrast, a long, tight, empty rectal vault with a stool "gush" when the finger is removed should raise suspicion of Hirschsprung's disease. During the rectal examination, it is important to run the finger along the sacrum to identify any masses that can lead to constipation, such as sacrococcygeal teratoma or anterior meningocoele. Finally, a careful neurologic examination is necessary to rule out subtle spinal cord lesions that may result in constipation, and an anal wink should be confirmed in all cases.

Diagnostic Tests

The clinical presentation and physical examination often determine the need for further laboratory or radiographic studies. Most children can be started on treatment if "idiopathic" constipation is suspected; however, a urinalysis and urine culture should be routinely performed because a significant number of these children have recurrent urinary tract infections.[8] An abdominal radiograph may help identify the extent of fecal impaction and may be useful in following the patient during management, but the same can generally be accomplished with careful examinations.

More extensive evaluations utilizing rectal manometry, rectal biopsy, and barium enema are reserved for patients failing medical therapy or suspected of having me-

TABLE 28–1.
Causes of Constipation

Medical
  Hypothyroidism
  Malnutrition
  Irritable bowel syndrome
  Intestinal pseudo-obstruction
  Celiac disease
  Electrolyte disturbances
  Neurofibromatosis
  Inspissated meconium
  Infant botulism
  Medications (e.g., iron, opiates)
  Toxins (e.g., lead)
  Pheochromocytoma
  Cystic fibrosis
  Multiple endocrine adenomatosis type II b
  Crohn's disease
Anatomic
  Anorectal anomalies
  Hirschsprung disease
  Sacrococcygeal teratomas
  Spinal cord injury
  Meningomyelocele
  Neonatal small descending colon syndrome

gacolon (see Chapter 29). This condition may be either congenital, as in Hirschsprung disease, or acquired secondary to a variety of proved or postulated causes. In the congenital form, the dilated bowel is proximal to a narrowed segment in which intramural ganglion cells are absent in the submucosal (Meissner's) and myenteric (Auerbach's) plexuses.[4] The importance of considering this disease in the evaluation of any neonate, child, or adult with constipation cannot be overemphasized. Early diagnosis prior to the onset of enterocolitis can greatly reduce the mortality from 33% to 4% or less.[9] Studies in children with chronic constipation since the first year of life and failing medical therapy have demonstrated Hirschsprung disease in 9% to 17% of those investigated (see Chapter 29).[5]

Treatment

When the constipation or encopresis (or both) is of functional origin, the treatment involves three stages: (1) education, (2) initial catharsis, and (3) maintenance.[2] The education of the patient and family begins with a discussion of normal variation in stool patterns. The family is usually greatly relieved to hear how common the problem of constipation and encopresis is among young children (1%–2% of first graders). This discussion will often alleviate the guilt and blame that the parents may feel and the embarrassment that the child is experiencing. The need for close follow-up, support, and reinforcement (especially by phone) to adjust diet and medications is emphasized.

Decisions regarding the initial catharsis must be made cautiously. Children with a less chronic course and those with less stool retention can be treated with oral mineral oil therapy alone. Those patients with significant stool retention may require rectal enemas for effective evacuation. If enemas are given, 500 to 750 ml of normal saline can be given to a child twice daily. More than 2 days of treatment should not be required. Older children may benefit from bisacodyl USP (Dulcolax) after the initial 2 days of saline enemas. Sodium phosphate (Fleet) enemas are usually not recommended because they may result in electrolyte disturbance. Hospitalization may be required for those patients who cannot be adequately treated at home.

The third stage of therapy involves developing and maintaining a pattern of regular bowel movements that are soft and passed without pain. This often requires a combination of dietary changes, laxative medication (Table 28–2), behavior modification, and, rarely, psychiatric intervention. The diet should include an adequate amount of fiber.[10] Dietary fiber is a complex mixture of compounds including cellulose, hemicellulose, mucilages, gums, pectin, and lignins. These substances vary in their water-holding properties and effects on bacterial fermentation. Concerns have been raised that a high-fiber diet may alter mineral balance in children, but there are few clinical data to support this objection.[11]

Unfortunately, the high-fiber foods and whole-grain products are often unappealing, and a significant percentage of children consume less than the recommended daily allowance for fruits, vegetables, and cereals.[11] Some parental education regarding the benefits of increasing fiber intake for the whole family may help alter these findings. The action of fiber is complex and varies with the chemical composition of the fiber. Fiber may be conveniently added to the diet through the use

TABLE 28–2.
Therapeutic Choices for Constipation

Fiber (bulk forming)	Lubricant
Dietary (bran, cellulose)	Mineral oil
Metamucil	
Osmotic agents	Stimulant
Prune juice	Bisacodyl (Dulcolax)
Karo syrup	Senna (Senokot)
Maltsupex	Phenolphthalein (Ex-Lax)
Lactulose	Castor oil
Magnesium salts	
Stool softeners	
Dioctyl sodium sulfosuccinate (Colace)	

of whole-grain (not whole-wheat) breads. Crude bran (tasteless) may be added to prepared and baked foods. Diced prunes, dates, and raisins are less objectionable when added to cookies or sprinkled over cereal. High-fiber cereals are also useful. Commercially prepared fiber preparations can be added to juice or frozen into popsicles to increase palatability. Adequate fluids should be taken with fiber products.

The vast multitude of over-the-counter prescription laxatives for treating constipation and encopresis make the choice of medication confusing. It is helpful to become familiar with three or four specific medications, including mineral oil, fiber, and one or two stimulant laxatives (Table 28–2). One can thus be prepared for the expected response, side effects, and difficulties of administering the medication.

Constipation during infancy generally responds to an increased fluid intake. Osmotic agents such as Karo syrup (5–15 ml/8-oz [24-dl] bottle) or malt soup extract (15–60 ml/day) are also beneficial. Glycerin suppositories exert their effect locally by lubricating the rectum and stimulating the passage of stool.

Stool softeners such as dioctyl sodium sulfosuccinate USP (Colace) are surface-active agents, increasing penetration of stool by water.[10] They also have some effect on gastrointestinal motor and secretory function. They may be most useful in the child who requires chronic stool softening but may be at risk of aspiration.

Mineral oil (liquid petrolatum) is a hydrocarbon mixture that produces a loose, frothy stool. Though not especially palatable, it may be mixed with fruit juice and ice cubes. Several commercially flavored mineral oil preparations are available, but some of these also contain a second cathartic. Doses as low as 5 to 10 ml may be effective in relieving constipation, but much larger doses are generally required for chronic constipation and encopresis. Fifteen milliliters/15 kg given twice daily is a good initial dose. The dose may then be increased by 7.5 ml every other day until the stools produced are quite loose, but not runny. Small amounts of mineral oil are absorbed systemically, producing deposits in liver, spleen, lymph nodes, and other tissues. The clinical importance of these deposits is unknown. Concerns for fat-soluble vitamin absorption have been raised, but this does not appear to be an important problem.[12] Reports of lipid pneumonia following aspiration of mineral oil are uncommon but contraindicate its use in infants or children with severe gastroesophageal reflux or in those with significant neurologic impairment. Mineral oil doses should not be given just before bedtime.

Irritant laxatives, such as bisacodyl and senna are useful in the evacuation of stool during the initial therapy for chronic constipation.[2] They may also be necessary in patients not having regular soft bowel movements despite high doses of mineral oil. Frequent use of cathartic laxatives, however, may cause significant fluid and electrolyte disturbances.

Behavioral modification can be helpful in conjunction with changes in diet and use of laxatives. Enlisting the older child in the treatment plan is essential and can be aided by various measures such as comparing bowel training with athletic training. Many treatment protocols include reward systems, such as a star chart. The goals to be achieved should be attainable and involve the patient. For example, this child and his parents agreed on a star system whereby stools in the toilet were rewarded with one red star; four red stars resulted in one new toy.

Toileting at specific times is beneficial. Chances of successful stooling are improved in the mornings and 1 hour after meals. The possibility of needing to use the toilet at an inopportune moment (school, shopping mall) is thus also minimized. Teachers need to be aware that the child may need to make an emergency visit to the toilet.

Psychiatric referral can prove helpful in children with major social or family dysfunction or in children strongly resisting medical intervention. Older children may be particularly bothered by the embarrassment, loss of self-esteem, and social isolation associated with soiling in their pants. On relieving the constipation and encopresis, a major improvement in the child's emotional status may be seen.

SUMMARY

Constipation is usually a symptom that is readily amenable to changes in diet, behavior modification, and psychologic support. In special cases, anatomic and physiologic testing of the rectum and rectal sphincters will reveal a neuroanatomic abnormality that requires surgical intervention. Familiarity with a few commonly used laxatives and close follow-up and support of most children with constipation will permit the successful treatment of this problem.

REFERENCES

1. Davidson M, Kugler MM, Bauer CH: Diagnosis and management in children with severe and protracted constipation and obstipation. *J Pediatr* 1963; 62:261–275.
2. Levine MD: The schoolchild with encopresis. *Pediatr Rev* 1981; 2:285–290.
3. Drossman DA, Sandler RS, McKee DC, et al: Bowel patterns among subjects not seeking health care. *Gastroenterology* 1982; 83:529–534.
4. Swenson O, Sherman JO, Fisher JH: Diagnosis of congenital megacolon: An analysis of 501 patients. *J Pediatr Surg* 1973; 8:587–592.
5. Orr JD, Scobie WG: Presentation and incidence of Hirschsprung's disease. *Br Med J* 1983; 287:1671.

6. Hendren WH: Constipation caused by anterior location of the anus and its surgical correction. *J Pediatr Surg* 1978; 13:505–512.
7. Leape LL, Ramenofsky ML: A common cause of constipation in children. *J Pediatr Surg* 1978; 13:627–629.
8. Neumann PZ, deDomenico IJ, Nogrady MB: Constipation and urinary tract infection. *Pediatrics* 1973; 52:241–245.
9. Klein MD, Coran AG, Wesley JR, et al: Hirschsprung's disease in the newborn. *J Pediatr Surg* 1984; 19:370–374.
10. MacCara ME: The uses and abuses of laxatives. *Can Med Am* 1982; 126:780–782.
11. Forbes GB (ed): *Pediatric Nutrition Handbook.* Elk Grove, Ill, American Academy of Pediatrics, 1985, pp 99–103.
12. Clark JH, Russell GJ, Nagamori KE, et al: Serum B-carotene retinol, and alpha tocophocol levels during mineral oil therapy for constipation. *Am J Dis Child* 1987; 141:1210–1212.

29   Hirschsprung Disease

Richard A. Schreiber, M.D.C.M., F.R.C.P.(C)

A 7.8-lb (3.54-kg) male product of an uncomplicated pregnancy was born full term by spontaneous vaginal delivery to a 34-year-old gravida IV, para III, abortus I woman. The Apgar scores were 9 and 9 at 1 and 5 minutes, respectively. On the first day of life, vomiting occurred following each formula feeding. This progressed to bilious vomiting by day 2 of life, associated with abdominal distention, and he was transferred to our hospital. He had passed meconium on two occasions within the first 24 hours of life and had a watery meconium stool on the second day of life. There was no history of fever, irritability, or respiratory distress and no maternal history of recent illness or medication use. There was no family history of intestinal disease.

On physical examination he was slightly mottled appearing with a temperature of 37°C, a pulse of 134 beats per minute, and a respiratory rate of 38/minute. The weight was 7.4 lb (3.36 kg). The fontanelle was soft. The chest was clear, and the cardiovascular examination was unremarkable. The abdomen was distended and tympanitic. No masses were appreciated, and the rectal examination revealed Hem-occult-negative stool. Results of the laboratory evaluation included hemoglobin 18 gm/dl, hematocrit 55%, white blood cell (WBC) count 3,200/mm³ with 50% poly-morphonuclear lymphocytes, 7% bands, 40% lymphocytes, and 2% monocytes; the platelet count was 160,000/mm³. The electrolyte values were normal, but the BUN level was 29 mg/dl, and the creatinine level was 1.1 mg/dl. A urinalysis showed a specific gravity of 1.018 with 10 WBCs/high-powered field. Cultures of blood, stool, urine, and cerebrospinal fluid were obtained. An abdominal radiograph showed dilated loops of bowel, and a barium enema showed no sign of obstruction or transition zone. An upper gastrointestinal (GI) series was unremarkable and showed no evidence of malrotation. A nasogastric tube was inserted for bowel decompression, and antibiotic therapy was started. After 24 hours a repeat abdominal radiograph showed residual barium. Bacterial cultures were negative. Because of the slow clearing of barium, a rectal manometry was done. A paradoxical rise of sphincter pressure following balloon distention of the rectum was observed, consistent with Hirschsprung disease. A suction rectal biopsy at 2.5 cm revealed no ganglion cells. A full-thickness rectal biopsy obtained in the operating room confirmed the agan-glionosis, the aganglionic segment was resected and a right transverse colostomy was performed. The child subsequently did well and was discharged home on regular formula with the plan for a colostomy closure and an endorectal pull-through pro-cedure at a later date.

DISCUSSION

Hirschsprung disease, first described in 1887, is a congenital anomaly of the bowel characterized by functional colonic obstruction and megacolon.[1] The incidence is estimated to be 1 in 5,000 live births with a male/female predominance of 4:1.[2] In approximately 15% of affected children there is a prior family history of Hirschsprung disease. A higher incidence is seen in association with trisomy 21 and with neurologic abnormalities, including cerebral palsy, congenital deafness, and mental retardation.[3]

Pathophysiology

The abnormal pathologic finding in Hirschsprung disease is the absence of intramural ganglion cells in the affected bowel segment.[1] These nerve cells, derived from neural crest tissue, are thought to migrate caudally along the bowel during normal development.[1] It is believed that the arrest of this migration leads to the clinical picture of Hirschsprung disease. The aganglionic segment becomes functionally obstructed, and the bowel proximal to this affected region dilates, resulting in the clinical features of constipation and abdominal distention. Hence, this disease is also referred to as congenital aganglionic megacolon.

In about 75% of patients with Hirschsprung disease, aganglionosis is restricted to the rectosigmoid region.[4] Another 15% may lack ganglion cells up to the transverse colon. Total colonic aganglionosis is seen in less than 10% of cases.[5] Rarely can the disease extend to the distal ileum. Ultrashort Hirschsprung disease is a poorly defined entity but generally refers to aganglionosis limited to the distal third of the rectum.[6]

Clinical Features

The clinical presentation of Hirschsprung disease can vary according to the age of the patient and the length of the aganglionic segment. In the child with typical rectosigmoid involvement the first clues to diagnosis are usually constipation and abdominal distention (Table 29–1).[1] Failure to thrive, intermittent intestinal obstruction, and intermittent diarrhea may also be seen, but these features are less common. In contrast, intestinal obstruction or enterocolitis are the usual presenting findings of congenital aganglionic megacolon in the newborn or young infant.[7] Encopresis is not common in classical Hirschsprung disease but can be seen with the rare ultrashort segment disease.[1]

One of the most helpful facts to obtain from the history is the time that the child passed his first stool. In normal neonates, the first meconium stool is usually passed within the first 24 hours of life, yet only 6% of neonates with Hirschsprung disease pass meconium by this time.[8] Early passage of meconium, however, does not exclude Hirschsprung disease since more than one half of children with aganglionosis have had a bowel movement by 48 hours of age.[7]

Examination of the abdomen may reveal nonspecific features such as palpable

TABLE 29–1.
Clinical Presentation of Hirschsprung Disease
by Age*

Age	Manifestations
Newborn	Common
	Intestinal obstruction
	Enterocolitis
	Rare
	Intestinal perforation
Older children	Common
	Constipation
	Abdominal distention
	Rare
	Failure to thrive
	Intermittent obstruction
	Intermittent diarrhea
	Encopresis

*Adapted from Blisard and Kleinman.[1]

fecal masses or abdominal distention. The physical findings that correlate best with Hirschsprung disease are absence of stool in the rectal vault and increased sphincter tone.[9] Sometimes, on digital rectal examination, the sphincter seems to grasp the examining finger, and following removal of the digit, there is a sudden gush of stool.

Diagnosis

Although the history and physical examination may raise the possibility of congenital aganglionic megacolon, various tests are used to help establish the diagnosis. These include the barium enema, rectal manometry, and rectal biopsy. The barium enema is useful in demonstrating the "transition zone," or area of dilatation adjacent to the contracted aganglionic segment. Although this radiologic finding has a high specificity, failure to visualize a transition zone is especially common in infants and does not exclude the diagnosis of Hirschsprung disease.[10]

Rectal manometric studies are reliable and can be performed in any age group. In the normal state, distention of the rectum leads to relaxation of the internal sphincter and a drop in internal sphincter pressure. In Hirschsprung disease not only may there be a high baseline sphincter pressure but there is also a paradoxical rise in sphincter pressure following rectal distention (Figure 29–1). For accurate recording of pressures, the patient should be cooperative, and mild sedatives such as chloral hydrate are sometimes required. The procedure is not painful and is usually less traumatic than a digital rectal examination. Because the distance between the anus and rectal sphincter is short, errors in pressure recording can occur, especially in the neonatal group. However, in experienced hands, rectal manometry has proved to be a valuable tool for the diagnosis of Hirschsprung disease.[11, 12]

The suction rectal biopsy can be used to obtain tissue for histologic analysis

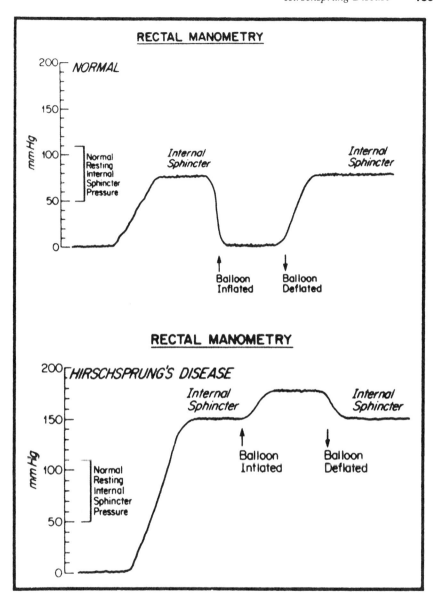

FIG 29–1.
Comparison of rectal manometry tracings from a normal child and a child with Hirschsprung disease.

and avoids the need for general anesthesia.[13] The histologic absence of ganglion cells is suggestive of, but not diagnostic for, Hirschsprung disease. Ganglion cells may be absent in one biopsy specimen, but this may represent a sampling error.[14] As a rule, at least two specimens are obtained for analysis. Histochemical staining of the suction rectal biopsy specimen for acetylcholinesterase can increase the diagnostic yield.[14] In the absence of intramural ganglion cells, a marked proliferation of nerve fibers occurs throughout the mucosa of the affected segment. Analysis of affected mucosal tissue with acetylcholinesterase staining can demonstrate this arborization of nerve fibers. Nevertheless, even with the most advanced techniques, the suction rectal biopsy can be either falsely positive or falsely negative for Hirschsprung disease.[15]

Since each laboratory study used for the diagnosis of Hirschsprung disease has limitations, most clinicians prefer to obtain more than one study to help confirm the diagnosis before proceeding with an operative procedure. The evaluation of Hirschsprung disease usually begins with a rectal manometric study. This is often accompanied by a suction rectal biopsy unless the manometric study is completely normal and a review of the history and physical examination is less suggestive for Hirschsprung disease. If, however, the history is suggestive but the rectal manometry is equivocal, a suction rectal biopsy is obtained. When both the manometric study and suction biopsy suggest Hirschsprung disease, a full-thickness rectal biopsy is obtained.

In the newborn and young infant, the diagnosis of Hirschsprung disease can be difficult because of the often atypical presentation. The American Academy of Pediatric Surgery review of 1,196 cases of Hirschsprung disease reported that physicians still fail to diagnose 85% of children by 1 month of age.[5] Early diagnosis of Hirschsprung disease is of particular importance to prevent the development of fatal enterocolitis. In a review of 47 patients with aganglionosis, 21 of the 24 children who developed enterocolitis had their onset in the neonatal period, and all who died from the acute episode of enterocolitis were neonates.[16] The authors concluded that the best treatment for the enterocolitis of Hirschsprung disease is prevention by early detection.

Some important points about the diagnosis of a child with suspected Hirschsprung disease in the newborn period are illustrated by this case report. The patient presented with features of intestinal obstruction characterized by bilious vomiting and abdominal distention but had passed meconium by 48 hours of age. In one study of 137 newborns who presented with signs and symptoms of intestinal obstruction, Hirschsprung disease was the second commonest cause.[7] This differs from the older age groups, where intestinal obstruction is a much less common presenting feature (see Table 29–1). When a newborn presents with the meconium plug syndrome, ileal atresia, or intestinal perforation, Hirschsprung disease should be considered in the differential diagnosis.[5, 17] Other conditions that should be considered include hypothyroidism, sepsis, the megacystis, microcolon, intestinal hypoperistalsis syndrome, and a variety of metabolic disturbances such as electrolyte disorders or adrenal insufficiency.

The barium enema study in our case did not show a transition zone, a radiologic feature that is more commonly seen in older children with Hirschsprung disease.

Although retention of barium at 24 hours is not a specific sign, it may be the only radiologic finding in some neonates.[7] Because of the presenting symptoms and the retained barium, a rectal manometry and biopsy were done. He was then taken to the operating room, where a full thickness biopsy confirmed the diagnosis.

Treatment

The treatment for Hirschsprung disease is surgical, and three techniques are currently popular: the Swenson, Duhamel, and Soave operations (Fig 29–2).[3] The Swenson operation involves resection of the aganglionic segment and direct end-to-end anastomosis of the proximal colon to the anorectal remnant. The major complication with this procedure is loss of sphincter control and fecal soilage. The Duhamel procedure involves a side-to-side anastomosis between the ganglion-containing colon and the aganglionic rectum. Difficulties with this operation have included fecalomas that formed in the aganglionic segment.[3] The Soave operation is the most frequently performed of these procedures at our institution and involves removal of the rectal mucosa while leaving the muscular wall intact. Ganglion-containing colon is then pulled through this muscular sleeve and anastomosed to the anorectal cuff. The major problems with the Soave procedure are the risk of developing an anastomotic stricture and increased stooling frequency.

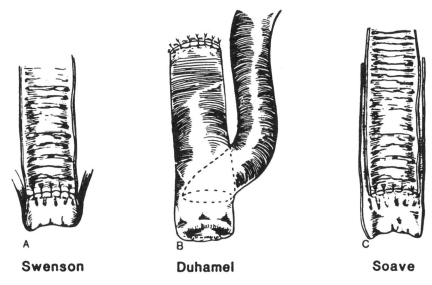

Swenson   **Duhamel**   **Soave**

FIG 29–2.
Three surgical techniques for Hirschsprung disease. **A,** Swenson: resection of aganglionic segment and direct end-to-end anastomosis. **B,** Duhamel: side-to-side anastomosis to blind-ending rectal stump. **C,** Soave: endorectal pullthrough after removal of the rectal mucosa. (From Martin LW, Torres M: Hirschsprung disease. *Surg Clin North Am* 1985; 65:1171–1179. Used with permission.)

SUMMARY

Hirschsprung disease, which is caused by an aganglionic segment of bowel, can have a variety of clinical presentations, which vary by age (see Table 29–1). The most severe diseases, enterocolitis and intestinal perforation, are seen in the neonatal period and can result in death if not recognized. A variety of tests are used to help diagnose Hirschsprung disease, but the final diagnosis rests on histologic evidence of absence of ganglion cells on rectal biopsy. The only therapy is surgical, and three operations are currently used in this country (see Fig 29–2). When this disease is recognized and treated early, the great majority of patients have a favorable outcome, as did the patient presented here.

REFERENCES

1. Blisard KS, Kleinman R: Hirschsprung's disease: A clinical and pathologic overview. *Hum Pathol* 1986; 17:1189–1191.
2. Lavery IC: The surgery of Hirschsprung's disease. *Surg Clin North Am* 1981; 63:161–175.
3. Martin LW, Torres M: Hirschsprung's disease. *Surg Clin North Am* 1985; 65:1171–1179.
4. Weinberg AG: Hirschsprung's disease—a pathologist's view. *Perspect Pediatr Pathol* 1975; 2:207–239.
5. Kleinhaus S, Boley SJ, Sheran M, et al: Hirschsprung's disease: A survey of the members of the surgical section of the American Academy of Pediatrics. *J Pediatr Surg* 1979; 14:588–596.
6. Chow CW, Campbell PE: Short segment Hirschsprung's disease as a cause of discrepancy between histologic, histochemical and clinical features. *J Pediatr Surg* 1983; 18:167–171.
7. Klein M, Coran AG, Wesly JR, et al: Hirschsprung's disease in the newborn. *J Pediatr Surg* 1984; 19:370–374.
8. Andrassy RJ, Isaacs H, Weitzmann JJ: Rectal suction biopsy for the diagnosis of Hirschsprung's disease. *Ann Surg* 1981; 193:419–424.
9. Swenson O, Sherman JO, Fisher JH: Diagnosis of congenital megacolon: An analysis of 501 patients. *J Pediatr Surg* 1973; 8:587–594.
10. Rosenfield NS, Ablow RC, Markowitz RI, et al: Hirschsprung's disease; accuracy of the barium enema examination. *Radiology* 1984; 150:393–400.
11. Tamate S, Shikawa C, Yamada C, et al: Manometric diagnosis of Hirschsprung's disease in the neonatal period. *J Pediatr Surg* 1984; 19:285–288.
12. Loening-Bauche V, Pringle KC, Ekwo EE: Anorectal manometry for the exclusion of Hirschsprung's disease in the neonate. *J Pediatr Gastroenterol Nutr* 1985; 4:596–603.
13. Noblett HR: A rectal suction biopsy for use in the diagnosis of Hirschsprung's disease. *J Pediatr Surg* 1969; 4:406–409.
14. Monkawa Y, Donahoe P, Hendren WH: Manometry and histochemistry in the diagnosis of Hirschsprung's disease. *Pediatrics* 1979; 63:865–877.
15. Cywes S: Hirschsprung's disease. Problems in diagnosis and management. *S Afr J Surg* 1975; 13:219–222.
16. Bill AH, Chapman ND: The enterocolitis of Hirschsprung's disease. *Am J Surg* 1962; 103:72–74.
17. Gauderer MWL, Rothstein FC, Izant RJ: Ileal atresia with long segment Hirschsprung's disease. *J Pediatr Surg* 1984; 19:15–17.

PART THREE

The Liver

30 Approach to the Neonate With Cholestasis

Eric S. Maller, M.D.

A 3-week-old male infant was found to be jaundiced at his first clinic appointment. He had been the 7.4-lb (3.4-kg) product of a full-term, uncomplicated pregnancy, labor, and delivery and was discharged from the nursery on day 3 of life with a peak total bilirubin value of 9.2 mg/dl while on breast milk. No direct bilirubin value was obtained. His mother reported that he was a vigorous exclusive breast-feeder with occasional small amounts of emesis and that his jaundice appeared to fade after a few days. There was no family history of liver disease or neonatal jaundice.

On physical examination he was an active, alert newborn infant. His weight, length, and head circumference were all at the 75th percentile. His skin was icteric without rash or petechiae. There was no adenopathy. The head showed no signs of trauma or cephalohematoma. Eye examination showed scleral icterus, presence of a red reflex, and no lens or other opacities. The nose, mouth, pharynx, neck, chest, and cardiac examinations were normal. The abdomen was soft and nondistended with a firm smooth liver edge 3 cm below the right costal margin, with a total span of 7 cm. The spleen was palpable 3 cm below the left costal margin. There were no other masses palpable. Rectal examination revealed pale, clay-colored stool that was negative for occult blood. His genitalia, extremities, and neurologic examination results were normal.

Laboratory evaluation revealed a hematocrit of 45% with normal white blood cell, differential cell, and reticulocyte counts. There was no evidence of hemolysis, and results of the direct Coombs' test were normal. The total bilirubin level was 8.9 mg/dl, with a direct-reacting fraction of 6.8 mg/dl. The albumin level was 3.1 gm/dl. The prothrombin time was 14.2 seconds (control 12.2 seconds), and the partial thromboplastin time was 49.2 seconds (control 35.4 seconds). The alanine aminotransferase (ALT) level was 95 mU/ml, the aspartate aminotransferase (AST) level was 110 mU/ml, the alkaline phosphatase level was 810 mU/ml, and the cholesterol level was 350 mg%, all elevated for age. The serum α_1-antitrypsin level was normal with MM protease inhibitor phenotype. The urine tested negative for reducing substances, bacteria, and protein. A sweat chloride determination was normal, as were serum thyroxine and thyroid-stimulating hormone levels. Ultrasound examination of the liver and biliary tree identified a small gall bladder, no dilated intrahepatic or extrahepatic ducts, and no cystic masses. A technetium 99m hepatobiliary scintigraphic scan was performed with good uptake of isotope by the liver but no excretion into the duodenum at 1, 6, or 24 hours after injection. A percutaneous needle liver biopsy showed interlobular bile duct proliferation with an inflammatory infiltrate in the portal area and preservation of lobular architecture. The patient was then prepared for exploratory laparotomy and intraoperative cholangiogram.

DISCUSSION

Approximately 1 in 500 infants will manifest neonatal cholestasis.[1] The patient described here demonstrates a fairly typical presentation of neonatal cholestasis or direct hyperbilirubinemia, which is defined by a direct bilirubin value greater than or equal to 2.0 mg/dl or accounting for greater than or equal to 15% of the total serum bilirubin value.[1] The most basic definition of "cholestasis" implies an absence or impairment of bile flow from the hepatocyte, where bile is formed, to the duodenum, where the excretory and digestive functions of bile are carried out. Disorders that interfere with this process at any point along a complex and, in many ways, poorly understood pathway may lead to the condition of cholestasis and associated jaundice. Therefore, it should come as no surprise that the causes of cholestasis in infancy are many and diverse.

Causes of Neonatal Cholestasis

Table 30–1 is a fairly comprehensive categoric listing of the known causes of cholestasis in the newborn and young infant.[2] The neonate with cholestasis presents both complex differential diagnostic possibilities as well as an urgent need to distinguish between them.

Of the many causes of neonatal cholestasis listed, approximately 60% to 80% are accounted for by either idiopathic neonatal hepatitis or biliary atresia, with α_1-antitrypsin being the next most common cause accounting for as many as 18% of cases in some series.[1]

TABLE 30–1.
Major Causes of Neonatal Cholestasis

I. Anatomic abnormalities
A. Extrahepatic (biliary atresia, choledochal cyst, biliary stenosis)
B. Intrahepatic abnormalities (idiopathic neonatal hepatitis, bile duct paucity syndrome [Alagille] and nonsyndromatic bile duct paucity)
II. Metabolic disorders (α_1-antitrypsin deficiency, tyrosinemia, galactosemia, hereditary fructose intolerance, glycogenosis type IV, cystic fibrosis)
III. Hepatitis
A. Infectious (toxoplasmosis, syphilis, rubella, cytomegalovirus, herpesvirus, echovirus, hepatitis B, etc.)
B. Toxic (total parenteral nutrition, sepsis)
IV. Genetic/chromosomal (Down syndrome, trisomy E group)
V. Miscellaneous (histiocytosis X, intestinal obstruction)

An increased direct serum bilirubin level is never benign, so the first step in evaluation is differentiating these children from infants with benign causes of increased unconjugated bilirubin levels, such as breast-feeding or the mobilization of sequestered blood from a large cephalohematoma. For children with conjugated hyperbilirubinemia, the evaluation of anatomic, infectious, or metabolic causes of cholestasis should proceed quickly since the results of the treatment may depend on the speed with which the diagnosis is made and treatment initiated. This urgency is especially important for biliary atresia, which accounts for 30% to 40% of the cases, because surgical therapy after 8 to 10 weeks of age has been associated with poorer outcome.[6]

Diagnosis

The overall diagnostic approach to the jaundiced neonate is outlined in Figure 30–1. As with all patients, any diagnostic approach begins with detailed maternal, family, and infant histories and a physical examination that may suggest particular causes of neonatal cholestasis. Laboratory and radiographic testing indicated by these findings are then pursued as summarized in Table 30–2.

In the maternal history, any unexplained illness during pregnancy or specific maternal exposures such as to raw meat or soiled cat litter (known to harbor the protozoan *Toxoplasma gondii*) may indicate a possible congenital infection. Paired serum titers from the mother or infant for toxoplasmosis, herpes simplex, rubella, cytomegaloviruses, and syphilis should always be drawn even in "uncomplicated" pregnancies. In addition, a maternal history of exposure to blood products or intravenous (IV) drug abuse should be sought, and hepatitis B surface antigen testing should be performed on the mother's and the infant's blood.

The family history may be of some importance particularly if other siblings or offspring of the parents' close relatives have had cholestatic jaundice in the newborn period. A positive history may indicate inherited metabolic disease such as cystic fibrosis, the cerebrohepatorenal syndrome of Zellweger, hereditary fructose intolerance, galactosemia, tyrosinemia, or α_1-antitrypsin deficiency (see Table 30–1). A positive family history may also indicate Alagille syndrome (arteriohepatic dysplasia), a form of intrahepatic biliary hypoplasia (see Chapter 34).[3] Metabolic disorders such as tyrosinemia (abnormal tyrosine degradation) and Zellweger's syndrome (absence of a subcellular organelle, the peroxisome) may be screened for by analysis of serum and urine amino and organic acids.[4] Hereditary fructose intolerance and galactosemia may be detected by testing the urine for reducing substances. Finally, α_1-antitrypsin deficiency, the commonest metabolic cause for cholestasis in the newborn, can be diagnosed by finding a low serum level of α_1-antitrypsin (see Chapter 35).

The infant's history may also provide some clues to the etiology of the cholestasis. Onset of jaundice within the first 24 hours of life or the early occurrence of acholic stools may indicate a greater likelihood of sepsis, a congenital process, or complete anatomic obstruction such as that due to a bile duct stricture or perforation. This patient, not atypically, appeared to have an early unconjugated hyperbilirubinemia, which then improved even as the onset of cholestasis supervened, though we cannot be sure since no direct bilirubin was initially drawn. Forceful and prolonged

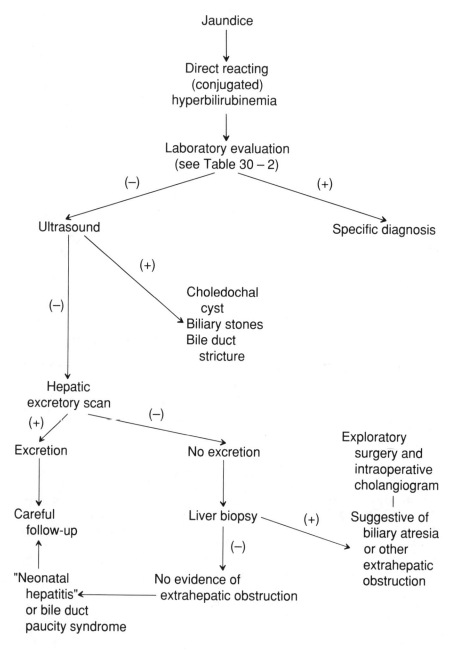

FIG 30–1.
Algorithm for evaluation of neonatal jaundice.

TABLE 30–2.
Evaluation of Jaundiced Neonate

1. Complete blood cell count, reticulocyte count, differential cell count, peripheral blood smear, infant and mother's blood types, and Coombs' test on infant's blood
2. Total and direct serum bilirubin values
3. Indices of hepatic synthetic function (prothrombin time, serum albumin level)
4. Indices of cholestasis or inflammation (alkaline phosphatase, aminotransferase, γ-glutamyl transpeptidase)
5. Cultures of urine (blood and spinal fluid as indicated)
6. Hepatitis B surface antigen (HBsAg); toxoplasmosis, rubella, cytomegalovirus, and herpes simplex (TORCH); Veneral Disease Research Laboratory (VDRL) titers
7. α_1-Antitrypsin serum level and phenotype
8. Metabolic screen (urine for reducing substances; urine and serum for amino and organic acids; galactose-1-phosphate uridyltransferase)
9. Thyroxine and thyroid-stimulating hormone levels
10. Sweat chloride concentration
11. Ultrasound
12. Hepatobiliary scintigraphy
13. Liver biopsy

emesis, compared to the mild regurgitation of our patient, should suggest the possibility of inherited metabolic disease such as galactosemia or tyrosinemia. In addition, a history of prolonged use of total parenteral nutrition use in the nursery has been implicated in cholestasis[5] but was clearly not an issue for this patient. Finally, the presence of acoholic stools for greater than 10 days and full-term gestation are epidemogically linked more to biliary atresia than neonatal hepatitis.[6]

It should be emphasized, however, that no risk factor is an absolute predictor of the etiology. The child with extrahepatic obstruction due to biliary atresia may have colored stools and can rarely be born prematurely, whereas a full-term infant with severe intrahepatic cholestasis of any cause may present with acholic stools.

The physical examination may provide additional diagnostic clues to the diagnosis of cholestasis. The fact that this patient was not small for gestational age, and did not have microcephaly, petechiae, adenopathy, or retinal lesions make a congenital infection less likely. This patient had no significant cardiac murmurs on examination, making Alagille syndrome unlikely since peripheral pulmonic stenosis is commonly present. Finally, physical examination of the liver may be of limited help in the diagnosis. A choledochal cyst may be palpable as a mass in the right upper quadrant. Also an irregular firm liver more likely indicates a fibrotic process such as biliary atresia. However, before 8 to 12 weeks of age, the size or consistency of the liver is rarely of help in differentiating the cause of cholestasis.

Laboratory Testing

The specific laboratory studies that should be obtained are included in Table 30–2. However, the most urgent determination to be made once cholestasis is diagnosed is whether bacterial infection in the form of systemic sepsis or even a localized urinary tract infection may cause an elevation in direct bilirubin values in the newborn.[7] The pathogenesis of the cholestasis is not known but may be mediated by circulating endotoxin, particularly from gram-negative organisms.[8] Although our patient appeared vigorous with no evidence of systemic disease or localized infections, a urine culture is always indicated, and cultures of the blood and spinal flood should also be obtained if there is any doubt regarding the infant's clinical status. Certain inherited metabolic causes of cholestasis such as galactosemia appear to place the newborn at considerably increased risk of gram-negative bacterial infection.[9] This disorder can be rapidly excluded by either direct assay of the enzyme galactose-1-phosphate uridyltransferase in red blood cells or by testing the urine for reducing substances if the infant is ingesting lactose (breast milk or lactose-containing formula). Finally, testing for thyroid function by determining serum thyroxine and thyroid-stimulating hormone may be helpful. Hypothyroidism alone usually produces a rise only in unconjugated bilirubin,[1] but it may be a marker for a more global pituitary defect (e.g., deficiencies in growth hormone or ACTH and cortisol secretion). These defects of pituitary function may occur alone or as part of the syndrome of deMorsier with atrophy of the optic disk and absent septum pellucidum.[10]

Radiography

If these laboratory investigations fail to reveal a cause for the cholestasis as they did in this patient, an ultrasound examination of the liver and biliary tree should be done. A choledochal cyst may be identified, or a dilated intrahepatic duct system may indicate that other causes of extrahepatic biliary obstruction such as a congenital bile duct stricture, bile duct perforation, or obstructing biliary mass or stone may be present. Though more than 50% of choledochal cysts are diagnosed in children less than 10 years of age, fewer than 5% are symptomatic before age 6 months (see Chapter 31).[11] However, should a cyst be demonstrated, the patient should proceed directly to surgery for immediate resection of the obstructing lesion.

If the ultrasound is not diagnostic, hepatobiliary scintigraphy using an IV dose of a ^{99m}Tc-labeled analogue of iminodiacetic acid (BIDA, PIPIDA, DISIDA, and others) should be performed.[12] Uptake by the liver and excretion of isotope into the duodenum proves the patency of the extrahepatic biliary tree and eliminates biliary atresia as a diagnostic possibility. However, absence of excretion of the isotope into the duodenum, even with good uptake by the liver, does not exclude the possibility of an intrahepatic disorder. Severe intrahepatic cholestatic processes such as idiopathic neonatal hepatitis or metabolic disorders can have no excretion of the isotope.

Liver Biopsy

If the screening laboratory tests, ultrasound, and scintigraphy have not established the diagnosis, the next step is a liver biopsy. A percutaneous liver biopsy is safe in experienced hands even in the smallest infants with normal coagulation studies and may help in avoiding an unnecessary open biopsy and laparotomy if findings suggestive of obstruction are absent. Table 30–3 summarizes the features found on liver biopsy that may suggest extrahepatic obstruction due to biliary atresia as opposed to neonatal hepatitis. Though sampling is a potential problem with needle biopsies, the findings of intralobular bile duct proliferation in a specimen containing five or more portal tracts, together with fibrosis and periductal inflammation, are presumptive evidence of extrahepatic obstruction if the possibility of α_1-antitrypsin deficiency has been eliminated.[13] Giant cells are usually considered as signs of neonatal hepatitis but can be present in patients with biliary atresia, especially if the patient is younger than 8 to 10 weeks of age at the time of biopsy. If biliary atresia is suggested, an exploratory laparotomy, wedge liver biopsy, and intraoperative cholangiogram of the biliary tree are then performed. If atresia of the extrahepatic biliary tree is found, surgical correction is undertaken (see Chapter 32).

Even when biliary atresia has been excluded, careful follow-up of the patient is mandatory because rare case reports have documented the progression of what was initially thought to be uncomplicated neonatal hepatitis to a condition with obliteration of the biliary tree and classic biliary atresia.[15] These cases indicate that neonatal hepatitis and biliary atresia may be different outcomes of a similar pathologic process.

SUMMARY

This case has provided the forum for a discussion of the approach to the child with neonatal cholestasis. The important facets of the history, physical examination, and laboratory evaluation have been reviewed. Guided by the principles of excluding known, treatable, life-threatening disorders and then excluding or surgically treating the patient with biliary atresia, the clinician can optimize the outcome and long-term survival of patients with neonatal cholestasis.

TABLE 30–3.
Liver Biopsy in Neonatal Cholestasis*†

Biliary Atresia	Hepatitis
Interlobular bile duct proliferation	Lobular disarray
Fibrosis or cirrhosis	Giant cell transformation
Periductular inflammation	Focal necrosis
with portal tract edema or expansion	Mononuclear cell infiltration

*Adapted from Spivak and Grand.[14]
†Percutaneous biopsy is 93%-95% accurate if ≥5 portal areas are present.[13]

REFERENCES

1. Mowat AP: Liver disorders in childhood, ed 2. New York, Butterworths, 1987, pp 24–71.
2. Balistreri WF: Neonatal cholestasis. *J Pediatr* 1985; 106:171–184.
3. Alagille D, Odievre M, Gautier M, et al: Hepatic ductular hypoplasia associated with characteristic facies, vertebral malformations, retarded physical, mental and sexual development, and cardiac murmur. *J Pediatr* 1975; 86:63–71.
4. Kelley RI: Reviews: The cerebrohepatorenal syndrome of Zellweger. *Am J Hum Genet* 1983; 16:503–517.
5. Chang CH, Brough AJ, Heidelberger P: Conjugated hyperbilirubinemia in infancy associated with parenteral nutrition. *J Pediatr* 1977; 90:361–367.
6. Alagille D: Cholestasis in the first three months of life. *Prog Liver Dis* 1979; 6:471–485.
7. Hamilton JR, Sass-Kortsak A: Jaundice associated with severe bacterial infection in young infants. *J Pediatr* 1963; 63:121–132.
8. Young RSK, Woods C, Towfighi J: Hepatic damage in neonatal rat due to *E. coli* endotoxin. *Dig Dis Sci* 1986; 31:651–656.
9. Levy HL, Seye SJ, Shih VE, et al: Sepsis due to *E. coli* in neonates with galactosemia. *N Engl J Med* 1977; 297:823–825.
10. Herman SP, Baggenstoss AH, Cloutier MD: Liver dysfunction and histologic abnormalities in neonatal hypopituitarism. *J Pediatr* 1975; 87:892–895.
11. Silverman A, Roy CC: *Pediatric Clinical Gastroenterology*, ed 3. St Louis, CV Mosby Co, 1983, pp 805–810.
12. Majd M, Reba RC, Altman RP: Hepatobiliary scintigraphy with ^{99m}technetium-PIPIDA in the evaluation of neonatal jaundice. *Pediatrics* 1981; 67:140–145.
13. Brough AJ, Bernstein J: Conjugated hyperbilirubinemia in early infancy: A reassessment of liver biopsy. *Hum Pathol* 1974; 5:507–516.
14. Spivak W, Grand RJ: General configuration of cholestasis in the newborn. *J Pediatr Gastroenterol Nutr* 1983; 2:381–392.
15. McDonald PH, Stehman FB, Stewart DR: Infantile obstructive cholangiopathy. *Am J Dis Child* 1979; 133:518–522.

31 Choledochal Cysts

Benjamin Shneider, M.D.
John D. Snyder, M.D.

A previously healthy 4-month-old girl presented with a 3-day history of inter-mittent nonbilious emesis and a 1-day history of jaundice. She had no history of fever, abdominal distention, or rash. Her stools were normally pigmented. The physical examination was remarkable for a mildly dehydrated infant with a tem-perature of 38.0°C. Slight scleral icterus was noted. Her abdomen had normal bowel sounds and was nontender, and no masses were palpated. The initial laboratory investigation was significant for an alanine aminotransferase (ALT) level of 88 mU/ml (normal <29 mU/ml), total bilirubin value of 4.6 mg/dl (normal <1.5 mg/dl) with a direct fraction of 2.8 and alkaline phosphatase value of 270 mU/ml (normal <150 mU/ml). Test results of serum electrolyte values, complete blood cell (CBC) count, albumin value, prothrombin time, partial thromboplastin time, ammonia value, amylase value, and urinalysis were unremarkable. Ultrasound revealed a dilated intrahepatic biliary tree and a large sacular dilatation of the common bile duct. Technetium scanning showed prompt hepatic uptake but no evidence of excretion into the biliary tree. An intraoperative cholangiogram demonstrated a large cystic dilatation of the common bile duct (Fig 31–1). One pigmented stone was found in the gallbladder, and another was found in the narrowed intrapancreatic portion of the common bile duct. The cyst, gallbladder, and common bile duct were resected. A hepaticojejunoduodenostomy was formed using an isolated jejunoconduit with an on-line intussusception. She did well postoperatively with normalization of the bil-irubin, transaminase, and alkaline phosphatase levels.

DISCUSSION

Although the differential diagnosis of an infant presenting with jaundice is extensive, only a handful of the diseases are potentially curable (see Chapter 30). Quick and accurate diagnosis is required to avoid complications and progression of the hepatic damage in these treatable conditions. Choledochal cyst, a term used to describe a wide variety of cystic dilatations of the biliary tree, is a prime example of a treatable cause of neonatal cholestasis. This chapter will review current clinical and experi-

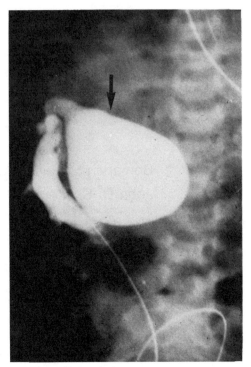

FIG 31–1.
Intraoperative cholangiogram demonstrating a large cystic dilatation *(arrow)* of the common bile duct.

mental evidence that supports the concept that this term actually represents a diversity of diseases with a common gross anatomic appearance.

The classification of choledochal cysts is based on their anatomic appearance. The original classification of Alonso-Lej et al.[1] has been expanded to include multiple cysts (2) (Fig 31–2).[2] Recently Lilly et al. proposed an additional category, a ''forme fruste'' choledochal cyst, that shares many of the clinical and pathophysiologic characteristics of choledochal cysts but has no dilatation of the biliary tree.[3]

Choledochal cysts are rare in the pediatric population; the incidence has been estimated at 1 in 13,000 hospital admissions.[2] This case is somewhat atypical in that there is a male predominance of this disease with ratios varying from 2:1 to 4:1.[4, 5] The majority of the reported cases are from Japan, although cases have been reported in virtually all racial groups.[6] The age of presentation varies widely from neonates to adults, but the commonest age of presentation is in the first decade of life.[7] The vast majority of the cysts are type I (see Fig 31–2).[6]

Pathophysiology

An understanding of the different hypotheses of the formation of choledochal cysts and their complications is essential to understanding the rationale of their therapy.

One of the most widely favored hypotheses is that choledochal cysts are a congenital lesion involving an unequal proliferation of epithelial cells in the fourth embryologic week when bile ducts are formed.[7] A weakened common bile duct wall results in dilation of the duct. Distal stenosis may also be required in the formation of the cyst, although most choledochal cysts do not have an associated stenosis. Such a process could have occurred in this child, who had a distal narrowing and obstruction secondary to a stone. The association of stones with choledochal cysts is well known.[7]

Recently, attention has been focused on abnormalities of the pancreaticobiliary junction. Reflux of pancreatic enzymes into the biliary tree has been suggested as a cause of inflammation and weakening of the bile duct wall.[8] This is supported by the finding of extremely high levels of amylase in choledochal cysts.[9, 10] Todani et al., using operative, transhepatic, or endoscopic retrograde cholangiopancreatography (ERCP), demonstrated an abnormally obtuse angle of the pancreaticobiliary junction in many patients with choledochal cysts.[9] This angle is believed to predispose to pancreatic enzyme reflux.

Another anatomic abnormality predisposing to pancreatic enzyme reflux is the

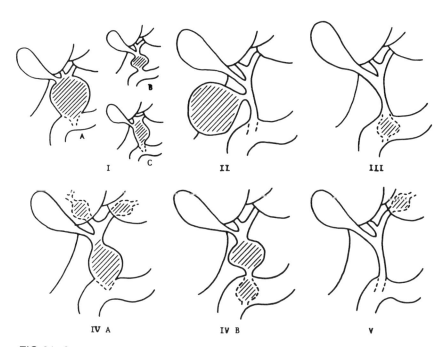

FIG 31–2.
Anatomical classification of choledochal cysts. I = extrahepatic cysts; II = extrahepatic diverticulum; III = intraduodenal cyst; IV A = intrahepatic and extrahepatic cysts; IV B = multiple extrahepatic cysts; and V = intrahepatic cyst(s). (From Crittenden SL, McKinley MJ: Choledochal cyst—clinical features and classification. *Am J Gastroenterol* 1985; 80:643–647. Reproduced by permission.)

"long common channel" described by Nagata et al.[11] Normally the pancreatic and biliary ducts converge in the tunica muscularis of the duodenum, and contraction of this musculature acts as a sphincter preventing reflux of their common effluents. The long common channel has no muscular sphincter, and pancreatic enzymes can reflux freely into the common bile duct.

Clinical Features

The classical presentation of a choledochal cyst is the triad of jaundice, pain, and an abdominal mass. As with many diseases, the classical presentation is the exception, with only 15% to 40% of patients presenting in this fashion.[5, 11] There are a wide variety of clinical signs and symptoms of choledochal cysts at presentation, and significant differences exist between children and adults (Table 31–1).

The clinical features in children are more attributable to acute obstruction, whereas adults are more likely to manifest signs of chronic hepatocellular damage. These findings support the hypothesis that the lesion is congenital and may be asymptomatic for many decades.

The infant presented here developed jaundice secondary to acute mechanical obstruction of the common bile duct. This is the commonest presentation in infants, and the laboratory values demonstrate evidence of cholestasis, biliary epithelial injury, and mild hepatocellular injury. Persistent obstruction can cause acholic stools and dark urine. Abdominal pain is thought to be secondary to stretching of the biliary or bowel mucosa. Occasionally the cyst can be large enough to present as a palpable abdominal mass. Care should be taken in examining the abdomen, because rough handling could cause rupture of the cyst. A large cyst could also cause bowel obstruction, and this patient's vomiting may have been secondary to a mass effect of the cyst. A child may also present with sepsis secondary to ascending cholangitis.

Persistent hepatocellular and biliary damage from bile stasis usually yields a different presentation in older patients. Insidious hepatocellular damage may become evident only once cirrhosis and portal hypertension are present. Pruritus, splenomegaly, bleeding varices, or hepatocellular dysfunction may be the first sign of a

TABLE 31–1.

Clinical Presentation*

Feature	Children, %	Adults, %
Jaundice	71	34
Abdominal pain	55	96
Hepatomegaly	46	14
Abdominal mass	42	14
Fever	34	41
Cholecystitis	13	—
Pancreatitis	12	35
Cholangiocarcinoma	0	24

*Adapted from Kim[6] and Nagorney et al.[15]

choledochal cyst. The increased incidence of cholangiocarcinoma in patients with choledochal cysts is well known and may present as weight loss and abdominal pain. Cholelithiasis is much more common in patients with choledochal cysts and accompanying cholecystitis or pancreatitis from acute obstruction can be the presentation.

Laboratory studies can be helpful in assessing the extent of disease associated with a choledochal cyst. Complete assessment of liver function tests is essential, including ALT, alkaline phosphatase, bilirubin, and ammonia values, clotting studies, and albumin levels. The serum amylase level should be checked, since it may be elevated in patients with pancreatic enzyme reflux.[9] Complete blood cell counts and blood cultures are important in excluding cholangitis.

Differential Diagnosis

Despite their rarity, the potential for surgical correction of choledochal cysts necessitates their consideration in the differential diagnosis of all forms of cholestatic jaundice (see Chapter 30). Prior to the development of advanced ultrasound techniques, choledochal cysts were most often diagnosed at surgery. The preoperative differential diagnosis included cholecystitis, cholelithiasis, abdominal tumor, obstructive jaundice, peritonitis, hepatic cyst or tumor, intestinal obstruction, pancreatic cyst, pancreatitis, intussusception, and duodenal ulcer.

Biliary cysts and biliary atresia can occur concurrently, and there is speculation that the pathogenesis of the two processes may be related.[4] Liver biopsy, hepatobiliary scanning, and intraoperative cholangiogram must be used to help exclude biliary atresia.

Diagnosis

Until recently the diagnosis of choledochal cyst was difficult. Historically, upper gastrointestinal x-ray studies and oral intravenous cholecystograms were used. Unfortunately, these two types of studies are not particularly sensitive. Endoscopic retrograde choledocopancreatography has been successful in defining the anatomy of the biliary tree in adults and is now being used more commonly in children. Percutaneous transhepatic cholangiography has also been successful in adults but has limited applications in the pediatric population.

The advent of ultrasound imaging and nuclear medicine scans has greatly improved the ability to diagnose choledochal cysts.[12] Few data establish the sensitivity and specificity of these techniques, yet they are currently the investigations of choice. In this case ultrasound demonstrated the cyst and its continuity with the biliary tree.

Hepatobiliary scanning compliments ultrasound by demonstrating the patency of the extrahepatic biliary tree. The scan in this patient showed evidence of complete obstruction after good uptake of the tracer by the hepatocytes. Computed tomography and magnetic resonance imaging have also been tried but do not add significantly to the diagnostic capabilities of ultrasound and hepatobiliary scanning.[13]

Therapy

Treatment of choledochal cysts is surgical. Medical therapy of a clinically significant lesion is associated with 97% mortality.[5] The potential complications, including calculi, cholangitis, sepsis, biliary cirrhosis, bile peritonitis, and cholangiocarcinoma, make nonsurgical therapy of symptomatic cysts untenable. The recommended therapy of an asymptomatic incidentally found cyst is usually surgery after weighing the risks of intervention with the potential complications of choledochal cysts.

The importance of excision of the choledochal cyst was recognized early in the history of its therapy, but high morbidity and mortality were associated with the technically difficult dissection of the fibrotic cyst from the underlying portal contents.[14] However, simple decompression by external drainage of the cyst yielded a high incidence of bile peritonitis and sepsis.[5] These difficulties led to the use of internal drainage procedures that resulted in initial success with decreased immediate morbidity and mortality. Unfortunately, there was a high incidence of long-term morbidity, including cholangitis, calculus formation, and pancreatitis.[5, 6, 15] Less commonly biliary cirrhosis and cholangiocarcinoma were seen.[6, 15] The cause of these problems was believed to be the persistent reservoir of bile or pancreatic enzymes.

Because of these complications, complete excision has been reexamined as a therapeutic option. In Japan in the last 15 years, complete excision has been accomplished with morbidity and mortality equivalent to internal drainage procedures.[15, 16] Lilly has developed a procedure that excises only the inside of the cyst, avoiding the difficult portal dissection.[4]

Currently the therapy of choice for a simple type I choledochal cyst is cyst excision with Roux-en-Y hepaticojejunostomy. Operative mortality is currently equivalent to internal drainage procedures.[14] The short-term morbidity of cholangitis, calculus formation, and pancreatitis has been significantly reduced.[6, 17] Data on the long-term complications of cholangiocarcinoma and biliary cirrhosis are not yet available.

In the child presented here an intussuscepted segment of jejunum was used to drain the hepatic tree. The intussusception acts to prevent reflux of intestinal contents into the porta hepatitis with the potential but as yet unproved advantage of preventing cholangitis.[18]

Recently, ERCP has been used in the treatment of a type I choledochal cyst and resulted in resolution of pain and vomiting and a decrease in the size of the cyst.[19] This procedure may be effective in simple distal obstruction but should be withheld for those patients with abnormal pancreaticobiliary junctions and potential reflux. Also, without excision of the cyst, the risks of the long-term complication of biliary cirrhosis and cholangiocarcinoma may still be present.

The surgical therapy of type II and III cysts is more straight-forward. Simple ligation and excision are the therapy of choice for a type II cyst.[2] Type III cysts have been treated with transduodenal excision.[2] Endoscopic retrograde cholangiopancreatography dilatation may become a nonsurgical alternative.

Type IVA cysts present a more difficult problem. When multiple intrahepatic cysts are present, complete resection is not always possible. Whether these cysts will resolve with the excision of the extrahepatic cyst is unclear. Currently the widest excision possible is recommended.[2] Type IVB cysts (multiple extrahepatic) are generally widely excised, although portoenterostomy is occasionally required.

Long-Term Complications

Kagawa et al. have reported a 3% risk of biliary carcinoma in patients with choledochal cysts that is at least 75 times greater than for other hospitalized patients.[20] The cause of the carcinoma is speculated to be bile stasis or refluxed pancreatic enzymes that could cause a degeneration-regeneration cycle that leads to anaplastic changes. This hypothesis is supported by the finding of an abnormal pancreaticobiliary junction in patients with cholangiocarcinoma without choledochal cysts.[11]

SUMMARY

Choledochal cysts are cystic dilatations of the biliary tree. They generally occur in boys less than 10 years old. The pathophysiology of their formation may involve several mechanisms, including abnormal pancreaticobiliary junctions. They usually present with cholestasis, cholangitis, and an abdominal mass. Choledochal cysts must be considered in the differential diagnosis of all cases of obstructive jaundice. The recommended therapy is complete excision and Roux-en-Y hepaticojejunostomy.

REFERENCES

1. Alonso-Lej F, Rever WB, Pessagno DJ: Congenital choledochal cyst, with a report of 2, and an analysis of 94 cases. *Int Abstr Surg* 1959; 108:1–30.
2. Crittenden SL, McKinley MJ: Choledochal cyst—clinical features and classification. *Am J Gastroenterol* 1985; 80:643–647.
3. Lilly JR, Stellin GP, Karrer FM: *Forme fruste* choledochal cyst. *J Pediatr Surg* 1985; 20:449–451.
4. Lilly JR. The surgical treatment of choledochal cyst. *Surg Gynecol Obstet* 1979; 149:36–42.
5. Flanigan DP: Biliary cysts. *Ann Surg* 1975; 182:635–643.
6. Kim SH: Choledochal cyst: Survey by the surgical section of the American Academy of Pediatrics. *J Pediatr Surg* 1981; 16:402–407.
7. Yamaguchi M: Congenital choledochal cyst. *Am J Surg* 1980; 140:653–657.
8. Babbitt DP: Congenital choledochal cysts: New etiological concept based on anomalous relationships of the common bile duct and pancreatic bulb. *Ann Radiol* 1969; 12:231–240.
9. Todani T, Watanabe Y, Fujii T, et al: Cylindrical dilatation of the choledochus: A special type of congenital bile duct dilatation. *Surgery* 1985; 98:964–966.
10. Yamashiro Y, Miyano T, Suruga K, et al: Experimental study of the pathogenesis of choledochal cyst and pancreatitis, with special reference to the role of bile acids and pancreatic enzymes in the anomalous choledocho-pancreatico ductal junction. *J Pediatr Gastroenterol Nutr* 1984; 333:721–727.
11. Nagata E, Sakai K, Kinoshita H, et al: Choledochal cyst: Complications of anomalous connection between the choledochus and pancreatic duct and carcinoma of the biliary tract. *World J Surg* 1986; 10:102–110.

12. Papanicolaou N, Abramson SJ, Teele RL, et al: Specific preoperative diagnosis of choledochal cysts by combined sonography and hepatobiliary scintigraphy. *Ann Radiol* 1985; 28:276–282.
13. Alexander MC, Haaga Jr: MR imaging of a choledochal cyst. *J Comput Assist Tomogr* 1985; 9:357–359.
14. Cheney M, Rustad DG, Lilly JR: Choledochal cyst. *World J Surg* 1985; 9:244–249.
15. Nagorney DM, McIlrath DC, Adson MA: Choledochal cysts in adults: Clinical management. *Surgery* 1984; 96:656–663.
16. Filler RM, Stringel G: Treatment of choledochal cyst by excision. *J Pediatr Surg* 1980; 15:437–442.
17. Takiff H, Stone M, Fonkalsrud EW: Choledochal cysts: Results of primary surgery and need for reoperation in young patients. *Am J Surg* 1985; 150:141–146.
18. Reynolds M, Luck SR, Raffensberger JG: The valved conduit prevents ascending cholangitis: A follow up. *J Pediatr Surg* 1985; 20:696–702.
19. Folsch UD, Weigel UR, Zappel H, et al: Choledochal cyst type 1: Successful endoscopic balloon dilatation of the distal common bile duct and sphincter of Oddi: a case report. *Gastroenterology* 1986; 24:195–199.
20. Kagawa Y, Kashihara S., Kuramoto S, et al: Carcinoma arising in a congenitally dilated biliary tract. *Gastroenterology* 1978; 74:1286–1294.

32 The Surgical Approach to Extrahepatic Biliary Atresia

Joseph P. Vacanti, M.D.

This girl was the product of a full-term pregnancy to a 28-year-old gravida IV, para III, abortus 1 woman and was born as a spontaneous vaginal delivery. Her birth weight was 6.5 lb (3 kg), and the Apgar scores were 9 at 1 and 5 minutes. The pregnancy was complicated by an abnormal Papanicolaou smear with severe dysplasia requiring colposcopy during the pregnancy. Otherwise the prenatal history was normal. One day after birth, jaundice was noted, with a total bilirubin value of 9.7 mg/dl and a direct component of 2.4 mg/dl. Over the first week of life the direct fraction rose to 4.3 mg/dl.

An evaluation for infectious causes, α_1-antitrypsin deficiency, cystic fibrosis, galactosemia, and other metabolic causes of cholestasis was negative. An abdominal ultrasound showed a small gallbladder with nonvisualization of the common hepatic duct and possible liver enlargement. A technetium 99m iminodiacetic nuclear scan showed poor uptake into the liver with no excretion. The patient was then treated for 1 week with phenobarbital but still had no excretion on restudy. She was therefore taken to the operating room at 7 weeks of age, where an exploration and intraoperative cholangiogram revealed extrahepatic biliary atresia. A Kasai portoenterostomy was performed. Her bilirubin level dropped from 18 to 7 mg/dl in the postoperative period but fell no further.

At 5 months of age she was evaluated for liver transplantation and was found to be a suitable candidate. Over the ensuing 13 months, her course was one of progressive hepatic deterioration, complicated by multiple episodes of sepsis often thought to be caused by ascending cholangitis. At 18 months of age, a suitable donor liver was found and a liver transplantation was performed. Her postoperative course was complicated by severe hepatic dysfunction for the first 36 hours and two episodes of steroid responsive rejection. However, she responded well to medical management, was discharged from the hospital, and is doing well.

DISCUSSION

Biliary atresia is a disease of unknown etiology in which the extrahepatic biliary ducts are nonpatent and thought to be actively destroyed over the first few weeks of life. It is a relatively rare disease, occurring in about 1 in 15,000 live births, but is seen in tertiary referral centers for children frequently enough to be a major problem in the care of children.[1] Biliary atresia occurs more frequently in girls, whereas the other major cause of cholestasis in infants, neonatal hepatitis, is seen more frequently in boys.[1] Neonatal hepatitis likewise occurs more commonly in low birth weight infants compared with children with biliary atresia, and the incidence of other congenital anomalies is significantly higher in children with neonatal hepatitis.

Pathophysiology

Most investigators now believe that biliary atresia is not a congenital malformation but rather a progressive sclerosis of biliary tissue that affects both the extrahepatic bile ducts, causing their gradual obliteration, and the intrahepatic bile ducts, causing damage more variable in nature. Since the entire extrahepatic remnant of the bile ducts is removed during the Kasai operation for biliary atresia, this tissue has been extensively studied. Complete fibrous obliteration is present at some level of the extrahepatic ducts in every case.[2] Most often, clusters of degenerating biliary epithelium are present in small remaining biliary radicles. They are surrounded by mononuclear inflammatory cells and reactive fibrosis. These changes advance to total fibrous obliteration unaccompanied by the inflammatory infiltrate seen in specimens from children operated on earlier in the disease process.[2] Results of liver biopsies performed at the time of surgery show cholestasis, giant cell transformation, portal fibrosis, and bile duct proliferation that accompanies the degenerative change in the intrahepatic bile duct epithelium.[2] There is often a mononuclear inflammatory cellular infiltrate in the portal areas, but it is not as intense as the inflammation seen in the extrahepatic portal scar.[2]

There is no generally accepted mechanism known to account for these changes. The evidence for progressive destruction of biliary tissue argues against defective embryogenesis as the major cause of biliary atresia. It has been hypothesized that an antenatal infection with reovirus type 3 may cause the biliary destruction of biliary atresia,[3] whereas others believe that an abnormal connection of the distal bile duct and pancreatic duct leads to reflux of pancreatic juice into the biliary tree causing epithelial sloughing.[4] Another hypothesis is that a dysfunction in immune regulation may lead to an autoimmune destruction of biliary epithelium, causing secondary obliteration of the extrahepatic biliary ducts and a variable insult to the intrahepatic ductal system.[5]

Clinical Features

In contrast to infants with neonatal hepatitis who may appear ill from birth, most children with biliary atresia do not show evidence for chronic illness in the first month to 6 weeks of life. However, they do develop increasing levels of conjugated hyperbilirubinemia. The child presented here was a bit atypical since her jaundice was noted on the first day of life. Except for jaundice, physical examination findings of liver disease may also be absent or mild in the first 6 weeks of life in biliary atresia.

Diagnosis

Jaundice in children with biliary atresia may be evident in the first week of life but is often not appreciated until 4 to 6 weeks of age. This jaundice may be an indication of biliary atresia or another serious, surgically treatable disorder such as choledochal cyst. If diagnosis and management are delayed, irreversible liver damage may result.

This jaundice must be differentiated from benign causes of jaundice including that found in a large percentage of healthy newborn infants who develop "physiologic jaundice of newborn" due to a temporary inability of the hepatocyte to excrete bilirubin. This condition can be worsened by breast milk feedings. It is the role of the pediatric surgeon to help identify those children with an obstructive component to their jaundice and to provide surgical drainage while the liver can still function. Since biliary drainage is more likely to be achieved with an operation before the age of 10 weeks, the workup of direct hyperbilirubinemia in the newborn period should be expeditious (see Chapter 30).[6] Most cases of infantile obstructive jaundice are due to the various causes of intrahepatic cholestasis or to extrahepatic obstruction of the biliary tree, either biliary atresia or choledochal cyst. Over the last 20 years, there have been many attempts to develop tests that would distinguish intrahepatic cholestasis from extrahepatic obstruction. Unfortunately, none have proved reliable and specific enough in most cases to avoid an exploratory laparotomy. Screening tests for infection, hematologic disease, or metabolic disease should be performed, but exploratory laparotomy should not be delayed while waiting for the results since favorable outcome is directly related to earlier age of surgical reconstruction in the case of biliary atresia.

Radiologic studies that have proved useful include ultrasonography, radioisotope imaging with technetium 99m iminodiacetic acid derivatives, or endoscopic retrograde cholangiopancreaticography (ERCP) in skilled hands. The presence of bile pigment in a 24-hour collection of duodenal fluid implies biliary continuity and therefore, intrahepatic cholestasis. Percutaneous liver biopsy at times may distinguish between extrahepatic obstruction and intrahepatic cholestasis[7] but can demonstrate an overlap of findings: giant cell transformation, ductular plugging, fibrosis, and ductular proliferation (see Chapter 30).[8]

Treatment

Operative Management.—Once the diagnosis of biliary atresia is suspected and cannot be ruled out by nonoperative means, operative exploration is undertaken to establish a diagnosis. If extrahepatic biliary atresia is found, the surgical team is prepared to proceed with a reconstructive Kasai portoenterostomy. The patient is explored through a small right subcostal incision. The gallbladder is visualized and, if present, is catheterized with a small feeding tube for an intraoperative cholangiogram. If free flow of contrast both distally into the duodenum and proximally into intrahepatic biliary radicles is not seen, the incision is then extended both laterally and medially across the midline. The porta hepatis is visualized, and the extent of extrahepatic fibrosis is assessed (Fig 32–1). In a small number of cases the common hepatic duct is patent and is continuous with intrahepatic radicles. In this situation,

DRAIN BY CHOLEDOCHOJEJUNOSTOMY

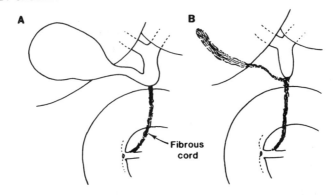

DRAIN BY PORTOENTEROSTOMY

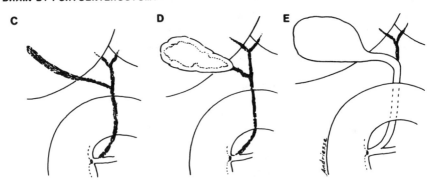

FIG 32–1.
Localization of the anatomic variants of extrahepatic biliary atresia. **A** and **B**, potential for drainage by choledochojejunostomy. **C–E**, potential for drainage by portoenterostomy.

a choledochojejunostomy can be performed. If the gallbladder, cystic duct, and distal common duct are patent, anastomosis of the fundus of the gallbladder to the under-surface of the liver can be accomplished, thereby decreasing the risk of ascending cholangitis. If no proximal ducts are visibly patent (so-called noncorrectable atresia), a Kasai portoenterostomy is constructed (Fig 32–2).

The Kasai procedure involves excision of the entire scarred remnant of the extrahepatic biliary tree and reconstruction using a Roux-en-Y limb of jejunum anastomosed to the hilum of the liver at the level of the hepatic capsule in the area of the biliary remnant (see Fig 32–2). The limb of intestine is usually 30 to 40 cm long. We prefer to anastomose it to the porta hepatis in an end-to-end fashion, but end-to-side reconstruction is also suitable. Many variations of this technique have been tried to decrease the complication of ascending cholangitis, but none has met with consistent success. A wedge biopsy of the liver is performed at the time of reconstruction.

Nutritional Management.—Thoughtful management of the nutritional status of children with liver disease and biliary atresia is important. The deficiency of bile acids resulting from poor flow of bile causes difficulty with the digestion and absorption of fats. This increase in fat malabsorption then causes the malabsorption of fat-soluble vitamins leading to deficiency states. Support of adequate protein and caloric intake can be accomplished with Portagen, which derives 85% of its fat calories from medium-chain triglycerides that do not require bile salts for absorption. Recently, concern has been raised over the potential for developing deficiencies in

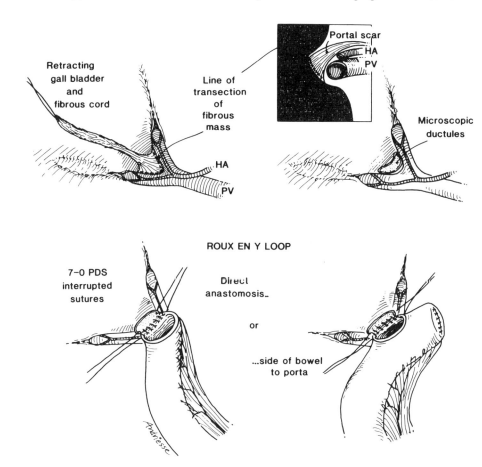

FIG 32–2.
Surgical technique for the portoenterostomy using a Roux-en-Y limb anastomosis to the hilum of the liver.

essential fatty acids if Portagen is used.[9] Pregestimil, which has 40% of fat as medium-chain triglycerides, and 60% as long-chain triglycerides, can provide the needed essential fatty acids while still being easily tolerated. The use of tube feedings may be important if anorexia occurs.

Supplementation for the fat-soluble vitamins, including vitamins A, D, E and K, is also necessary. Diuretic therapy may be necessary to control ascites.[9]

Results

Although Kasai et al. first reported the Kasai operation for biliary atresia in the American medical literature in 1968,[10] the results of the procedure and its role in the management of children with biliary atresia remain controversial. On one hand, Kasai has reported an 80% to 90% "cure" of biliary atresia with a properly performed portoenterostomy and careful postoperative management of cholangitis and nutrition.[11] In contrast, Starzl recommends listing a child for liver transplantation immediately after the diagnosis of biliary atresia is made, thus avoiding the portoenterostomy totally.[12] He believes the results of the Kasai operation do not warrant the increased morbidity and mortality it may cause for later liver transplantation. A review of several large series of patients in the United States and Japan show that approximately two thirds of patients will achieve bile drainage after a portoenterostomy. Of this group, approximately one half (or about one third of all patients) may never need liver transplantation, and many of the remaining patients will achieve growth before transplantation is necessary.[13]

Given the severe shortage of pediatric donor organs and the fact that 15% to 25% of children will die while awaiting a suitable donor, we agree that the Kasai operation should be offered to children with biliary atresia.[14] To help identify patients who will not do well with the Kasai procedure, a recent report suggested that intraoperative biopsy results can be correlated with bile output measured from the Kasai limb of intestine.[15] These findings may predict early failure of the Kasai and, therefore, which children require early listing for transplantation. Progress in the ability to discriminate which group of children with biliary atresia will benefit from the Kasai operation should improve our ability to manage this difficult group of patients.

SUMMARY

Extrahepatic biliary atresia is a disease of unknown etiology, which likely results from progressive sclerosis of biliary tissue. The diagnosis must be confirmed early in life since surgery is the only effective therapy and must be carried out by 10 weeks of age to have the best chance for success. The Kasai portoenterostomy (see Fig 32–2) is almost always the surgical procedure of choice. Nutritional management is an important arm of therapy and emphasizes supplying easily absorbed forms of fat, including essential fatty acids and fat-soluble vitamins. For children who have progressive liver disease following the Kasai procedure, liver transplantation now provides hope for long-term survival.

REFERENCES

1. Lilly JR: Biliary atresia: The jaundiced infant, in Welch KJ, Randolph JG, Ravitch MM, et al (eds): *Pediatric Surgery*, ed 4. Chicago, Year Book Medical Publishers, 1986, vol II, pp 1047–1056.
2. Chandra R: Histopathology of the liver and fibrous remnant in biliary atresia, in Ohi R (ed): *Biliary Atresia*. Professional Postgraduate Services, Tokyo, Japan, 1987, pp 55–61.
3. Morecki R, Glaser J, Cha S, et al: Biliary atresia and reovirus type 3 infection. *N Engl J Med* 1982; 307:481–484.
4. Miyano T, Suruga K, Suda K: Abnormal choledocho-pancreatic coductal junction related to the etiology of infantile obstructive jaundice disease. *J Pediatr Surg* 1979; 14:16–26.
5. Vacanti JP: Serum antibodies to biliary epithelium in children with biliary atresia. Paper presented at the 17th Meeting of the Am Pediatr Surg Assoc, May 1986.
6. Altman RP, Stolar CJH: Pediatric hepatobiliary disease. *Surg Clin North Am* 1985; 65:1245–1267.
7. Manolaki G, Larcher VF, Mowat AP, et al: The prelaparotomy diagnosis of extrahepatic biliary atresia. *Arch Dis Child* 1983; 58:591–594.
8. Shiraki K, Takayoshi O, Kaname T: Evaluation of various diagnostic methods in biliary atresia, in Ohi R, (ed): *Biliary Atresia*. Professional Postgraduate Services, Tokyo, Japan, 1987, pp 85–94.
9. Kaufman SS, Murray ND, Wood RP, et al: Nutritional support for the infant with extrahepatic biliary atresia. *J Pediatr* 1987; 110:679–686.
10. Kasai M, Kimura S, Asakura Y, et al: Surgical treatment of biliary atresia. *J Pediatr Surg* 1968; 3:665–675.
11. Kasai M: Personnel communication, 1987.
12. Starzl T: Personal communication, 1987.
13. Ohi R, Chiba T, Ohkochi N, et al: The present status of surgical treatment for biliary atresia: Report of the questionnaire of the main institutions in Japan, in Ohi R (ed): *Biliary Atresia*. Professional Postgraduate Services, Tokyo, Japan, 1987, pp 125–132.
14. Lilly JR, Hall RJ, Altman RP: Liver transplantation and Kasai operation in the first year of life: Therapeutic dilemina in biliary atresia. *J Pediatr* 1987; 110:561–562.
15. Vazquez-Estevez J, Stewart B, Shikes RH, et al: Biliary Atresia: Early determination of prognosis. *J Pediatr Surg* 1989; 24(1):48–51.

33 Total Parenteral Nutrition Cholestasis

Nancy Sheard, Sc.D., R.D.
Veronique A. Pelletier, M.D., F.R.C.P.(C)

The patient was the 1,840-gm female product of a 33-week gestation to a 26-year-old gravida 1, para 0 mother. The pregnancy had been complicated by a maternal urinary tract infection the week before delivery and premature rupture of membranes, accompanied by fever and an elevated white blood cell count. Following spontaneous vaginal delivery, the child had normal Apgar scores, and gavage formula feedings were begun. At 36 hours of life she developed apnea, bradycardia, acidosis, thrombocytopenia, and increasing abdominal girth. An abdominal radiogram revealed pneumatosis intestinalis but no evidence of perforation, and a diagnosis of necrotizing enterocolitis (NEC) was made. She stabilized on endotracheal respiratory ventilation, bowel rest, intravenous antibiotics, and central venous parenteral nutrition. She then did well except for evidence of a patent ductus arteriosus, which was ligated at 20 days of age.

At 1 month of age a barium enema was done to assess the extent of her NEC, and an extraluminal collection of barium was found. At surgery, large segments of necrotic small and large bowel, including the ileocecal valve, were resected, leaving 65 cm of small bowel and approximately one half of the colon.

She then was stable until 6 weeks of age, when direct hyperbilirubinemia and elevated liver aminotransferase levels developed. Her evaluation included a normal abdominal ultrasound and a hepatoiminodiacetic acid (HIDA) scan that revealed normal excretion from the biliary tree. Results of serologic screening for neonatal infection were negative, as was testing for galactosemia, amino acid abnormalities, α_1-antitrypsin deficiency, thyroid disease, and cystic fibrosis.

Because of chronic diarrhea secondary to short gut syndrome, total parenteral nutrition (TPN) was continued. Her bilirubin level rose to 12 mg/dl total, 10 mg/dl conjugated, and her aspartate aminotransferase (AST) level rose to 81 mU/ml and her alanine aminotransferase (ALT) level to 105 mU/ml. A percutaneous liver biopsy was performed (Fig 33–1), and histology revealed canalicular and hepatocellular bile stasis, fibrosis, and giant cell proliferation, consistent with TPN cholestasis.

At 2 months of age the patient began to tolerate an elemental formula (Pregestimil). By 6 months of age, almost all nourishment came from her enteral feedings, and her bilirubin and transaminase levels had returned to normal. Subsequent clinical evaluation and laboratory testing have revealed no evidence for liver disease.

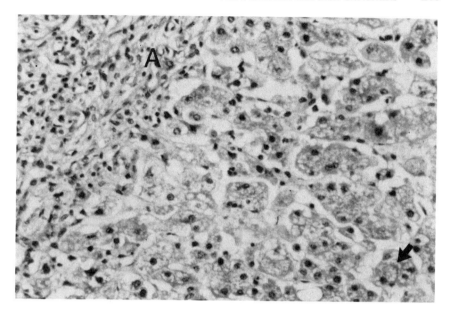

FIG 33–1.
Liver biopsy demonstrating moderate periportal inflammation *(A)* microvesicular fat, and intracanalicular bile plugs *(arrow)* (× 150).

DISCUSSION

Total parenteral nutrition–related liver disease can be a common occurrence in infants who receive parenteral nutrition. The incidence of liver disease associated with parenteral nutrition varies widely among institutions from 7% to 42%.[1–3]

The development of TPN liver disease is related to birth weight. Beale et al. reported an incidence of 7% in infants with a birth weight of 3.3 to 4.4 lb (1.5–2 kg), 18% in those weighing 2.2 to 3.3 lb (1–1.5 kg) at birth, and a 50% incidence in infants weighing less than 2.2 lb (1 kg) at birth.[4]

The occurrence of liver disease also increases with the duration of parenteral nutrition therapy. Approximately one half of the cases can be detected as early as 2 weeks following the initiation of parenteral nutrition.[1–6] Nearly all cases are diagnosed within 2 to 10 weeks of starting parenteral nutrition.

Several studies have demonstrated specific subgroups of patients who are at greater risk for developing cholestasis (Table 33–1). The lack of enteral feedings is the most common risk factor.[3, 4] Other factors include premature birth, abdominal surgery, hypoxia, and bacterial sepsis.[1, 3, 6–8]

TABLE 33–1.

Risk Factors Associated With
Total Parenteral Nutrition
Cholestasis

Lack of enteral feedings
Prematurity
Abdominal surgery
Sepsis
Hypoxic episode
Parenteral nutrition > 2 wk

Pathophysiology

The cause of TPN liver disease is multifactorial with prematurity, hypoxia, infection, and abdominal surgery being major risk factors. As previously discussed, the lack of enteral feedings may also be a significant causative factor in the development of this disorder. It is hypothesized that the decrease in vagal stimulation along with decreased gastrin and glucagon excretion during prolonged fasting result in diminished bile flow and a concomitant increase in serum bile acid and serum bilirubin levels. Gastrointestinal hormones in patients receiving parenteral nutrition are also in the fasting range. It has been suggested that cholecystokinin levels are insufficient to induce gallbladder contraction, resulting in a "physiologic" cholestasis.

Specific components of the parenteral nutrition solutions (i.e., amino acids, glucose, lipid, vitamins, minerals) have also been implicated in the etiology of TPN-related liver disease, although no clear cause and effect relationship has been documented (Table 33–2). A deficiency of one or more nutrients, which are not routinely included in parenteral nutrition solutions, may also contribute to the development of liver disease. Currently, the true etiology of this disorder remains unknown.

Several studies have suggested a relationship between the quantity of amino acids infused and the development of TPN cholestasis.[2, 10] The specific composition of amino acid solutions has also been implicated in the etiology of TPN-related liver disease. Newer amino acid solutions have been designed to more closely meet the requirements of pediatric patients. Although preliminary data confirm their efficacy in promoting growth and positive nitrogen balance, their efficacy in preventing TPN-related liver disease has not been determined.[11]

The amino acid tryptophan is unstable in commercial amino acid solutions perhaps due to exposure to light or to the presence of the antioxidant bisulfite, commonly found in amino acid solutions. The infusion of degradation by-products of tryptophan in rats results in periportal fatty changes in the liver.[12] It is not clear what role such compounds might have in the etiology of cholestasis in humans. The development of such degradation by-products is prevented by mixing and using the parenteral solutions within a 24- to 48-hour period and protecting them from bright light.

The oversupply of calories has been implicated in the etiology of hepatic dysfunction in adults receiving parenteral nutrition.[13, 14] Excessive energy intake results in increased fatty acid synthesis in the liver, leading to steatosis and increased glycogen and water content of the liver.[13] The consequent swelling of hepatocytes may lead to canalicular obstruction and cholestasis. The source of the excess calories (i.e., fat or glucose) does not appear to be a critical factor in the genesis of TPN-related liver disease.[2, 4, 8, 9]

Because metabolic pathways are immature in the newborn, certain nutrients may become essential components of the infant's diet. Several of these, including taurine, choline, and carnitine, may play a role in the development of TPN cholestasis.

Taurine is involved in a number of important metabolic reactions in the body, including the conjugation of bile salts. In the first months of life, bile acids are conjugated primarily with taurine rather than glycine.[15] Taurine-conjugated bile acids stimulate bile salt secretion as well as aid in fat digestion.[16] When taurine intake is low, more bile acids are conjugated with glycine.[15] In the adult guinea pig and rat, cholestasis can be induced by lithocholic acid, a by-product of the glycine conjugate.[5] Taurine supplementation can protect against this.[17] Similar findings in humans have not been reported.

Both choline and carnitine are required for normal lipid metabolism.[18, 19] In animals, a deficiency of either compound produces liver dysfunction.[19, 20] During development, the ability of the liver to synthesize these compounds is limited.[21] Total parenteral nutrition solutions do not contain these nutrients, and thus, deficiencies may lead to or aggravate TPN liver disease.

Clinical Features

Commonly, TPN liver disease presents in the first 2 to 8 weeks of therapy. It occurs most often in low birth weight infants and is frequently associated with sepsis, ischemia, or surgery of the gastrointestinal (GI) tract. Lack of enteral feedings is a universal finding. Clinically, the direct bilirubin level rises gradually, as does the alkaline phosphatase level. Increases in serum transaminase levels occur later in the course of the disease. Histopathologic changes occur over time as well. Discontinuation of parenteral nutrition or initiation of enteral feedings will result in improvement in liver function and histologic changes. If parenteral nutrition therapy persists, with continued lack of enteral stimulation, cirrhosis and death can occur.

TABLE 33–2.
Possible Etiologies of Total
Parenteral Nutrition Cholestasis

Excess calories
Amino acid excess or imbalance
Tryptophan degradation products
Nutrient deficiency
Taurine
Carnitine
Choline

Diagnosis

There is no specific or sensitive test currently available to diagnose TPN-associated liver disease. Usually, other causes of cholestasis must first be ruled out, as was done for this patient. These include infections, inborn errors of metabolism and obstruction of the extrahepatic biliary system. An elevated direct bilirubin level is the earliest abnormality seen in pediatric patients.[1, 6] Increases in serum amino acid transferases (ALT, AST) may not be observed until later in the progression of liver disease. γ-Glutamyl transpeptidase, 5'nucleotidase, and alkaline phosphatase levels are often elevated as the disease progresses but are no more sensitive or specific than bilirubin and transaminase levels. Some patients will develop synthetic dysfunction, and a small number of these will progress to hepatic failure.[8, 22] Early in the course, there is no way to determine which patients will develop irreversible disease.

Since the infant liver has only a limited number of ways to respond to insults, the liver biopsy demonstrates features common to a number of cholestatic disorders. Canalicular and hepatocellular bile stasis, giant cell transformation, Kupffer cell hyperplasia, cellular infiltrates (which sometimes include eosinophils), and bile duct proliferation may be present.[21, 23] In a small percentage of infants, fibrosis or cirrhosis may also be present. Steatosis of varying degrees is a common finding. None of these findings is specific for TPN cholestasis, and therefore, the liver biopsy is useful mostly to assess the degree of damage and to exclude certain other known causes of infantile cholestasis.[24]

Treatment

Liver disease that results from parenteral nutrition is usually reversible once this therapy is discontinued.[3, 9] In certain instances, however, it is not possible to withdraw parenteral nutrition completely. Because the lack of enteral feedings has been linked to the development of TPN cholestasis, it seems feasible to encourage the use of the GI tract to mechanically stimulate the flow of bile. One study in adults demonstrated a decreased incidence of cholestasis in patients who received as little as 500 kcal/day enterally.[24]

Because excessive calories have been implicated as a causative factor in the development of TPN liver disease, it is important to provide adequate but not excessive energy. A balance of glucose and fat should be provided. Protein intakes should approximate 2 to 3 gm/kg/day.

Maini et al. have suggested that cycling parenteral nutrition solutions in adults over a 12- to 16-hour period may decrease the incidence of liver disease.[25] As yet, similar data in pediatric patients have not been collected.[25] Finally, nutrients such as carnitine, taurine, and choline, which are not considered essential in older children and adults, may need to be provided in the parenteral nutrition solutions of infants.

SUMMARY

Cholestatic liver disease is a frequent complication in infants who receive parenteral nutrition. The etiology of this disorder is probably multifactorial. Although the composition of parenteral nutrition solutions may play a role in the development of cholestasis, at this time there are limited data to suggest how to change parenteral solutions to alter the course of this disease. However, early initiation of enteral feedings can lead to prompt reversal of findings. Even patients who have evidence for fibrosis, such as the patient presented here, can often have a good outcome when enteral feedings are started.

REFERENCES

1. Bell RL, Ferry GD, Smith EO, et al: Total parenteral nutrition-related cholestasis in infants. *J Parent Enteral Nutr* 1986; 10:356–359.
2. Vileisis R, Inwood RJ, Hunt CE: Prospective controlled study of parenteral nutrition-associated cholestatic jaundice: Effect of protein intake. *J Pediatr* 1980; 96:893–897.
3. Rodgers BM, Hollenbeck IL, Donnelly W, et al: Intrahepatic cholestasis with parenteral alimentation. *Am J Surgery* 1976; 131:149–155.
4. Beale EF, Nelson RM, Bucciarelli RL, et al: Intrahepatic cholestasis associated with parenteral nutrition in premature infants. *Pediatrics* 1979; 64:342–347.
5. Sondheimer JM, Bryan H, Andrews W, et al: Cholestatic tendencies in premature infants on and off parenteral nutrition. *Pediatrics* 1978; 62:984–989.
6. Merritt RJ: Cholestasis associated with total parenteral nutrition. *J Pediatr Gastroenterol Nutr* 1986; 5:9–22.
7. Pereira GR, Sherman MS, DiGiacomo J, et al: Hyperalimentation-induced cholestasis. Increased incidence and severity in premature infants. *Am J Dis Child* 1981; 135:842–845.
8. Postuma R, Trevenen CL: Liver disease in infants receiving total parenteral nutrition. *Pediatrics* 1979; 63:110–115.
9. Black DD, Suttle EA, Whitington PT, et al: The effect of short-term total parenteral nutrition on hepatic function in the human neonate: A prospective randomized study demonstrating alteration of hepatic canalicular function. *J Pediatr* 1981; 99:445–449.
10. Sankaran K, Berscheid B, Verma V, et al: An evaluation of total parenteral nutrition using Vamin and Aminosyn as protein base in critically ill pre term infants. *J Parent Enteral Nutr* 1985; 9:439–442.
11. Hay WW, Storm MC: Evaluation of a new pediatric amino acid formulation in low birthweight infants. Paper presented at the Second Scientific Symposium on Fetal and Neonatal Nutrition and Metabolism, Denver, 1984.
12. Grant JP, Cox LE, Kleinman LM, et al: Serum hepatic enzyme and bilirubin elevations during total parenteral nutrition. *Surg Gynecol Obstet* 1977; 145:573–580.
13. Stein TP, Mullen JL: Hepatic fat accumulation in man with excess parenteral glucose. *Nutr Res* 1985; 5:1347–1351.
14. Lowry SF, Brennan MF: Abnormal liver function during parenteral nutrition: Relation to infusion excess. *J Surg Res* 1979; 26:300–307.
15. Jarvenpao AL, Rassin OK, Kuitunen P, et al: Feeding the low-birthweight infant: III. Diet influences bile acid metabolism. *Pediatrics* 1983; 72:677–683.
16. Malgelada JR, DiMagno EP, Summerskill WHJ, et al: Regulation of pancreatic and gallbladder functions by intraluminal fatty acids and bile acids in man. *J Clin Invest* 1976; 58:493–499.
17. Dorvil NP, Yausef M, Tuchweber B, et al: Taurine prevents cholestasis induced by lithocholic acid sulfate in guinea pigs. *Am J Clin Nutr* 1983; 37:221–232.

18. Zeisel SH: Dietary choline: Biochemistry, physiology, and pharmacology. *Annu Rev Nutr* 1981; 1:95–121.
19. Borum P: Carnitine. *Annu Rev Nutr* 1983; 3:233–259.
20. Lombardi B: Pathogenesis of fatty liver. *Fed Proc* 1965; 24:1200–1205.
21. Zeisel SH, Wurtman RJ: Developmental changes in rat blood choline concentration. *Biochem J* 1981; 198:565.
22. Peden VH, Witzleben CL, Skeleton MA: Total parenteral nutrition. *J Pediatr* 1971; 78:180–181.
23. Dahms BB, Halpin JC: Serial liver biopsies in parenteral nutrition-associated cholestasis of early infancy. *Gastroenterology* 1981; 81:136–144.
24. Pallares R, Stigres-Serra A, Fuentes J, et al: Cholestasis associated with parenteral nutrition. *Lancet* 1983; 1:758–759.
25. Maini B, Blackburn GL, Bistrian BR, et al: Cyclic hyperalimentation: An optimal technique for preservation of visceral protein. *J Surg Res* 1976; 19:515–535.

34 Syndromic and Nonsyndromic Paucity of Bile Ducts

Richard H. Sandler, M.D.

A 2-month-old boy was referred for evaluation of cholestatic jaundice. He was born full term by a normal spontaneous vaginal delivery after an unremarkable pregnancy. On day 1 of life, mixed hyperbilirubinemia was noted, without physical examination or laboratory evidence of congenital infection or hemolytic anemia. The child otherwise looked well and was discharged home on day 3 of life with the diagnosis of physiologic jaundice. On day 10 of life the child presented with vomiting and jaundice. Results of a sepsis workup were normal. However, a total bilirubin level of 8 mg/dl, with a direct bilirubin level of 4 mg/dl was noted, along with an alanine aminotransferase (ALT) level of 300 mU/ml (normal (29 mU/ml) and an alkaline phosphatase level of 380 mU/ml (normal <150 mU/ml). Hepatitis serology results were normal for the infant and the mother. Neither a liver biopsy nor a nuclear medicine technetium 99m diisopropyl iminodiacetic (DISIDA) biliary excretion scan was done. Over the next 10 days the vomiting resolved, and the child was discharged with the diagnosis of "neonatal hepatitis."

At 2 months of age he was growing well, had a good appetite, seemed alert and comfortable, and had normal-colored stools, but since he remained icteric, he was referred to Children's Hospital for further evaluation.

On admission the child appeared icteric, though comfortable and alert, with height and weight at the 30th percentile for age. The child's appearance was similar to his mother's, both having prominent foreheads, moderate hypertelorism, small chins, and flattened nasal bridges. The patient's lungs were clear. The heart examination revealed a grade II/VI systolic murmur, heard best at the left upper sternal border. His abdomen was not distended, he had normal bowel sounds, the spleen tip was barely palpable, and the liver edge was 4.5 cm below the right costal margin in the midclavicular line. The total liver span was 7 cm to percussion. The liver was smooth, mildly firm, but not hard. The rectal examination showed soft, yellow, heme-negative stool.

The initial laboratory examination included an aspartate aminotransferase (AST) level of 73 mU/ml (normal <25 mU/ml), ALT level of 90 mU/ml, alkaline phosphatase level of 150 mU/ml, an albumin level of 4.6 gm/dl, a total bilirubin level of 4.3 mg/dl, and a conjugated bilirubin level of 2.2 mg/dl. The prothrombin time and partial thromboplastin time were normal. Triglyceride and cholesterol levels were elevated at 401 mg/dl (normal <100 mg/dl) and 200 mg/dl (normal <180 mg/dl), respectively. His leukocyte count was 10,000/mm³ with a normal differential, and his hemoglobin level was 10 gm/dl. The fasting glucose level was 95 mg/dl, creatinine level 0.5 mg/dl, and the blood urea nitrogen value (BUN) 18 mg/dl. The urine was negative for reducing substances.

Ultrasound of the liver showed normal-appearing hepatic parenchyma and vasculature. No dilated ducts were seen. The gallbladder could not be identified. A DISIDA nuclear medicine scan showed delayed uptake by the liver but good excretion through the biliary system. A liver biopsy was then done, which showed paucity of intrahepatic bile ducts, cholestasis, and periportal iron deposition (Fig 34–1).

DISCUSSION

The general approach to infants with conjugated hyperbilirubinemia is presented in detail in Chapter 30; this discussion will center on intrahepatic causes of cholestasis associated with paucity of bile ducts.[1, 2] There are two categories recognized for patients having paucity of bile ducts: the syndromic and the nonsyndromic types.[2] The syndromic form (Alagille syndrome) was first recognized in the early 1970s and accounts for about 50% of the pediatric patients with bile duct paucity and cholestatic jaundice. In 1975, Alagille and co-workers first reported their experience with chil-

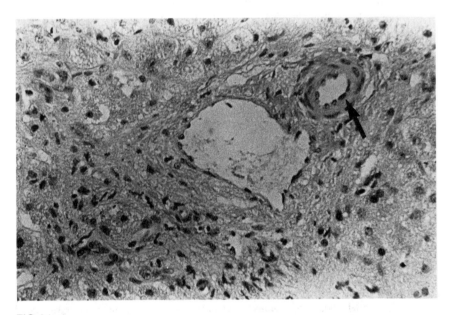

FIG 34–1.
Liver biopsy showing portal area with portal vein *(center)* and branch of hepatic artery *(arrow).*
No bile ducts are present (× 400).

dren having the constellation of facial, occular, cardiac, and vertebral abnormalities associated with hepatic ductular hypoplasia and normal extrahepatic bile ducts.[1] Since then several case reports and reviews have appeared,[3, 4] and most recently Alagille and co-workers reported their experience on 80 children with syndromic bile duct paucity.[5] Nonsyndromic paucity of bile ducts refers to children having only intrahepatic biliary ductular hypoplasia.

Pathophysiology

The cause of intrahepatic bile duct hypoplasia is unknown, but Valencia-Mayoral et al. have reported on a possible defect of the bile secretory apparatus in patients with Alagille syndrome.[6] They identified several electron microscopic changes of the liver in these patients compared with the findings in children with other forms of chronic intrahepatic and extrahepatic cholestasis. Bile pigment retention was found in the cytoplasm, especially in the lysosomes, and in the vesicles of the Golgi apparatus (*cis*-Golgi). However, bile pigment retention was rarely found in bile canaliculi or the immediate pericanalicular region. In contrast, the bile canalicular and pericanalicular changes usually observed in other forms of cholestasis were infrequently found in patients with Alagille syndrome. These results suggested to the authors that the defect in patients with this syndrome might be a block in the Golgi apparatus or in the pericanalicular cytoplasm.

Alagille syndrome is thought to be inherited as an autosomal dominant with variable penetrance.[5] Genetic counseling is complicated by the variable severity of the liver disease and associated abnormalities.

Clinical Features

Patients with both the syndromatic and nonsyndromatic forms of bile duct hypoplasia have signs and symptoms of chronic cholestasis that usually present during the first 3 months of life (Table 34–1). The major features in patients with Alagille syndrome include peculiar (although not pathognomonic) facies,[7] chronic cholestasis, peripheral pulmonary artery hypoplasia or stenosis, posterior embryotoxon (an abnormality posterior to the lens), and vertebral arch defects.[5]

The facial characteristics include prominent forehead, deepset eyes, mild hypertelorism, straight nose, and small pointed chin.[1] A recent study has demonstrated that the predictive value of the characteristic facies is about 50% and that they seem to be a general feature of several forms of congenital intrahepatic cholestatic liver disease.[7]

The chronic cholestasis of Alagille syndrome is often manifested by a more intense pruritus than the moderate elevations in bilirubin levels might indicate.[1] The pruritus might be due, at least in part, to the marked elevation in serum bile acid levels.[8] The AST, ALT, and alkaline phosphatase levels are usually only modestly elevated, whereas the serum lipid levels can rise to 15 to 20 times the normal values. This hyperlipidemia may cause xanthomas to develop on the palms, extensor surfaces, and body creases.[1] Hepatomegaly is always present, but splenomegaly is a variable finding.[1, 5]

TABLE 34–1.
Characteristics of Syndromic Paucity of Bile Ducts

Usually present
  Paucity of bile ducts (average < 0.4 bile ducts per portal area)
  Chronic cholestasis
  Characteristic facies
  Hepatomegaly
  Cardiac murmur (usually peripheral pulmonic stenosis)
  Vertebral anomolies (usually butterfly vertebrae)
  Posterior embryotoxon (anterior chamber anomaly seen with slit lamp examination)
  Xanthomas (especially of finger extensor surfaces, and palmer creases)
  Elevated triglyceride, cholesterol, and phospholipid values
Less frequent associated abnormalities
  Growth retardation
  Splenomegaly
  Renal glomerular abnormalities (usually mesangiolipidosis)
  Mental retardation
  Skeletal abnormalities (especially other vertebral)
  High-pitched voice
  Hypogonadism

The most common cardiovascular abnormality of Alagille syndrome is asymptomatic, nonprogressive pulmonary artery stenosis.[4, 5] Pulmonary hypoplasia, intracardiac defects, and tetrology of Fallot have also been described.[5]

The vertebral defects, although present from the first few months of life, are more easily recognized in older children. The vertebral changes usually consist of a failure of the anterior arch to fuse (butterfly deformity), resulting in single or multiple spina bifida defects without scoliosis.[1]

Less frequently associated abnormalities include other skeletal anomolies, growth retardation, hypogonadism, developmental delays, high-pitched voice, and glomerular renal involvement.[5] The mesangiolipidosis found in the renal lesions appear to be specific for this syndrome.[5]

Microscopic examination of liver biopsy specimens in patient's with Alagille syndrome typically shows an absence of bile ducts in most portal triads. However, a few portal triads may contain hypoplastic biliary ductules, frequently without a visible lumen. The ratio of interlobular bile ducts to portal areas, normally 0.9:1.8 in children, is greatly decreased to 0.0:0.4.[9]

Treatment

Treatment at present for patients with bile duct paucity syndromes is mainly supportive, emphasizing optimal nutritional management.[10] Patients with cholestatic jaundice have decreased intraluminal bile salt values, the latter being needed for proper digestion of fat-soluble vitamins and long chain triglycerides. To maximize fat absorption, infant formulas should contain a significant proportion of their fat as medium chain triglycerides (MCTs). Because of the concern for essential fatty acid deficiency on a high-MCT diet, Pregestimil is now recommended because it provides adequate long chain essential fatty acids while usually being well tolerated.[11]

Fat-soluble vitamin therapy is of the utmost importance. The routine vitamin supplementation recommendations include 100,000 international units (IU) of vitamin A every 2 months, 10 mg/kg (up to 200 mg) of vitamin E as α-tocopherol every 2 weeks, 10 mg of vitamin K every 2 weeks, and 5 mg of vitamin D_3 every 3 months.[5]

The considerable discomfort of pruritus often experienced by patients with bile duct paucity can be combatted with the use of cholorrhetic agents such as phenobarbitol (5–10 mg/kg/day) to increase bile flow.[5] Cholestyramine, which binds to bile acids, may also be helpful with pruritus.[5] The usual dose is 4 to 12 gm/day. A review by Garden et al. discusses other approaches to pruritus such as phototherapy.[8]

Liver transplantation is another therapeutic option for those patients progressing to liver failure.

Course and Prognosis

The prognosis for patients with the syndromic form is more favorable than that for nonsyndromic intrahepatic cholestasis.[2, 3, 5] The nonsyndromic patients often die before 2 years of age from rapidly progressive liver failure or biliary cirrhosis.[2]

In the largest reported series of patients with Alagille syndrome (mean follow-up of 10 years), 21 of the 80 patients had died, but only 4 died of liver complications.[5] Infections and cardiovascular abnormalities were the cause of death in the majority of cases. Cholestasis was severe and unremitting in 28 of the patients during the first 4 years of life, but in the oldest patients cholestasis decreased progressively after about 5 years of age. The prognosis in this series depended most on the severity of initial cholestasis (and secondary malnutrition), the severity of the cardiovascular disease, and the presence or absence of portal hypertension or liver failure.

Typically children with Alagille syndrome experience intense pruritus by about the fourth month of life, with relatively moderate cholestatic bilirubin elevation (with the conjugated fraction equaling about one half of the total bilirubin value), and very high serum cholesterol and triglyceride values.[5] In about one third of patients, cholestasis is relatively severe, resulting in some degree of malnutrition.[5] Even though portal fibrosis may be present, cholestasis tends to decrease after about 5 years of age, usually with only persistence of biochemical signs of jaundice.[2, 5] Pruritus usually resolves by adolescence.[2] Many of the patients in Alagille's series have reached adulthood, and several have borne children.[5] The long-term sequelae of Alagille syndrome are unknown, but one case of hepatocellular carcinoma has been reported in a child with the syndrome.[12]

SUMMARY

Intrahepatic paucity of bile ducts, a rare cause of cholestasis in young children, may present as part of a recognized syndrome (Alagille syndrome) or may be nonsyndromatic. The clinical course is generally better for those with the syndromic form but is influenced by the severity and duration of the initial cholestasis, severity of the cardiovascular disease, and the presence of portal hypertension and liver failure. The treatment is supportive and focuses on nutritional issues.

REFERENCES

 1. Alagille D, Odievre M, Gautier M, et al: Hepatic ductular hypoplasia associated with characteristic facies, vertebral malformations, retarded physical, mental and sexual development and cardiac murmur. *J Pediatr* 1975; 86:63–71.
 2. Silverman A, Roy CC: *Pediatric Clinical Gastroenterology.* St Louis, CV Mosby Co, 1983, pp 527–535.
 3. Riely CA, Cotlier E, Gensen PS, et al: Arteriohepatic dysplasia: A benign syndrome of intrahepatic cholestasis with multiple organ involvement. *Ann Intern Med* 1979; 91:520–527.
 4. Levin SE, Zarvos P, Milner S, et al: Arteriohepatic dysplasia: Association of liver disease with pulmonary arterial stenosis as well as facial and skeletal abnormalities. *Pediatrics* 1980; 66:876–883.
 5. Alagille D, Estrada A, Hadchouel M, et al: Syndromic paucity of interlobular bile ducts: Review of 80 cases. *J Pediatr* 1987; 110:195–200.
 6. Valencia-Mayoral P, Weber J, Cutz E, et al: Possible defect in the bile secretory apparatus in arteriohepatic dysplasia (Alagille's syndrome): A review with observations on the ultrastructure of liver. *Hepatology* 1984; 4:691–698.
 7. Sokol RJ, Heubi JE, Balistreri WF: Intrahepatic "cholestasis facies": Is it specific for Alagille syndrome? *J Pediatr* 1983; 103:205–208.
 8. Garden JM, Ostrow JD, Roenigk HH Jr: Pruritus in hepatic cholestasis. *Arch Dermatol* 1985; 121:1415–1420.
 9. Kahn E, Saum F, Markowitz J, et al: Nonsyndromatic paucity of interlobular bile ducts: Light and electron microscopic evaluation of sequential liver biopsies in early childhood. *Hepatology* 1986; 6:890–901.
10. Alagille D: Management of paucity of interlobular bile ducts. *J Hepatol* 1985; 1:561.
11. Kaufman SS, Murray ND, Wood RP, et al: Nutritional support for the infant with extrahepatic biliary atresia. *J Pediatr* 1987; 110:679–686.
12. Kaufman SS, Wood P, Shaw BW Jr, et al: Hepatocarcinoma in a child with the Alagille syndrome. *Am J Dis Child* 1987; 141:698–700.

35 α_1-Antitrypsin Deficiency

Veronique A. Pelletier, M.D., F.R.C.P.(C)
John D. Snyder, M.D.

A 13.5-year-old girl had persistent splenomegaly and recently developed hematuria. She had been the full-term product of an uncomplicated pregnancy and had no neonatal problems. She grew and developed normally but was found to have splenomegaly on a routine physical examination at 3 years of age. There was no history of infection, including hepatitis, liver dysfunction, hematochezia, or hematemesis. Her initial laboratory workup, including liver function tests and liver-spleen scan, was unrevealing, and because she was growing well, no further evaluation was done.

She continued to do well without signs of illness for 10 years until 2 weeks prior to seeking medical care when she developed hematuria. Because of her continued splenomegaly, she was seen by a gastroenterologist who found mildly elevated liver aminotransferase and bilirubin levels and a slightly low albumin level on laboratory examination. The workup included normal hepatitis serology values, urine and serum amino acid values, abdominal ultrasound, and sweat chloride test results, but the serum α_1-antitrypsin level was 15 mg/ml (normal range 85–213 mg/ml) and the protease inhibitor (Pi) typing was ZZ. A percutaneous liver biopsy specimen revealed macronodular and micronodular cirrhosis and numerous intracytoplasmic periodic acid–Schiff (PAS)–positive, diastase-resistant, granules consistent with α_1-antitrypsin deficiency (Fig 35–1).

Her renal workup included a normal urine analysis except for red blood cells; no casts were seen. Her blood urea nitrogen level, creatinine, and creatinine clearance values were normal.

DISCUSSION

In 1963, Laurell and Ericksson described an association between the deficiency of the serum protease inhibitor, α_1-antitrypsin and chronic obstructive lung disease.[1] Six years later, Sharp et al. reported the relationship of α_1-antitrypsin and juvenile cirrhosis.[2] α_1-Antitrypsin deficiency is now recognized as the commonest metabolic cause of neonatal cholestasis.[3]

α_1-Antitrypsin is an α_1-globulin synthesized in hepatocytes and secreted into the

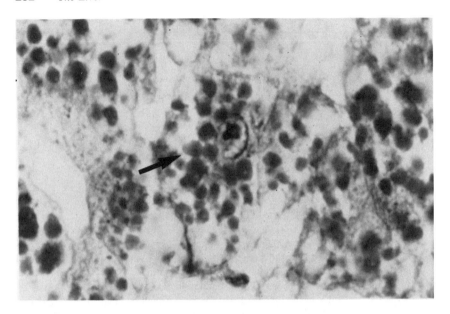

FIG 35-1.
Distended hepatocytes containing numerous intracytoplasmic PAS-positive, diastase-resistant hyalin droplets *(arrow)* (×450).

serum, where it acts as the major inhibitor of trypsin and also inhibits a number of other proteolytic enzymes, including chymotrypsin, elastase, collagenase, and urokinase.[4] The diagnosis is made by measuring serum levels of the enzyme, which are greatly reduced in patients with the deficiency. More than 24 genetic variants (phenotypes) have been determined by use of starch gel electrophoresis; samples from deficient patients give the faintest bands that have the slowest electrophoretic mobility.[4] The protease inhibitor (Pi) system has been developed for labeling the various phenotypes. The slowest proteins are designated Z, the proteins migrating at normal speed are designated M, and the fastest proteins are designated by earlier letters in the alphabet. The M phenotype is the commonest, and the S and Z isotypes are associated with decreased serum concentrations of α_1-antitrypsin.[4] The homozygote for α_1-antitrypsin deficiency is designated Pi ZZ, and the normal homozygote is Pi MM.

The epidemiologic features of α_1-antitrypsin deficiency have been well studied in several large populations (Table 35-1).[5-7] In a prospective study of 200,000 Swedish newborns, 122 Pi ZZ homozygotes and 51 heterozygotes were identified.[5] The incidence of the Pi ZZ phenotype in American infants is about one third as great as in Swedish infants.[6] Approximately 10% to 20% of α_1-antitrypsin-deficient individuals will develop signs and symptoms of liver dysfunction.[8] Cholestatic jaundice developed in 11% of the Pi ZZ Swedish infants and in 6% of the Pi ZZ American infants.[5, 6] In the Swedish study, 50% of the asymptomatic Pi ZZ patients had occasional elevations of values.[5] Clinically evident liver disease is rarely found in children of the Pi SZ phenotype even though their plasma α_1-antitrypsin concentrations average only about 40% of normal.[9] There is no reported difference in the likelihood of males or females developing α_1-antitrypsin deficiency, but males with α_1-antitrypsin deficiency are twice as likely to develop clinical and biochemical signs of cholestasis.[8]

Pathophysiology

The mechanism by which α_1-antitrypsin deficiency causes liver damage is unknown. Recent studies indicate that a genetic defect in secretion of the α_1-antitrypsin protein may be present in affected individuals.[10] Deposits of an amorphous material that contains α_1-antitrypsin precursors are found in hepatocytes of patients with α_1-antitrypsin deficiency.[4] However, these deposits are found in both healthy and ill homozygotes as well as healthy heterozygotes, indicating that they are not the sole cause of damage. Several possible synergistic or additive factors have been proposed. Since there is a male predominance of liver disease in patients with α_1-antitrypsin deficiency, some endogenous factors may play a role.[5] Udall et al. have recently postulated that diet or bowel flora may influence the onset of hepatitis in infants with α_1-antitrypsin deficiency.[11] They reported decreased severity of liver disease in α_1-antitrypsin-deficient infants who received breast milk compared with infants who received formula. The protective effect of breast milk may be due to its protease inhibitors (absent in α_1-antitrypsin deficiency), which could prevent potential damage to the liver from intestinal enzymes.[12] These observations indicate that the pathogenic mechanism may, indeed, be multifactorial.

Clinical Features

Deficiency of α_1-antitrypsin has been associated with both pulmonary and hepatic disease. The pulmonary disease, which is more commonly seen, is obstructive and is usually manifested as emphysema or bronchiectasis.[12] Most individuals will develop their pulmonary symptoms as young adults, although infants and children can be affected.

The liver disease in α_1-antitrypsin deficiency often presents as a neonatal hepatitis-like syndrome with severe symptoms in the first or second week of life (see Chapter 30). The disease probably begins during intrauterine life; 45% of clinically affected infants in one series were small for gestational age.[14]

TABLE 35–1.
Clinical Features Of α_1-Antitrypsin Deficiency

	Hemozygote (ZZ)	Heterozygote (MZ, SZ, Z Null)
Liver dysfunction, %	20%	Rare
Neonatal hepatitis	Yes	Never
Onset later in life	Yes	Yes
Cirrhosis	Often in late adolescence	Rare

The natural course of liver disease associated with α_1-antitrypsin deficiency is very variable. The initial reports described a high likelihood of progression to cirrhosis and liver failure,[15] but the prognosis is not as poor as was first believed.[14] Most infants enter an asymptomatic phase after the initial period of conjugated hyperbilirubinemia resolves.[13] However, hepatomegaly and laboratory evidence of mild hepatic dysfunction usually persist.[7, 16] A few infants will progress to cirrhosis and early death, but the majority lead healthy-appearing lives through childhood,[7] as has this patient. The clinical signs of cirrhosis, if it develops, are often manifested in these patients by late adolescence, followed by a predictably downhill course.[13, 16] A clearer understanding of the long-term course of liver disease in α_1-antitrypsin deficiency will be provided by the prospective studies on the large cohort of patients identified by Svegar; these patients have now been followed for 11 years.[8]

Liver disease can also develop at a later age in α_1-antitrypsin-deficient individuals who had no evidence of neonatal hepatitis or childhood liver disease.[13] A range of liver involvement from mild portal fibrosis to cirrhosis or hepatoma has been described.[17, 18] Cirrhosis rarely becomes clinically apparent in these patients before the age of 50 years.[18] A small percentage of heterozygotes (Pi MZ or Pi SZ) can also develop chronic liver disease, but they are not at risk for neonatal cholestasis.[18]

Adults with α_1-antitrypsin deficiency and cirrhosis have a very high risk of hepatomas.[19] The risk of these Pi ZZ homozygotes developing cirrhosis and hepatoma is not altered by environmental factors such as drinking.[19]

Pancreatic fibrosis and membranoproliferative glomerulonephritis have also rarely been associated with α_1-antitrypsin deficiency.[20, 21] This patient had evidence for nephritis (hematuria, proteinuria) but has not yet undergone a renal biopsy.

Diagnosis

The diagnosis of α_1-antitrypsin deficiency should be considered in all infants with cholestatic jaundice and in older children who present with evidence of chronic liver abnormalities (see Chapter 30). Serum levels of α_1-antitrypsin are diagnostic but may be falsely elevated in heterozygotes in conditions such as intercurrent infections.[3] Pi phenotyping should be done to confirm the diagnosis, although homozygous individuals are incapable of raising their levels in response to stress.

When liver biopsy specimens are obtained, PAS staining demonstrates amorphous intracellular globules that are resistant to diastase digestion (see Fig 35–1).[3] The material appears to be precursor of α_1-antitrypsin but lacks sialic acid, and collections are found especially in the periportal areas.[14] These collections may be found in the livers of all α_1-antitrypsin-deficient patients with or without liver disease.[3]

When liver biopsy specimens are obtained from symptomatic infants, giant cells, altered lobular architecture, bile duct abnormalities, and portal fibrosis are often seen.[3, 14] Eventual progression to cirrhosis occurs in almost all affected patients.

Treatment

Treatment for liver disease associated with α_1-antitrypsin deficiency is currently limited to supportive care, and liver transplantation is the only known cure.[22] However, a recent study indicates that breast-feeding may offer some protection against liver disease.[12] The mechanism for this protection may be related to protease inhibitors, which are known to be present in breast milk but are absent in α_1-antitrypsin deficiency. These proteins could prevent potential damage to the liver caused by the proposed increased uptake of intestinal enzymes from the neonatal intestine.[18] In the one series reported, severe liver disease was found in 40% of bottle-fed and 8% of breast-fed infants with α_1-antitrypsin deficiency; all eight infants who died were bottle-fed.[12]

Liver transplantation is curative for α_1-antitrypsin deficiency.[22] After transplantation, the metabolic defect appears to be permanently corrected as the phenotypes of the recipients become those of the donors and the α_1-antitrypsin levels become normal.[22]

The long-term prognosis for patients with α_1-antitrypsin deficiency awaits reports from the ongoing follow-up of large prospectively identified populations. However, for patients such as this patient with chronic liver disease, the progression to cirrhosis and early death appears unavoidable. For this reason, this patient is now being evaluated for liver transplantation.

SUMMARY

α_1-Antitrypsin deficiency is an important cause of metabolic liver disease in children and should be suspected in every child with cholestasis. The diagnosis is made by measuring serum α_1-antitrypsin levels and is confirmed by liver biopsy. Treatment is limited to supportive care, but liver transplantation now offers a chance for cure.

REFERENCES

1. Laurell CB, Eriksson S: The electrophoretic alpha-1-globulin pattern of serum in alpha-1-antitrypsin deficiency. *Scand J Clin Lab Invest* 1963; 15:132–140.
2. Sharp HL, Bridges RA, Krivit W, et al: Cirrhosis associated with alpha-1-antitrypsin deficiency: A previously unrecognized inherited disorder. *J Lab Clin Med* 1969; 73:934–939.
3. Mowat AP, Psacharopoulos HT, Williams R: Extrahepatic biliary atresia versus neonatal hepatitis. *Arch Dis Child* 1976; 51:763–770.
4. Morse JO: Alpha₁-antitrypsin deficiency. (First of two parts.) *N Engl J Med* 1978; 299:1045–1048.
5. Svegar T: Liver disease in alpha₁-antitrypsin deficiency detected by screening of 200,000 infants. *N Engl J Med* 1976; 294:1316–1321.
6. O'Brien ML, Burist NRM, Murphy H: Neonatal screening for alpha-1-antitrypsin deficiency. *J Pediatr* 1978; 92:1006–1010.
7. Cottrall K, Cook PJL, Mowat AP: Neonatal hepatitis syndrome and alpha-1-antitrypsin deficiency: An epidemiological study in south-east England. *Postgrad Med J* 1974; 50:376–380.
8. Svegar T: Prospective study of children with alpha-1-antitrypsin deficiency: Eight-year-old follow up. *J Pediatr* 1984; 104:91–94.

9. Wilkinson EJ, Rabb K, Browning CA, et al: Familial hepatic cirrhosis in infants associated with alpha-1-antitrypsin SZ phenotype. *J Pediatr* 1974; 85:159–164.

10. Perlmutter DH, Kay RM, Cole FS, et al: The cellular defect in alpha$_1$-proteinase inhibitor (alpha$_1$-PI) deficiency is expressed in human monocytes and in *Xenopus* oocytes injected with human liver mRNA. *Proc Natl Acad Sci* 1985; 82:6918–6922.

11. Udall JN, Dixon M, Newman AP, et al: Liver disease in alpha-1-antitrypsin deficiency: A retrospective analysis of the influence of early breast- vs bottle-feeding. *JAMA* 1985; 253:2679–2682.

12. Udall JN, Block KJ, Walker WA: Transport of proteases across neonatal intestine and development of liver disease in infants with alpha-1-antitrypsin deficiency. *Lancet* 1982; 1:1441–1443.

13. Morse JO: Alpha$_1$-antitrypsin deficiency (second of two parts). *N Engl J Med* 1978; 299:1099–1105.

14. Svegar T: Alpha$_1$-antitrypsin deficiency in early childhood. *Pediatrics* 1978; 62:22–25.

15. Sharp HL: Alpha-1-antitrypsin deficiency. *Hosp Pract* 1971; 6(5):83–96.

16. Odievre M, Martin J-P, Hadchovel M, et al: Alpha$_1$-antitrypsin deficiency and liver disease in children: Phenotypes, manifestations, and prognosis. *Pediatrics* 1976; 57:226–231.

17. Moroz SP, Cutz E, Cox DW, et al: Liver disease associated with alpha$_1$-antitrypsin deficiency in childhood. *J Pediatr* 1976; 88:19–25.

18. Berg NO, Eriksson S: Liver disease in adults with alpha$_1$-antitrypsin deficiency. *N Engl J Med* 1972; 287:1264.

19. Eriksson SG: Liver disease in alpha$_1$-antitrypsin deficiency: Aspects of incidence and prognosis. *Scand J Gastroenterol* 1985; 20:907–911.

20. Freeman HJ, Weinstein WM, Shnitka TK, et al: Alpha-1-antitrypsin deficiency and pancreatic fibrosis. *Ann Intern Med* 1976; 85:73–76.

21. Moroz SP, Cutz E, Blate JW, et al: Membranoproliferative glomerulonephritis in childhood cirrhosis associated with alpha-1-antitrypsin deficiency. *Pediatrics* 1976; 57: 232–238.

22. Hood JN, Koep LJ, Peters RL, et al: Liver transplantation for advanced liver disease with alpha-1-antitrypsin deficiency. *N Engl J Med* 1980; 302:272–275.

36   Vertical Transmission of Hepatitis B

Alan M. Leichtner, M.D.

Prior to receiving his third injection of hepatitis B vaccine, a 6-month old boy was noted to have a positive test result for serum hepatitis B surface antigen (HBsAg). He had been a 7.4-lb (3.4-kg) product of a full-term gestation of a gravida II, para II, woman of Vietnamese descent who had come to the United States 1 year prior to his birth. Because her previous child had died at 3 months of age from an illness that ''turned his eyes yellow,'' the mother had been screened for HBsAg in the prenatal clinic. Her serum result was positive for hepatitis B e antigen (HBeAg) as well as for HBsAg. Therefore, this child received both hepatitis B immune globulin (HBIG) and his first dose of hepatitis B vaccine at 12 hours after birth.

On examination, the infant was alert and vigorous. His weight and length were both at the 25th percentile for age. The sclerae were not icteric. The abdomen was not distended. A soft liver edge was palpable 1 cm below the right costal margin, and the liver measured 4 cm by percussion in the midclavicular line. The spleen tip was palpable below the left costal margin. The infant had no cutaneous stigmata of chronic liver disease.

Results of a laboratory evaluation revealed an elevated aspartate aminotransferase (AST) level of 65 mU/ml but normal levels of bilirubin, alkaline phosphatase, and albumin and a normal prothrombin time. The third dose of hepatitis B vaccine was not given, and a return appointment to reassess the child's hepatic status was scheduled in 3 months.

DISCUSSION

Prevention of transmission of hepatitis B infections from infected mothers to their infants is of critical importance. Although most neonatally acquired hepatitis B infections are clinically mild, severe and even fatal cases have been reported.[1] Also of great concern is the development of chronic antigenemia with a markedly increased lifetime risk of chronic hepatitis, cirrhosis, and primary hepatocellular carcinoma.[2]

Transmission

Vertical transmission of hepatitis B virus most commonly results from exposure of the infant to maternal blood or vaginal secretions at the time of delivery. Evidence for this hypothesis is largely indirect, however, and is based on the fact that the incubation period of hepatitis B is approximately 70 days and that most infected infants present at between 1 and 3 months of age. In a recent study, none of 51 Senegalese neonates born to chronic carrier mothers tested positive for IgM anti–hepatitis B core antigen at birth, suggesting that in utero transmission of the virus did not occur in these infants.[3] Since a few infants already have clinically evident hepatitis B at birth, in utero transmission probably does occasionally occur. It is also thought to account for infection of infants of mothers who had acute hepatitis B early in pregnancy but cleared their antigenemia before delivery.[4]

Both mothers who are acutely infected with hepatitis B and those who are chronic carriers (serum HBsAg positive for 6 months or longer) may transmit the virus to their offspring. The risk of transmission from mothers with acute hepatitis depends on when during pregnancy the infection occurs. With infection in the first or second trimester, vertical transmission occurs in less than 10% of cases, whereas third trimester illness transmits the virus with 40% to 50% efficiency.[5]

More significant epidemiologically is vertical transmission of hepatitis B to infants of chronic carrier mothers. There are an estimated 200 million carriers worldwide,[6] and the number of women of child-bearing age who are serum HBsAg positive is very substantial. Transmission of hepatitis B to infants of carrier mothers in the United States and Western Europe is unusual, but in areas where there is a high prevalence of infection, transmission occurs at a high rate. Stevens et al. reported 40% of infants of carrier mothers became HBsAg carriers in a study in Taiwan.[7] Carrier mothers from high-prevalence areas who immigrate to the United States or Western Europe retain this propensity to transmit the virus vertically.[8]

The most important risk factor for vertical transmission of hepatitis B virus is the presence in the mother of serologic markers indicating active viral replication, such as HBeAg, DNA polymerase, or hepatitis B virus DNA. Greater than 95% of infants whose carrier mothers were HBeAg positive became HBsAg positive in another study from Taiwan.[9] Although the risk when the carrier mother is positive for antibody to HBeAg (anti-HBe) is substantially lower, transmission may still occur. A previously identified risk factor, that of already having transmitted hepatitis B to other children, is probably just indicative of active viral replication and a large burden of circulating viral particles. Presumably, these mothers would be identified by these serologic markers if tested at the present time.

Clinical Features

As in older patients, the hepatitis B virus causes a spectrum of disease in the neonate. However, most infants infected in the neonatal period are asymptomatic and a high percentage become chronic carriers, especially if the mother is HBeAg positive. In the Stevens et al. Taiwan study, more than 85% of infants of such mothers not only became HBsAg positive but became chronic carriers as well.[9] Histologically, the usual pattern is one of minimal changes or of chronic persistent hepatitis, and commonly a mild, fluctuating elevation of the serum aminotransferase levels is noted.[10] Occasionally, however, chronic active hepatitis may develop and progress rapidly to cirrhosis before 1 year of age.[11] Rarely, hepatitis B virus can cause fulminant hepatitis with a fatal outcome in infancy.[2] Even though rare, fulminant hepatitis B acquired by vertical transmission in the neonatal period may account for a sizeable percentage of all cases of fulminant hepatitis in childhood.[12]

The very significant association of chronic hepatitis B infection and hepatocellular carcinoma is not an issue to be ignored by the pediatrician. The predisposing chronic hepatitis B infection is frequently contracted via vertical transmission in the neonatal period. Furthermore, the latency period may be quite short because hepatocellular carcinoma associated with hepatitis B infection has been reported in a child only 7 years of age.[2]

Prevention

The first step in the prevention of vertical transmission of hepatitis B is to identify which mothers are at high risk of being HBsAg positive. The Committee on Infectious Diseases of the American Academy of Pediatrics recommended that the following women be screened: (1) women of Asian, Pacific Islander, or Alaskan Eskimo descent; (2) women born in Haiti or sub-Saharan Africa; and (3) women with a history of (a) having acute or chronic liver disease, (b) having worked or been treated in a hemodialysis unit, (c) having household or sexual contact with a hemodialysis patient, (d) having occupational or residential exposure in an institution for the mentally retarded, (e) having been rejected as a blood donor, (f) receiving blood transfusions on repeated occasions, (g) having frequent occupational exposure to blood in medicodental settings, (h) having household contact with a hepatitis B virus carrier, (i) having multiple episodes of venereal disease, and (j) using illicit drugs percutaneously.[13] Recent studies have suggested that even this exhaustive list may not identify all HBsAg-positive mothers at risk to transmit hepatitis B to their offspring.[14, 15] It is likely that future recommendations will include screening of all pregnant women.

Before the advent of a hepatitis B vaccine, passive immunoprophylaxis, using standard immune globulin or hepatitis B immune globulin (HBIG), was the only method available to attempt to disrupt vertical transmission. Hepatitis B immune globulin is prepared from pooled donors having very high titers of anti-HBs, the protective antibody. Beasley and co-workers demonstrated that the major effects of HBIG were to prolong the incubation period and, more significantly, to decrease the rate of development of chronic carriage.[16] One dose of HBIG administered within 48 hours of birth decreased the incidence of chronic infection from 92% to 54% of infected infants.[16] Three doses reduced the chronic carriage rate to 26%. No decrease in the incidence of overall infection was seen in this study, however, despite more promising results from other groups.

Even if HBIG were successful in preventing vertical transmission resulting from exposure at birth, the problem of infection in infancy would not be solved. Twenty-six percent of infants of carrier mothers not infected at birth acquire infection by 1 year of age.[17] Breast-feeding has not been shown to increase this high risk for postpartum transmission of hepatitis B virus and should probably not be discouraged. However, the need for active, long-lasting prophylaxis as afforded by vaccination is very apparent.

An early report documenting the efficacy of a plasma-derived hepatitis B vaccine in neonates was published in 1982. Greater than 90% of neonates showed a specific anti-HBs response after three doses at 1-month intervals.[18] Subsequent studies demonstrated the benefit of combined active and passive immunization, which is the basis for current recommendations for immunoprophylaxis (Table 36–1).[21] Trials reexamining the role of HBIG by comparing vaccine administration with and without HBIG have generally confirmed the utility of HBIG.[19, 20] Hepatitis B vaccine and HBIG may be given simultaneously if injected at different sites in separate syringes. The side effects of such immunoprophylaxis are minimal.

Recently, a recombinant hepatitis B vaccine manufactured in yeast has become commercially available for use in the United States. This vaccine has been demonstrated to be as highly immunogenic in neonates as are plasma-derived vaccines.[21] Hopefully, the increased availability and decreased cost of production of the recombinant vaccines will allow large vaccination programs to be undertaken.

Because the hepatitis B virus can survive for significant periods of time even on environmental surfaces, infants born to HBsAg-positive mothers should be carefully washed by a gloved attendant. Prophylaxis, as outlined in Table 36–1, should be administered as soon as possible after birth, certainly within 48 hours.[21] The schedule includes recommendations for serologic testing. The detection of HBsAg positivity at 6 or 9 months indicates that the immunoprophylaxis failed and that the infant has active hepatitis B infection. Conversely, the detection of anti-HBs at 9 months indicates immunity. Yet to be assessed is the possible future need for booster doses of vaccine.

SUMMARY

This case illustrates a number of important points regarding the vertical transmission of hepatitis B. The infant's mother was from an endemic area and, hence, at high

TABLE 36–1.
Hepatitis B Virus Prophylaxis and Monitoring of Infants of HBsAg-Positive Mothers

Age	HBIG	Hepatitis B Vaccine*	Hepatitis B Virus Marker Screening
As soon as possible after birth	0.5 ml, IM	0.5 ml, IM	—
1 mo.	—	0.5 ml, IM	—
6 mo.	—	0.5 ml, IM	HBsAg
>9 mo.	—	—	HBsAg, anti-HBs

*Plasma-derived vaccine contains 20 μg/ml, and recombinant vaccine contains 10 μg/ml.

risk to be HBsAg positive. Both the probable history of having had a previous infant with hepatitis B and the presence of HBeAg suggested a high risk of vertical transmission. However, even following the guidelines for immunoprophylaxis does not guarantee successful disruption of transmission since as many as 14% of treated infants may become infected.[20] These infants infected in the neonatal period are usually asymptomatic and have no evidence of liver disease on physical examination. They may, however, have mild serum aminotransferase elevation, as did this child. Such infants should be followed closely to monitor their antigenemia and to permit early detection of significant liver disease, including the possible late development of hepatoma. Future use of the hepatitis B vaccine may ultimately break the cycle of vertical transmission of this dangerous virus.

REFERENCES

1. Delaplane D, Yogev R, Crussi F, et al: Fatal hepatitis B in early infancy: The importance of identifying HBsAg-positive pregnant women and providing immunoprophylaxis to their newborns. *Pediatrics* 1983; 72:176–180.
2. Beasley RP, Shiao I-S, Wu T-C, et al: Hepatoma in an HBsAg carrier—seven years after perinatal infection. *J Pediatr* 1982; 101:83–84.
3. Goudeau A, Lesage G, Denis F, et al: Lack of anti-HBc IgM in neonates with HBsAg carrier mothers argues against transplacental transmission of hepatitis B virus infection. *Lancet* 1983; 2:1103–1104.
4. Schweitzer IL: Vertical transmission of the hepatitis B surface antigen. *Am J Med Sci* 1975; 270:287–291.
5. Stevens CE, Krugman S, Szmuness WA, et al: Viral hepatitis in pregnancy: Problems for the clinician dealing with the infant. *Pediatr Rev* 1980; 2:121–125.
6. Szmuness W: Recent advances in the study of the epidemiology of hepatitis B. *Am J Pathol* 1975; 81:629–650.
7. Stevens CE, Beasley RP, Tsui J, et al: Vertical transmission of hepatitis B antigen in Taiwan. *N Engl J Med* 1975; 292:771–774.
8. Derso A, Boxall EH, Tarlow MI, et al: Transmission of HBsAg from mother to infant in four ethnic groups. *Br Med J* 1978; 1:949–952.
9. Stevens CE, Neurath RA, Beasley RP, et al: HBeAg and anti-HBe detection by radioimmunoassay: correlation with vertical transmission of hepatitis B virus in Taiwan. *J Med Virol* 1979; 3:237–241.
10. Tong MJ, Thursby M, Rakela J, et al: Studies on the maternal-infant transmission of the viruses which cause acute hepatitis. *Gastroenterology* 1981; 80:999–1004.
11. Shinozaki T, Saito K, Shiraki K: HBsAg-positive giant cell hepatitis with cirrhosis in a 10-month-old infant. *Arch Dis Child* 1981; 56:64–74.
12. Chang M-H, Lee C-Y, Chen D-S, et al: Fulminant hepatitis in children in Taiwan: The important role of hepatitis B virus. *J Pediatr* 1987; 111:34–39.
13. Brunell PA, Bass JW, Daum RS, et al: Prevention of hepatitis B virus infections. *Pediatrics* 1985; 75:362–364.
14. Kumar ML, Dawson NV, McCullough AJ, et al: Should all pregnant women be screened for hepatitis B? *Ann Intern Med* 1987; 107:273–277.
15. Jonas MM, Schiff ER, O'Sullivan MJ, et al: Failure of Centers for Disease Control criteria to identify hepatitis B infection in a large municipal obstetrical population. *Ann Intern Med* 1987; 107:335–337.

16. Beasley RP, Hwang L-Y, Stevens CE, et al: Efficacy of hepatitis B immune globulin for prevention of perinatal transmission of the hepatitis B virus carrier state: Final report of a randomized double-blind, placebo-controlled trial. *Hepatology* 1983; 3:135–141.

17. Beasley RP, Hwang L-Y: Postnatal infectivity of hepatitis B surface antigen-carrier mothers. *J Infect Dis* 1983; 147:185–190.

18. Barin F, Denis F, Chiron JP, et al: Immune response in neonates to hepatitis B vaccine. *Lancet* 1982; 1:251–253.

19. Beasley RP, Lee G C-Y, Roan C-H, et al: Prevention of perinatally transmitted hepatitis B virus infections with hepatitis B immune globulin and hepatitis B vaccine. *Lancet* 1983; 2:1099–1102.

20. Lo K-J, Tsai Y-T, Lee S-D, et al: Immunoprophylaxis of infection with hepatitis B virus in infants born to hepatitis B surface antigen-positive carrier mothers. *J Infect Dis* 1985; 152:817–822.

21. Stevens CE, Taylor PE, Tong MJ, et al: Yeast-recombinant hepatitis B vaccine: Efficacy with hepatitis B immunoglobulin in prevention of perinatal hepatitis B virus transmission. *JAMA* 1987; 257:2612–2616.

22. Centers for Disease Control: Update on Hepatitis B prevention. *Ann Intern Med* 1987; 107:353–357.

37 Autoimmune Chronic Active Hepatitis

Tien-Lan Chang, M.D.

A 15-year-old girl was noted to have splenomegaly by her pediatrician during a routine school physical examination. She had no previous symptoms of a viral illness, including coryza, cough, sore throat, vomiting, diarrhea, or fever. She also denied lethargy, anorexia, or weight loss. There was no history of recent travel, contact with people with viral illness, or jaundice, and she had been taking no medications. Her past medical history was unremarkable except that 2 years earlier another pediatrician in the same practice had also noted an enlarged spleen during a similar school physicial examination. Also, she had missed her menstrual period for 4 months. Results of her initial laboratory evaluations showed hemoglobin 12.2 mg%, platelet count 49,000/mm³, aspartate aminotransferase (AST) 79 mU/ml (normal <25 mU/ml), alanine aminotransferase (ALT) 71 mU/ml (normal <22 mU/ml), alkaline phosphatase level 160 mg/dl, total bilirubin level 2.7 mg/dl, total protein level 8.4 mg/dl, and albumin level 3.5 mg/dl. Because of splenomegaly and thrombocytopenia, she was first referred to an oncologist. Results of a bone marrow biopsy and aspiration showed normal cellularity except for an increased number of megakaryocytes A hepatitis screen was negative for hepatitis B surface antigen (HBsAg), hepatitis A antigen, anti–hepatitis B core antigen, Epstein-Barr virus (EBV), and cytomegalovirus (CMV). Her serum ceruloplasmin level, urinalysis, serum copper level and opthalmologic examination results were normal. She was then referred to the gastroenterology clinic where her examination revealed stable vital signs, but spider angiomata were scattered on her face and upper extremities, and bruises were present on her legs. She was anicteric, and results of the head, ear, eye, nose, and throat; pulmonary; and cardiac examinations were normal. No adenopathy was present, and her abdomen was flat; the liver edge was not palpable, but the spleen was palpated 4 cm under the left costal margin extending from the sternum to the left lateral axillary line. Rectal examination findings were normal, and the stool guaiac was negative. Further laboratory test results showed a prothrombin time of 17.4 seconds (control 13.2 seconds), partial thromboplastin time 41.9 seconds (control 31.4 seconds), IgG 3,600 mg/dl (normal <1,300 mg/dl, IgM 226 mg/dl, IgA 213 mg/dl α_1-antitrypsin 160 mg/ml (normal 85–213 mg/ml) with a protease inhibitor (Pi) type MM. The antinuclear antibody (ANA) result was positive at 1:40. A liver biopsy was performed after transfusions of fresh frozen plasma and platelets. The biopsy revealed cirrhosis and piecemeal and bridging necrosis consistent with chronic active hepatitis (Fig 37–1). Since infectious and metabolic etiologies had been ruled out and since she had a positive ANA result and elevated immunoglobulin levels, the patient was diagnosed as having autoimmune chronic active hepatitis (CAH) and was started on prednisone therapy.

DISCUSSION

This case is typical of the presentation of many patients with autoimmune CAH. Approximately 70% to 80% of the patients are women, one half are 11 to 30 years of age, and only 30% present with symptoms of acute disease.[1] A genetic predisposition is suggested by a strong association of autoimmune CAH with the major histocompatibility complex antigens HLA-B8 and HLA-DR3 and with the immunoglobin allotype Gm a + .[2]

Pathogenesis

The pathogenesis of autoimmune CAH remains poorly understood. Support for an autoimmune mechanism of injury has come from studies of the liver-specific protein

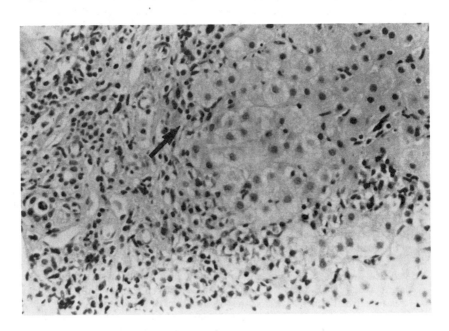

FIG 37–1.
Portal area and adjacent hepatic lobule demonstrating evidence of chronic active hepatitis. Portal tract contains a mononuclear cell infiltrate that extends in an irregular pattern into the adjacent hepatic parenchyma *(arrow)* (× 400).

(LSP), which is a complex glycoprotein with many antigenic determinants, only some of which are specific to the liver.[2] Despite this lack of specificity, the titer of the anti-LSP antibody has been correlated with CAH disease activity.[2, 3] In vitro studies have shown that peripheral mononuclear non–T cells of patients with CAH are cytotoxic against autologous hepatocytes obtained by biopsy, and this cytotoxicity appears to be mediated by the anti-LSP antibody bound to the surface of the liver cells.[2] A similar cytotoxic phenomenon has also been observed in cases of HBsAg-positive CAH. In contrast T cell–mediated cytotoxicity against autologous hepatocytes has been observed in HBsAg-positive cases but only infrequently in autoimmune CAH. Although defects in immunoregulation are surely involved, as evidenced by the decrease in non-antigen-specific T suppressor function,[4] the nature of these defects and their link to the HLA-B8 and HLA-DR3 loci remain to be worked out.

Clinical Features

The clinical presentation of CAH may take one of several forms. Patients may be completely asymptomatic and discovered only during a routine checkup; they may have certain nonspecific complaints such as anorexia, lethargy, and low-grade fever; or they may present with acute onset of hepatitis, with jaundice, fever, and hepatomegaly. Amenorrhea is often present in females. Other associated complaints can include arthritis, ulcerative colitis, thyroiditis, glomerulonephritis, and diabetes. The physical examination may reveal evidence of chronic liver disease, including spider angiomata, bruises, digital clubbing, and erythema nodosum. Jaundice or icterus is often present. There may be bounding pulses and a high-output murmur on cardiovascular examination. The abdomen may be enlarged from either hepatomegaly, splenomegaly, or ascites. If cirrhosis is present, the liver may be shrunken, and the left lobe may be compensatorily enlarged.

The laboratory evaluation of patients with autoimmune CAH reveals evidence of varying degrees of hepatocyte inflammation or dysfunction. The gamma globulin portion of the total serum protein is usually greatly elevated, as was true for this patient. A number of abnormalities found in common with other diseases of autoimmune etiology are frequently seen in autoimmune CAH.[5] Elevated levels of antinuclear antibodies (ANA) are present in as many as 80% of the patients, whereas the lupus erythematosus cell is found in approximately 10%, which has led to the use of the term lupoid hepatitis. Other autoantibodies have also been identified, including anti-liver, kidney microsomal (LKM), antismooth muscle, and less frequently, antimitochondrial antibodies.[2, 5] The antimitochondrial antibody is seen more frequently in patients with primary biliary cirrhosis and has been suggested as a distinguishing marker between the two conditions.[5]

Diagnosis

Chronic active hepatitis is a diagnosis based on both clinical and pathologic criteria. The chronicity is usually defined in adults by a period of 6 months or greater from the onset of signs or symptoms. This period is important in the decision to perform the liver biopsy since the clinical features and the pathology of a resolving acute hepatitis may be difficult to distinguish from that of CAH.[7] The presence of an elevated gamma globulin fraction and autoimmune markers are clues to the diagnosis of autoimmune CAH (Table 37–1).

The liver biopsy is also crucial in distinguishing CAH from other types of chronic hepatitis, including chronic persistent hepatitis and chronic lobular hepatitis, which carry a good prognosis and need not be treated. The histopathologic appearance of the liver in CAH is characterized by a disruption of the normal lobular structure, with piecemeal necrosis and periportal infiltration with mononuclear inflammatory cells (see Fig 37–1).[7] Bridging necrosis and fibrosis or cirrhosis can be seen in the more severe cases. In comparison, the lobular structure is intact, and piecemeal necrosis is not seen in chronic persistent or lobular hepatitis.[7]

Autoimmune CAH is but one of several possible etiologies in the differential diagnosis of CAH (see Table 37–1). Chronic active hepatitis due to other causes can be broadly categorized as drug induced, viral induced, and metabolic. Although numerous drugs are known to cause elevations in the liver enzymes with or without hepatocellular injury, at least four drugs have been definitely associated with the development of CAH, namely, methyldopa, oxyphenisatin, nitrofurantoin, and isoniazid.[8] Since the pathology is often nondiagnostic in CAH, and autoantibodies may be seen in drug-induced hepatitis, the history becomes of paramount importance for the diagnosis. Improvement in symptoms and laboratory values usually occurs on withdrawal of the suspected drug.

TABLE 37–1.

Differential Diagnosis of Chronic Active Hepatitis

Etiologies	Distinguishing Features
Drug-related	
Methyldopa	Temporal association, im-
Oxyphenisatin	provement off medication
Nitrofurantoin	
Isoniazid	
Virus-related	
Hepatitis B	Serologic markers
CMV	Serologic markers
EBV	Serologic markers
Non-A, non-B hepatitis	Epidemiologic features
Metabolic	
α_1-Antitrypsin deficiency	Serum level of α_1-antitrypsin
Wilson disease	Ceruloplasmin, liver copper
Cystic fibrosis	Sweat test
Anatomic	
Choledochal cyst	Ultrasound
Polycystic disease	Ultrasound
Idiopathic	
Autoimmune	Gammaglobulin, autoantibodies

Viral causes include hepatitis B, CMV, EBV, and non-A, non-B hepatitis, the latter probably representing more than one type of virus. Serology is helpful in these cases except for non-A, non-B hepatitis. In contrast to the improvement in survival seen in patients with autoimmune CAH, steroid treatment of patients with HBsAg-positive CAH may actually increase mortality and should not be used.[9]

The metabolic disorders producing a CAH-like picture include α_1-antitrypsin deficiency and Wilson disease. Both of these disorders can be difficult to distinguish from autoimmune CAH clinically and pathologically. α_1-Antitrypsin deficiency is diagnosed by a low serum level of the protein and by the characteristic findings on liver biopsy (see Chapter 35). However, a normal level of α_1-antitrypsin does not rule out the disorder, since the protein is an acute-phase reactant and can approach normal levels in illness. Obtaining Pi phenotyping is essential to make the diagnosis because only phenotypes ZZ, null, and SZ have been associated with illness. Wilson disease should be considered in any young patient with chronic hepatitis (see Chapter 40). Laboratory features of elevated urine copper and low ceruloplasmin levels in combination with the finding of Kaiser-Fleischer rings on physical examination are very suggestive of this diagnosis. Very elevated levels of liver copper help to confirm the diagnosis. Since Wilson disease is a treatable form of liver disease, this diagnosis should not be missed. Other chronic disorders in the pediatric age group that can cause elevation in the liver enzymes with or without cellular injury include metabolic disorders such as cystic fibrosis, hereditary fructose intolerance, Indian childhood cirrhosis, glycogen storage diseases, disorders of the biliary tree including choledochal cyst, congenital hepatic fibrosis, polycystic disease of the liver, and intrahepatic biliary hypoplasia, and infiltrative tumors such as leukemia and reticuloendothelioses.

This list is not exhaustive but is intended to point out that a number of disorders can present just as subtly as CAH. The diagnostic evaluation should therefore include studies to help rule out these disorders (see Table 37–1).

Therapy

Glucocorticosteroid therapy has been shown to be effective in the management of autoimmune CAH. Studies by the Mayo Clinic, Royal Free Hospital, and King's College Hospital in mostly adult patients have shown a definite improvement in survival for those taking prednisone or prednisone plus azathioprine compared with those taking placebo or azathioprine alone.[10] The difference in survival holds true even for patients with histologic evidence of severe hepatitis and cirrhosis.[10–13] However, the same studies also have shown that steroid treatment did not halt the progression to cirrhosis and that relapses in clinical symptoms and laboratory values occur in a majority of patients when they are withdrawn from treatment.[12]

Similar findings have been reported in smaller studies in children (Table 37–2).[14–18] Although the initial therapeutic regimen was not the same in each of the studies, prednisone or prednisolone was used alone or in combination by each of the investigators. Initial improvement in clinical and laboratory values on therapy was seen in a high percentage of the patients. Long-term remissions occurred in about one half of all the patients but long-term remission off medications occurred in only

TABLE 37–2.
Treatment of Chronic Active Hepatitis in Children

Study	Patients, No. (% Female)	Age Range, yr	Initial Medication*	Initial Clinical and Biochemical Improvement (%)	Remission off Medications†
Page et al.[14] 1969	21 (76)	3–18	A, C, P, or 6-MP	15 (71)	1
Dubois and Silverman[15] 1974	38 (79)	3–17	P	33 (87)	15
Arasu et al.[17] 1979	26 (81)	3–16	P	26 (100)	19
Maggiore et al.[16] 1984	17 (82)	1–15	A + P	15 (88)	2
Vegnente[18] 1984	28 (71)	3–13	PI (25) A + PI (2) A (1)	26 (93)	8

*A = azathioprine; C = cortisone; P = prednisone; PI = prednisolone; 6-MP = 6-mercaptopurine.
†At least 2 months.

about one third of the patients.[14-18] The best results from therapy were reported by Arasu et al. who claimed long-term remissions off medication in 73% of their patients.[17] The authors speculated that their results were better because they initiated therapy earlier.

The effect of therapy on cirrhosis was difficult to assess since about one third of these patients reported had cirrhosis before starting therapy. Some patients showed histologic improvement of their cirrhosis on therapy, whereas other patients progressed to cirrhosis. The use of steroids appeared to decrease the risk of death from liver disease in children with CAH although no control studies have been done. The risk of death was much greater in nonresponders to therapy than in responders.

Our approach to treating autoimmune CAH is to initiate therapy early if a high suspicion for the diagnosis is present. If the workup for infectious (including hepatitis B) and metabolic causes of liver disease is negative, and if autoimmune markers or a high globulin level are present, a liver biopsy is done before the classic 6-month period used to diagnose chronic hepatitis.

Prednisone is started at 2 mg/kg/day up to 40 mg/day for 6 weeks to 2 months, then tapered gradually. Azathioprine can be added at 1 to 2 mg/kg/day (up to 100 mg/day) if no improvement is seen within 1 month or if side effects of the steroids become intolerable (including glucose intolerance, Cushingoid appearance, hypertension, striae, and bone demineralization). The decision to stop treatment should be made with caution since the chance of relapse is quite high.

The evidence for remission is based on clinical well-being, laboratory values, and liver histology obtained by a percutaneous liver biopsy; however, the possibility of sampling error must be considered when a liver biopsy is evaluated. If the medications are discontinued, the patient should continue to be followed regularly for evidence of relapse. Since cirrhosis is very likely to occur despite treatment success, the patient should also be observed for occurrence of possible complications, such as bleeding from esophageal varices, infections, peritonitis, and gallstones.

A significant percentage of patients may fail to respond to conventional therapy and progress to liver failure. For these patients the only alternative that offers some hope of improved survival is liver transplantation. However, even a successful transplantation may not be the final answer, since recurrence of autoimmune CAH has been reported after orthopic liver transplantation.[19]

SUMMARY

Autoimmune chronic active hepatitis in children is usually found in girls and can follow a slow, insidious pattern. Medical treatment with immunosuppressive agents can improve survival, but the regimens currently available do not prevent the eventual development of cirrhosis. Delay in diagnosis and treatment may worsen the patient's prognosis. Further studies are needed to determine whether earlier institution of therapy may lead to improvement in the prognosis for these patients.

REFERENCES

1. Mistilis SP, Blackburn CRB: Active chronic hepatitis. *Am J Med* 1970; 48:484–495.
2. MacKay IR: Immunological aspects of chronic active hepatitis. *Hepatology* 1983; 3:724–728.
3. Chisari FV: Liver-specific protein in perspective. *Gastroenterology* 1980; 78:168–170.
4. Nouri-Aria KT, Hegarty JE, Alexander GJM, et al: Effect of corticosteroids on suppressor-cell activity in "autoimmune" and viral chronic active hepatitis. *N Engl J Med* 1982; 307:1301–1304.
5. Eddleston ALWF: Immunology of chronic active hepatitis. *Q J Med* 1985; 55:191–198.
6. Gurian LE, Rogoff TM, Ware AJ: The immunologic diagnosis of chronic active "autoimmune" hepatitis: Distinction from systemic lupus erythematosus. *Hepatology* 1985; 5:397–402.
7. DeGroote J et al: A classification of chronic hepatitis. *Lancet* 1968; 2:626–628.
8. Boyer JL, Miller DJ: Chronic hepatitis, in Schiff L, Schiff ER (eds): *Diseases of the Liver*, ed 6. Philadelphia, JB Lippincott Co, pp 687–723.
9. Lam KC: Deleterious effect of prednisolone in HBsAg-positive chronic active hepatitis. *N Engl J Med* 1981; 304:690–695.
10. Wright EC, Seefe LB, Berk PD, et al: The treatment of chronic active hepatitis: An analysis of three controlled trials. *Gastroenterology* 1977; 73:1422–1430.
11. Czaja AJ, Beaver SJ, Shiels MT: Sustained remission after corticosteroid therapy of severe hepatitis B surface antigen-negative chronic active hepatitis. *Gastroenterology* 1987; 92:215–219.
12. Kirk AP, Jain S, Pocock S, et al: Late results of the Royal Free Hospital prospective trial of prednisolone therapy in hepatitis B surface negative antigen chronic active hepatitis. *Gut* 1980; 21:78–83.
13. Murray-Lyon IM: Controlled trial of prednisone and azathioprine in active chronic hepatitis. *Lancet* 1973; 1:735–737.
14. Page AR, Good RA, Pollara B: Long-term results of therapy in patients with chronic liver disease associated with hypergammaglobulinemia. *Am J Med* 1969; 47:765–774.
15. Dubois RS, Silverman A: Treatment of chronic active hepatitis in children. *Postgrad Med J* 1974; 50:386–391.
16. Maggiore G, Bernard O, Hadchouel M, et al: Treatment of autoimmune chronic hepatitis in childhood. *J Pediatr* 1984; 104:839–844.
17. Arasu TS, Wyllie R, Hatch TF, et al: Management of chronic aggressive hepatitis in children and adolescents. *J Pediatr* 1979; 95:514–522.
18. Vegnente A, Larcher VF, Mowat AP: Duration of chronic active hepatitis and the development of cirrhosis. *Arch Dis Child* 1984; 59:330–335.
19. Neuberger J, Portman B, Calne, et al: Recurrence of autoimmune chronic active hepatitis following orthotopic liver grafting. *Transplantation* 1984; 37:363–365.

38 Toxic Hepatitis: Acetaminophen Ingestion

Talyn Hanissian, M.D.

John D. Snyder, M.D.

An 18-year-old girl who suffered from anorexia nervosa, bulimia, and depression admitted ingesting 20 tablets (equivalent to 10 gm) of acetaminophen (Tylenol) and 10 tablets of despiramine, a tricyclic antidepressant, in a suicide gesture. She developed vomiting and dizziness but did not seek medical attention for 2 days. On the day of admission, she had a scheduled follow-up visit during which she admitted to the ingestion of the two drugs. She had no complaints of bleeding, bruising, or diaphoresis but felt tired.

Her physical examination was remarkable only for her slender, malnourished appearance. Her abdomen was soft, nontender, and without hepatosplenomegaly. The admission laboratory values included normal hemaglobin (13 mg/dl), white blood cell count, platelet count, erythrocyte sedimentation rate, electrolytes, BUN level, creatinine level, total protein, albumin, bilirubin, ammonia, alkaline phosphatase, prothrombin time (PT), and partial thromboplastin time (PTT) and urinalysis. Her initial aspartate aminotransferase (AST) level was 342 mU/ml (normal <21 mU/ml) and alanine aminotransterase (ALT) level was 470 mU/ml (normal <22 mU/ml). Her toxic screen done 60 hours after ingestion showed no detectable level of acetaminophen and a nontoxic level of despiramine.

She received only supportive care because too much time had elapsed since her ingestion to give N-acetylcystine (NAC); her psychiatric counseling continued. She complained of nausea and lethargy but had no further vomiting. Her aminotransferase levels peaked on the third hospital day (day 5 after ingestion) at 2,420 mU/ml for AST and 2,560 mU/ml for ALT; the maximum total bilirubin level was 2.3 mg% with 1.6 mg% conjugated. The PT and PTT continued to be normal. By the fifth hospital day the bilirubin level was normal, the AST level had fallen to 170 mU/ml, and the ALT level had fallen to 233 mU/ml; she was discharged. When seen in clinic 1 week later, she was feeling well, and her liver functions had returned to normal.

DISCUSSION

Toxic damage to the liver can occur with several drugs commonly used in pediatric practice, including acetaminophen, aspirin, and phenytoin (Dilantin). This discussion will focus on acetaminophen hepatic toxicity because acetaminophen is so widely used in pediatric practice, and its use is expected to increase due to concern for the statistical link between salicylate use and Reye syndrome (see Chapter 39).

Two distinct clinical presentations of acetaminophen overdose are described in Table 38-1. Acetaminophen hepatoxicity is more commonly seen and appears to be more severe in the adolescent.[2] In the great majority of cases, acetaminophen hepatotoxicity has been caused by a suicide attempt, but liver damage from accidental overdoses or large single or multiple therapeutic doses do occur in younger children.[1] Overdose from acetaminophen has become a popular means of attempting suicide, especially in England where nearly 1,000 overdoses were reported in adolescents in 1978.[3] The incidence in the United States appears to be less than in England but is rising.[3]

Pathophysiology

Acetaminophen is a mild analgesic and antipyretic agent that is rapidly absorbed after oral administration with peak serum levels achieved usually within 1 hour after ingestion.[4] The drug is metabolized almost exclusively in the liver, with less than 2% being excreted unchanged in the urine. In adults and adolescents, greater than 90% of acetaminophen is metabolized to the glucuronide or sulfate conjugate.[5] The remaining 5% is metabolized through the cytochrome P-450 mixed function oxidase system and is conjugated with glutathione to produce mercapturic acid.[5] In contrast, in younger children, the percentage of acetaminophen metabolites associated with the P-450 system appears to be less than one half of those seen with adult patients.[6]

In an overdose of acetaminophen, the P-450 system is the pathway associated with hepatotoxicity. The first molecules passing through the system are conjugated with hepatic stores of glutathione and are excreted as the nontoxic compound mercapturic acid.[5] However, as the stores of glutathione are depleted, buildup of a highly reactive intermediate metabolite occurs, which can bind with proteins of the cytosol and endoplasmic reticulum in the centrilobular zone of the liver leading to centrizonal

TABLE 38-1.
Acetaminophen Ingestion in the Pediatric Population

Features	Age Group	
	Children <6 yr Old	Older Children
Cause of ingestion	Accidental	Suicide attempt
Toxic plasma levels	Rare	More common
Hepatotoxicity	Very rare	6 times more common
Recovery	Complete	Complete

necrosis.[7] The development of hepatic toxicity depends on the rate of biotransformation of the drug to the active metabolite and on the tissue content and rate of regeneration of glutathione.[7, 8]

Young animals have a higher turnover of glutathione, indicating that more may be available for detoxification.[9] This may account in part for the less severe hepatotoxicity seen in children, but studies in humans to evaluate this possibility have not been done.

Clinical Features

Two distinct clinical patterns of acetaminophen overdose have been described in the pediatric population (see Table 38–1). In children less than 6 years old, the ingestion is almost always accidental and rarely results in significant hepatotoxicity.[10] In contrast, older children, especially adolescents, are more likely to ingest an overdose of acetaminophen as a suicide gesture and are six times more likely to develop hepatotoxicity and twice as likely to develop potentially toxic blood levels than younger children.[1] The clinical course in older children and adolescents is identical to adults.[10]

In children less than 6 years old, the likelihood of developing any significant degree of hepatotoxicity is very small. Only 55 of 417 young children who ingested a potentially toxic dose of acetaminophen developed plasma levels in the toxic range and only 3 of these patients had AST levels greater than 1,000 mU/ml; all three recovered.[1] In another series of 2,787 overdosed younger children, none developed toxic plasma levels, and none had elevated AST levels.[1]

The clinical course in children can be divided into four stages (Table 38–2).[3, 10] Symptoms usually develop only in children who have toxic levels, but almost all children less than 6 years old will have vomiting regardless of the serum levels.[10] Children who have plasma levels of acetaminophen in the toxic range have a mean onset of symptoms by 6 hours after ingestion, and all will show symptoms by 14 hours.[10] The laboratory evaluation is normal during this stage. In stage 2, the child experiences a feeling of well-being that can last for 1 or 2 days.[3, 10] The peak abnormalities (stage 3) occur 2 to 4 days after ingestion and are related primarily to the hepatotoxicity. Fulminant hepatic injury, which is very rare in young children, can occur during this period.[10] The final stage is the recovery phase when the liver function abnormalities return to normal. Fortunately, no clinical or histologic hepatic sequelae develop in patients who recover from the acute insult.[10]

Renal abnormalities, including renal failure, have been reported.[11] However, the renal problems are never as severe as the hepatic insult.[10]

Diagnosis

A nomogram (Fig 38–1) has been developed by Rumack and Matthews that relates the risk of toxicity to the plasma acetaminophen level for the first 24 hours after ingestion.[12] Because it has been impossible to distinguish between potentially toxic and nontoxic patients based on the history of the amount ingested, a plasma acet-

TABLE 38–2.

Clinical Course of Acetaminophen Overdose*

Stage 1 (day 1)
  Acute gastrointestinal (GI) symptoms
    Anorexia
    Nausea
    Vomiting
    Diaphoresis
    Malaise
    Normal liver function tests

Stage 2 (day 2)
  Relative state of well-being
  Early biochemical evidence for hepatic injury

Stage 3 (day 2–4)
  Clinical evidence of hepatic damage

AST level	200–400 × normal
ALT level	150–300 × normal
Bilirubin level	4–10 × normal
Prothrombin time	2–4 × normal

  Possible fulminant hepatic failure

Stage 4 (day 5–8)
  Resolution of hepatic abnormalities
  No sequelae

*Adapted from Meredith et al.[3] and Rumack.[10]

aminophen level should always be drawn but no sooner than 4 hours after ingestion.[10] Other baseline laboratory values that should be obtained include AST, ALT, bilirubin, prothrombin time, and creatinine clearance.[10] These determinations should be repeated at 24-hour intervals.

A toxic metabolic screen should also be obtained because other drugs may have been ingested. An altered mental status in the patient cannot be attributed to acetaminophen ingestion and indicates that another substance or substances have been ingested.[10]

Alcohol is the most commonly coingested agent and has been found to be hepatoprotective.[1] The AST levels in children with toxic acetaminophen levels were significantly lower in those who had ingested alcohol and acetaminophen together than those who ingested acetaminophen alone.[1] The protective effect of alcohol is probably secondary to competition at the P-450 site.[10]

Treatment

The first step in the treatment of acetaminophen ingestion is to remove as much of

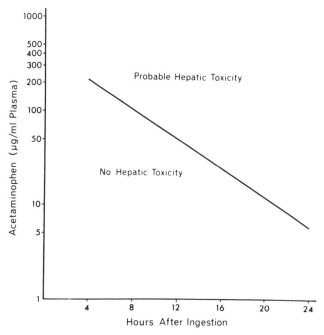

FIG 38–1.
Prediction of probable hepatic toxicity from a semilogarithmic plot of plasma acetaminophen levels and hours after ingestion. (From Rumack BH, Matthew H: Acetaminophen poisoning and toxicity. *Pediatrics* 1975; 55:871–876. Reproduced by permission.)

the acetaminophen as possible. This is best accomplished by inducing vomiting, especially in the first 2 hours after ingestion, which can produce a mean recovery of about 30% of an ingested dose.[11] In adults, gastric lavage with a large bore catheter has been advocated as an effective means of emptying the stomach.[13] The administration of charcoal or cholestyramine to bind acetaminophen has not proved beneficial in pure acetaminophen ingestion.[12] However, since other agents are often coingested, charcoal should be given after emesis has been achieved.

The antidote for acetaminophen overdose is NAC, which binds to the toxic metabolite and prevents hepatotoxicity.[10] Oral NAC has proved to be very effective if administered within the first 16 hours after ingestion.[13] When it is administered within 10 hours after ingestion, only 7% of patients with toxic-range acetaminophen levels developed transient AST elevations, whereas 29% of such patients treated between 10 and 16 hours after ingestion had AST elevations. In patients treated between 16 and 24 hours after ingestion, 62% of those with toxic levels developed AST elevations. Since the drug is relatively free of side effects, administration of NAC is recommended up to 24 hours after ingestion to provide the chance for protective binding.[10]

Oral NAC is diluted from acetylcysteine (Mucomyst) concentrate to a final concentration of no more than 5% (weight/volume).[10] The initial dose is 140 mg/kg, with subsequent doses of 70 mg/kg. Doses are given every 4 hours for 3 days.[13]

Intravenous NAC is used in Europe and Canada because of the foul taste of NAC, but the oral route appears to be superior.[10] Cystamine has also been used extensively in Great Britain but has been associated with a high rate of side effects.[13] *N*-Acetylcystine has the additional advantage of demonstrating a protective effect when administered at later time intervals.[13]

Although children less than 6 years old are unlikely to have any toxicity, NAC administration is recommended for all patients with plasma concentrations in the toxic range.[10] If toxic levels are not found, the great majority of patients can be managed at home with close telephone follow-up.[10]

Forced diuresis and hemodialysis have been considered as possible therapies in the past but have not been found effective.[12] Forced diuresis is especially contraindicated because of the renal damage that can occur in acetaminophen overdose and because of the antidiuretic effect of acetaminophen.[12]

Outcome

The great majority of patients with acetaminophen overdose, especially children, recover completely from the insult. Even in the severely poisoned patients, liver function should begin to improve by day 7 or 8 (see Table 38–2). Patients such as the one presented here, who do not receive NAC, are also likely to recover. No long-term sequelae of acetaminophen overdose are known.[9]

SUMMARY

Acetaminophen overdose is a common event in the pediatric age group. The development of toxic plasma levels and hepatoxicity is extremely rare in young children (see Table 38–1) probably because of greater glutathione synthesis. In older children the early administration of NAC has proved to be very effective therapy. Fulminant hepatitis can develop in untreated patients, so all patients with toxic plasma levels should be treated. Fortunately, almost all patients recover, and no long-term sequelae have been reported.

REFERENCES

1. Rumack BH: Acetaminophen overdose in young children: Treatment and effects of alcohol and other additional ingestants in 417 cases. *Am J Dis Child* 1984; 138:428–433.
2. Zimmerman HJ: Effects of aspirin and acetaminophen on the liver. *Arch Intern Med* 1981; 141:333–342.
3. Meredith TJ, Vale JA, Goulding R: The epidemiology of acute acetaminophen poisoning in England and Wales. *Arch Intern Med* 1981; 141:397–400.
4. Peterson RG, Rumack BH: Pharmacokinetics of acetaminophen in children. *Pediatrics* 1978; 62:877–879.

5. Mitchell JR, Jollow DJ, Potter WZ, et al: Acetaminophen-induced hepatic necrosis: I. Role of drug metabolism. *J Pharmacol Exp Ther* 1973; 187:185–194.

6. Lieh-Lai MW, Saronaik AP, Newton JF, et al: Metabolism and pharmacokinetics of acetaminophen in a severely poisoned young child. *J Pediatr* 1984; 105:125–128.

7. McJunkin B, Barwick KM, Little WC, et al: Fatal massive hepatic necrosis following acetaminophen overdose. *JAMA* 1976; 236:1874–1875.

8. Mitchell JR, Thorgeirsson SS, Potter WZ, et al: Acetaminophen-induced hepatic injury: Protective role of glutathione in man and rationale for therapy. *Clin Pharmacol Ther* 1974; 16:676–684.

9. Rauterburg BH, Vaishnow Y, Stillwell WG, et al: The effect of age and glutathione depletion on hepatic glutathione turnover determined by acetaminophen probe analysis. *J Pharmacol Exp Ther* 1980; 213:54–58.

10. Rumack BH: Acetaminophen overdose in children and adolescents. *Pediatr Clin North Am* 1986; 33:691–701.

11. Corby DG, Decker WJ, Moran MJ, et al: Clinical comparison of pharmacologic emetics in children. *Pediatrics* 1968; 42:361–364.

12. Rumack BH, Matthews H: Acetaminophen poisoning and toxicity. *Pediatrics* 1975; 55:871–876.

13. Rumack BH, Peterson RC, Koch GG, et al: Acetaminophen overdose: 662 cases with evaluation of oral acetylcysteine treatment. *Arch Intern Med* 1981; 141:380–385.

39 Reye Syndrome

Samuel Nurko, M.D.
John D. Snyder, M.D.

A 13-year-old boy was in excellent health until 7 days prior to admission when he developed upper respiratory tract symptoms and a flulike illness. He complained of mild headaches, a temperature of 38°C, coryza, and frequent sneezing. His symptoms gradually improved over the next 4 days, but he suddenly developed nausea, decreased oral intake, and severe vomiting. His vomiting increased in frequency, and he then became lethargic and disoriented. Because of increasing lethargy he was taken to Children's Hospital for evaluation. His past medical history was unremarkable. He lived in a suburb of Boston. There were no other family members ill, and his family denied the ingestion of any medications or drugs, although during his respiratory illness he took 650 mg of aspirin every 4 hours for 2 days. In the emergency room he was found to be combative and lethargic; he was afebrile, and his respiratory rate was 28. His heart rate and blood pressure were normal. His pupils were equal, 3 mm, and reacted sluggishly to light. His neck was supple. His deep tendon reflexes were brisk. He was able to move his extremities, and he responded to painful stimuli. Results of the rest of his examination were normal.

His initial laboratory values included a normal complete blood cell count, aspartate aminotransferase (AST) level 116 mU/ml, alanine aminotransferase (ALT) level 228, total bilirubin level 0.8 mg/dl, arterial ammonia 439, a blood gas of pH 7.32, Pco_2 23, Po_2 190, and $NaHCO_3$ 22. His prothrombin time (PT) was prolonged at 15.9 seconds, and his partial thromboplastin time was prolonged at 34.4 seconds.

Because of signs of increasing intracranial pressure, he was intubated and hyperventilated. Fluid restriction and mannitol administration were instituted, and his intracranial pressure was monitored with an intracranial pressure transducer. His initial intracranial pressure (ICP) was 12 to 15. On the second day of his hospitalization his ICP could not be controlled with this therapy, and pentobarbital coma was instituted as his ICP rose to more than 50. His ammonia level peaked on day 3 at 590, and at that time his AST level was 951 mU/ml, ALT level was 1,170 mU/ml, bilirubin level was 0.5 mg/dl, and PT was 20.2 seconds. His ICP continued to remain increased, and he died on the fourth day of hospitalization.

His autopsy showed an enlarged liver with microvesicular fat accumulation and no inflammation. His brain was swollen, with flattening of the gyri. He had evidence of uncal herniation. The histopathology showed diffuse cerebral edema. His kidneys revealed swollen proximal tubules, and his pancreas had evidence of hemorrhagic necrosis.

DISCUSSION

Reye syndrome, which was first described in 1963,[1] is characterized by an acute noninflammatory encephalopathy associated with fatty degeneration of viscera, especially liver and kidneys, and hyperammonemia.[2] The syndrome occurs most commonly in infants and children with cases occurring both sporadically and in epidemics[3]; Reye syndrome rarely occurs in adults.

Epidemiologic investigations of Reye syndrome have indicated that the incidence is less than 1 case/100,000 children less than 17 years old[4] and that the syndrome tends to occur in white, middle-class school-age children who live in suburban and rural areas.[5] However, cases in infants are more likely to occur in ethnic minorities and poor, inner city dwellers.[6] The peak season for the syndrome is winter when cases are often associated with epidemics of influenza and varicella.[5]

The pathogenesis of Reye syndrome remains unknown, but numerous studies have helped to define a characteristic clinical presentation. The syndrome is a biphasic illness initiated usually by an influenza or varicella viral prodrome.[7] At the time of recovery from this prodromal illness, recurrent vomiting develops, which progresses to encephalopathy within 24 to 48 hours.[5]

Because influenza and varicella infections are so common and Reye syndrome is uncommon, genetic predisposition probably plays a role.[8] Further evidence for probable genetic vulnerability is the similarity of the clinical and pathologic findings in Reye syndrome and known inheritable metabolic defects. Commonly found biochemical abnormalities include hypoglycemia, elevated serum ammonia, AST, ALT, and creatine phosphokinase levels, short- and medium-chain fatty acids, amino, lactic, and uric acid values, and evidence of metabolic acidosis. Microvesicular fat deposition and noninflammatory liver changes can also be found in these disorders. However, significant metabolic defects have not been found in Reye syndrome; urea cycle enzymes are not absent, and carnitine levels are elevated in patients with Reye syndrome.

Because of the fairly distinctive epidemiologic features of Reye syndrome, including the predilection for rural or suburban school-age children and geographic clustering of outbreaks, environmental factors associated with the syndrome have been vigorously sought. Viral illnesses, especially influenza and varicella, commonly precede Reye syndrome, but no histologic evidence of inflammation or recovery of virus from involved organs has been seen. Environmental toxins such as pesticides have been extensively sought but only rarely associated with Reye syndrome cases. Two naturally occurring toxins, alflatoxins and hypoglycin, can cause Reye syndrome–like illness, but these toxins have been found in no greater levels in affected patients compared with controls.[9]

The use of salicylates during the antecedent illness by patients who develop Reye syndrome has been shown to be a significant risk factor by epidemiologic studies.[10, 11] Fewer cases than controls took acetaminophen products, combination products not containing acetylsalicylate or acetaminophen, or antibiotics.[11] Based on these and other confirmatory studies, the Centers for Disease Control (CDC), the Surgeon General, and the American Academy of Pediatrics have recommended that salicylates should not be used to treat children with varicella and influenza.[11–13]

Interestingly, the incidence of reported cases of Reye syndrome has fallen in the past several years beginning just as the public health recommendations on aspirin use were announced.[14, 15] The reasons for the declining incidence are not known but are not explained by declining rates of influenza or varicella infections.[16] A falling incidence of Reye syndrome has also been noted in Australia where aspirin is used much less frequently than acetaminophen in the pediatric population and in children with Reye syndrome.[17]

The classic clinical features of Reye syndrome are well demonstrated by this case. Patients are usually of school age and from a suburban area. They usually have a mild antecedent "flu" like illness, and as they begin to improve, intractable vomiting develops 3 to 5 days after onset without significant fever. Although patients are usually well-oriented and irritable when the vomiting begins, their condition can progress to lethargy, and later coma (Table 39–1). Some patients have no change in consciousness and remain only lethargic without any further progression. The physical examination is usually remarkable for the changes in consciousness and hyperreflexia. Hepatomegaly can be found. This patient did not experience seizures, but they are often encountered in younger children. The laboratory evaluation demonstrates elevated serum transaminase values and serum ammonia, variable degrees of prolongation in the PT, and a normal bilirubin. Testing for infectious and toxic etiologies is unrevealing. These findings, the acute onset of noninflammatory encephalopathy associated with sterile spinal fluid, elevated serum aminotransferase levels, abnormal PT, and elevated blood ammonia level in the absence of other diagnostic possibilities, fulfill the criteria for diagnosis established by the CDC (Table 39–2).[16]

The diagnosis can usually be made on clinical grounds, and liver biopsies are now obtained only when the history, physical, and laboratory findings do not provide a clear-cut diagnosis. The management of the patient is strongly influenced by the clinical staging of coma at the time of admission. Most centers use the clinical staging scheme proposed by Lovejoy et al. (Table 39–1).[2] Stages I and II represent the precoma state, whereas stages III, IV, and V represent gradations of coma.[2]

What controls the rate of progression is unknown. It has been difficult to predict which children will progress to deeper coma. A recent prospective study showed that a combination of PT prolonged more than 3 seconds compared with the control value and a serum ammonia level on admission more than 100 mg/dl predicted with a sensitivity of 100% and a specificity of 97.6% which patients will progress.[18]

The principles of management focus on intensive supportive care, correction of metabolic abnormalities, and treatment of increased ICP.[3, 18, 19] Any child suspected of having Reye syndrome should be admitted to a pediatric intensive care unit. Children in stage I or II Reye syndrome generally receive a hypertonic glucose solution and are monitored and observed closely.[20]

For children in stages III, IV, or V, endotracheal tubes are electively inserted along with arterial lines, nasogastric tubes and Foley catheters.[3, 18, 19] The patients are paralyzed and placed on mechanical ventilation. Intracranial pressure is monitored by a manometer placed in the subarachnoid or intraventricular spaces. Improved supportive care, especially in preventing increased ICP, has led to improved survival figures.[18] Factors known to increase pressure, including hypercarbia, hypoxia, hy-

TABLE 39–1.

Clinical Staging in Reye Syndrome*

Stage I
  Vomiting, lethargy, sleepiness, laboratory evidence of
    hepatic dysfunction, and type 1 EEG (slowing with
    dominant theta and rare delta waves)
Stage II
  Disorientation, delirium, combativeness, hyperventila-
    tion, hyperreactive reflexes, appropriate response to
    painful stimuli, evidence of hepatic dysfunction, and
    type 2 EEG (dysrhythmic slowing with dominant
    delta and some theta waves)
Stage III
  Obtundation, coma, hyperventilation, decorticate rigid-
    ity, preserved light reflexes and oculovestibular re-
    flexes, liver dysfunction, and type 2 EEG continue
Stage IV
  Deepening coma, decerebrate rigidity, loss of oculoce-
    phalic reflexes (often asymmetrical) large fixed pup-
    ils, dysconjugate eye movements in response to
    caloric stimulation, minimal liver dysfunction, EEG
    type 3 or 4 with evidence of brainstem dysfunction
    (disorganized or isoelectric EEG)
Stage V
  Seizures, loss of deep tendon reflexes, respiratory ar-
    rest, flaccidity, and type 4 EEG (isoelectric); liver
    function tests are often normal at this stage

*Adapted from Lovejoy et al.[2]

potension, hyperosmolar state, overhydration, painful stimuli, and hypoglycemia, are avoided.[17, 19] When ICPs rise, hyperventilation and osmotic diuretics like mannitol are used. Patients refractory to treatment for increased ICP and those who rapidly progress to deeper stages of coma and increased ICP carry the worst prognosis.[2, 3, 18, 19]

Earlier therapy for Reye syndrome attempted to reduce circulating toxins by exchange transfusion, peritoneal dialysis, and plasmapheresis.[3, 20] However, these treatments have not proved successful and in some cases have been associated with poorer prognosis,[2] so they are no longer used.

The prognosis in Reye syndrome correlates most closely with the final depth of coma and level of blood ammonia elevation.[21] Patients who did not progress beyond stage II and whose blood ammonia levels remained less than 300 μg/dl uniformly did well.[22]

The mortality rate for Reye syndrome has fallen in recent years probably from the dual effect of improved supportive care and greater recognition of milder cases.[21] Most survivors do well, but morbidity figures of 10% to 30% are found especially in patients who remain in deeper levels of coma for long periods or who have poorly controlled ICP.[23] Younger children are more susceptible to neuropsychologic sequelae including changes in cognitive, academic, and psychiatric function.[23]

TABLE 39–2.
Criteria for Diagnosing Reye Syndrome*

1. Acute noninflammatory encephalopathy documented clinically or by cerebrospinal fluid or histologic criteria.
2. Hepatic involvement documented by a threefold or greater rise in the levels of either the AST, ALT, or serum ammonia values or by a liver biopsy considered to be diagnostic of Reye syndrome.
3. No more reasonable explanation for the cerebral or hepatic abnormalities.

*Adapted from *MMWR*.[15]

The most important factor in obtaining a successful outcome for the patient with Reye syndrome is making an early diagnosis so that the appropriate supportive care can be instituted. Transfer to a tertiary center where expert pediatric critical care can be administered is essential. The outlook for most patients with Reye syndrome treated in this manner is good, but the outcome of our patient is a reminder that rapid progression to stage V coma carries a grim prognosis.

SUMMARY

The etiology of Reye syndrome remains unknown, but the disease is often preceded by an influenza or varicella viral prodrome. The laboratory findings of elevated serum transaminase and ammonia levels, a prolonged PT, and a normal bilirubin level are consistent with Reye syndrome. No specific therapy is available, but early identification of patients and institution of appropriate supportive care has helped to improve the overall survival rate. The epidemiologic evidence in the United States linking aspirin ingestion with the development of Reye syndrome strongly supports the recommendation that salicylates should be withheld from children with a viral illness.

REFERENCES

1. Reye RDK, Morgan G, Baral J: Encephalopathy and fatty degeneration of the viscera: A disease entity in childhood. *Lancet* 1963; 2:749–752.
2. Lovejoy FH, Smith AL, Bresnan MJ, et al: Clinical staging in Reye syndrome. *Am J Dis Child* 1974; 128:36–41.
3. Trauner DA: Reye syndrome. *West J Med* 1984; 414:206–209.
4. National Surveillance for Reye Syndrome, 1981: Update, Reye syndrome and salicylate usage. *MMWR* 1982; 31:53–56.
5. Corey L, Rubin RJ: Reye syndrome 1974: An epidemiological assessment, in Pollack JD (ed): *Reye Syndrome*. New York, Grune & Stratton, 1975, pp 179–187.
6. Huttenlocher PR, Trauner DA: Reye syndrome in infancy. *Pediatrics* 1978; 62:84–90.
7. Glick TH, Likosky WH, Leavitt LP, et al: Reye syndrome: An epidemiologic approach. *Pediatrics* 1970; 46:371–377.

8. Romshe CA, Hilty MD, McClung HJ, et al: Amino acid pattern in Reye syndrome: Comparison with clinically similar entities. *J Pediatrics* 1981; 98:788–790.
9. Nelson DB, Kimbrough R, Landrigan PS, et al: Aflatoxin and Reye syndrome: A case control study. *Pediatrics* 1980; 66:865–869.
10. Starko KM, Ray CG, Dominquez LB, et al: Reye syndrome and salicylate use. *Pediatrics* 1980; 66:859–864.
11. Hurwitz ES, Barrett MJ, Bergman D, et al: Public Health Service study on Reye syndrome and medications: Report of the pilot phase. *N Engl J Med* 1985; 313:849–857.
12. Food and Drug Administration Drug Bulletin. Washington, DC, Department of Health and Human Services, FDA, 1982, no. 12, p 9.
13. Surgeon General's advisory on the use of salicylates and Reye syndrome. *MMWR* 1982; 31:289.
14. Barrett MJ, Hurwitz ES, Schonberger LB, et al: Changing epidemiology of Reye syndrome in United States. *Pediatrics* 1986; 77:598–602.
15. Arrowsmith JB, Kennedy DL, Kuritasky JN, et al: National patterns of aspirin use and Reye syndrome reporting, United States, 1980 to 1985. *Pediatrics* 1987; 79:858–863.
16. Reye Syndrome—United States, 1985. *MMWR* 1986; 35:66–68, 73–74.
17. Orlowski JP, Gillis J, Kilham HA: A catch in the Reye. *Pediatrics* 1987; 80:638–642.
18. Boutros AR, Esfandiaris S, Orolowski JD, et al: Reye syndrome: A predictably curable disease. *Pediatric Clin North Am* 1980; 27:539–552.
19. Rockoff MA, Pascucci RC: Reye syndrome. *Emerg Med Clin North Am* 1983; 1:87–100.
20. Heubi JE, Daugherty CL, Partin JS, et al: Grade I Reye syndrome—outcome and predictions of progression to deeper coma grades. *N Engl J Med* 1984; 311:1539–1542.
21. Lichtenstein PK, Heubi JE, Daugherty CC, et al: Grade I Reye syndrome—a frequent cause of vomiting and liver dysfunction after varicella and upper-respiratory-tract infection. *N Engl J Med* 1983; 309:133–139.
22. Corey L, Rubin RJ, Hartwick MAW: Reye's syndrome: Clinical progression and evaluation of therapy. *Pediatrics* 1977; 60:708–714.
23. Shaywitz SE, Cohen PM, Cohen DJ, et al: Long-term consequences of Reye syndrome: A sibling-matched, controlled study of neurologic, cognitive, academic, psychiatric function. *J Pediatr* 1982; 100:41–46.

40 Wilson Disease

Victor L. Fox, M.D.
John D. Snyder, M.D.

A 16-year-old girl had developed lethargy and jaundice 10 months earlier. Previously she had been in excellent health and had no known contact with hepatitis, blood products, toxins, or recent use of medications. Results of an evaluation revealed elevated liver aminotransferase levels, bilirubin level 3.1 mg/dl, alkaline phosphatase level 180 mg/dl (normal <110 mg/dl), and normal prothrombin (PT) and partial thromboplastin (PTT) times. There was no evidence of infection with hepatitis A or B virus, Epstein Barr virus, or cytomegalovirus. The serum α_1-antitrypsin level was normal and no autoantibodies were detected. A liver biopsy specimen showed piecemeal necrosis and a periportal lymphocyte and plasma cell infiltrate consistent with a diagnosis of chronic active hepatitis. Steroid therapy was initiated. The patient showed no change in her liver function for 6 months but then developed slowly rising liver aminotransferase levels, bilirubin level, PT, and PTT over the course of 3 months. Three weeks earlier, she was admitted to her local hospital in liver failure with a normal neurologic examination. Her laboratory evaluation revealed evidence for mild hemolysis on peripheral smear, aspartate aminotransferase (AST) level 356 mU/ml (normal <21 mU/ml), alanine aminotransferase (ALT) level 383 mU/ml (normal <22 mU/ml), bilirubin level 5.6 mg/dl, albumin level 2.1 mg/dl, and PT and PTT that were twice the control value. The urine copper was 1,028 µg/24 hour (normal <64 µg/24 hour), and the serum ceruloplasmin was 18 mg/dl (normal >22 mg/dl). A liver biopsy revealed findings consistent with chronic active hepatitis. The copper stain was positive and the liver copper level was 1,256 µg/gm of dry weight (normal <50 µg/gm dry weight) confirming the diagnosis of Wilson disease. The patient was treated with 1 gm/day of D-penicillamine and transferred to this hospital, where her course rapidly deteriorated. She died on the third hospital day.

DISCUSSION

Wilson disease (WD) represents a rare autosomal recessive disorder of copper metabolism resulting in abnormal accumulation of copper, leading to lenticular degeneration and cirrhosis of the liver.[1] The disease frequently presents in childhood as chronic hepatitis but may also present as a neurologic, psychiatric, or skeletal disorder.[2]

Cases are distributed worldwide with a prevalence of approximately 1 per 50,000

264

persons.[3] The prevalence increases in populations with higher rates of consanguinity. The frequency of heterozygous carriers is approximately 5 per 1,000.[4] Greater than 50% of all patients have symptoms before reaching their middle teenage years.[5]

Pathophysiology

The primary defect in WD remains unknown. A single mutant gene is assumed to be causative, and recent studies have localized the gene to chromosome 13.[4] Epstein and Sherlock have postulated that the abnormal gene in WD is a mutant regulatory gene that fails to promote the transition from fetal copper metabolism, which resembles that of WD, to normal mature copper metabolism.[6]

Although the defect is unknown, circumstantial evidence points to an hepatic lysosomal defect which interferes with the excretion of copper from lysosomes to bile. Copper accumulation occurs in numerous organs, including brain, liver, eye, and kidney.

The low levels of ceruloplasmin found in WD patients were originally believed to play some pathophysiologic role. However, there is no correlation between ceruloplasmin levels and severity of disease. Ceruloplasmin levels often fall during successful treatment, and heterozygous individuals with no evidence of disease may have very low levels.[7] In addition, as many as 28% of WD patients may have normal levels at presentation.[8]

The progressive accumulation of copper and resultant tissue injury may be viewed in stages as proposed by Deiss et al.[9] Stage I represents the asymptomatic period during which copper accumulates primarily in the liver without evidence of overt liver injury. Stage 2 begins as the liver reaches saturation with copper and more copper is released to the systemic circulation. Clinical hepatitis and hemolytic anemia may occur. Greater amounts of copper accumulate in extrahepatic tissues during stage 3, resulting in the onset of neurologic symptoms, Kayser-Fleischer (KF) rings (a golden brown or greenish discoloration of Descemet's membrane in the limbic region of the cornea), renal disease, or other organ dysfunction. Stage 4 is characterized by fully manifest, life-threatening neurologic, hepatic, and multiorgan system disease. Patients receiving effective treatment enter a period of presumed negative copper balance designated stage 5.

The mechanism of tissue-specific injury by copper is largely unknown. In the case of hemolysis, the elevated erythrocyte copper content level is thought to both directly oxidize glutathione and inhibit the activity of glutathione-reducing enzymes.[10] This net effect on glutathione activity may subject erythrocytes to greater oxidative stress, resulting in accelerated hemolysis.

Clinical Features

The varied clinical presentation of WD reflects the diversity of organ involvement. The most common presentation in children is either acute or chronic liver disease, which can mimic acute hepatitis, chronic active hepatitis, cirrhosis, or fulminant hepatitis.[1, 11, 12] Although hepatic copper accumulation begins during infancy, hepatic manifestations rarely appear before 5 or 6 years of age.[2] The youngest reported case was 4 years old.[13] The clinical course of the liver disease varies but is often silent. Asymptomatic patients are often evaluated only because they are siblings of a known WD patient.[8] Patients have progressed to cirrhosis without clinical evidence of hepatic disease. Extrahepatic involvement is believed to occur only when the liver binding sites have been saturated.[9]

The neurologic manifestations of WD often begin with subtle changes such as decreased school performance and deteriorating fine motor coordination.[5] More discrete abnormalities of movement and tone, including dysarthria, dysphagia, rigidity, tremors, chorioathetosis, spasticity, and ataxia may follow.[14] These findings usually begin after the age of 10 to 12 years and are almost always associated with the presence of KF rings.[15] Kayser-Fleisher rings may be absent in patients with only hepatic disease[5] and can be present in other forms of chronic cholestatic liver disease besides WD.[11]

Patients with WD may also have psychiatric disturbances ranging from subtle behavioral and affective disorders to frank psychoses.[16] These manifestations have been recognized since the disease was first described, but the incidence of these symptoms remains unknown. In older children and adolescents, behavioral disorders are often confused with commonly observed psychologic problems of adolescents. Appropriate treatment for WD usually results in only partial psychiatric recovery.[5]

Although the great majority of children with WD present with liver or neurologic disease,[2] skeletal abnormalities, hemolytic anemia, or renal disease may also be the presenting problem.[1] Skeletal abnormalities include osteopenia, chondrocalcinosis, and arthropathy. The anemia is usually self-limited and is thought to be caused by an abrupt rise in plasma copper, which causes oxidative damage to red blood cell membranes and hemoglobin.[5] The association of acute anemia with acute hepatic failure correlates with a poor prognosis for recovery.

Renal abnormalities in WD include renal tubular disorders and decreased glomerular filtration rate.[17] The severity of the renal defect ranges from mild proteinuria to the Fanconi syndrome.

Diagnosis

Few diseases are mistaken for WD in a patient presenting with the classic triad of neurologic disease, KF rings, and liver dysfunction. However, because WD can present as hepatic, neurologic, psychiatric, skeletal, hematologic, or renal disease, the differential diagnosis may be extensive. To prevent the tragedy of failing to make the diagnosis of a potentially fatal but treatable disease, the clinician must consider WD in any child, adolescent, or young adult with liver disease.

The diagnosis of WD has classically rested on the findings of deficient serum ceruloplasmin levels, marked increase in urine copper excretion, KF rings, and marked elevation of hepatic copper levels.[2] However, none of these criteria individually is sufficient to make the diagnosis of WD.

Table 40–1 compares the important clinical features used to distinguish WD from the acute and chronic forms of liver disease with which it may be confused. Some patients with chronic active hepatitis (CAH) and idiopathic fulminant hepatitis (IFH) unrelated to WD can also have low ceruloplasmin levels.[5] Urinary copper

TABLE 40–1.
Comparative Features of Liver Disorders Resembling Wilson Disease

Features	WD	CAH	Idiopathic Fulminant Hepatitis	Idiopathic Cirrhosis
Familial	Autosomal recessive	–	–	–
Age onset	>3 yr	>1.5 yr	Any	Any
Extrahepatic disease	Yes	Yes	–	–
KF rings	+/–	+/–	–	+/–
Liver copper	↑↑	+/– ↑	+/– ↑	+/– ↑
Ceruloplasmin	↓	+/– ↓	+/– ↓	Normal
Urine copper	↑↑	↑	↑	↑

excretion may be increased in CAH, IFH, and cirrhosis but usually not to such a high level as found in WD.[8] Kayser-Fleisher rings should always be sought but are often not present in children with only hepatic involvement.[2] The hepatic copper concentration is the single most important value for diagnosing WD. The upper limit of normal hepatic copper values is 50 μg/gm of dry liver weight; values greater than 250 to 300 μg/gm are usually found with WD.[8] The serum copper, bilirubin, transaminase, and alkaline phosphatase levels are not helpful in distinguishing between these diseases. Very elevated gamma globulin levels and autoantibodies may help to identify patients with autoimmune CAH.

The histologic changes on liver biopsy may be suggestive but are not pathognomonic of WD. Findings commonly seen include fatty vacuolization of hepatocytes, glycogen-filled nuclei, and Mallory bodies (cytoplasmic hyalin).[18] A variety of other lesions including macrolobular or post necrotic cirrhosis, portal lymphocytic infiltration, and periportal and perilobular necrosis have been reported.[3] Because the liver histology can mimic acute, chronic active, chronic persistent, or fulminant hepatitis, the diagnosis of WD cannot be made on pathologic criteria alone.[18]

The diagnostic studies listed in Table 40–2, accompanied by the history and physical findings are required to make the diagnosis. The constellation of low serum ceruloplasmin level, elevated urine copper level, and elevated hepatic copper level in association with hemolytic anemia, skeletal changes, KF rings, and discrete behavioral and neurologic changes is found only in WD.

Treatment

The treatment of WD relies on the use of copper chelating agents and a low-copper diet, with liver transplantation available for fulminant cases. The therapy is usually successful when initiated early in the course of the disease.

D-Penicillamine, which chelates copper as well as mercury, lead, and zinc, remains the mainstay of therapy.[19] The mode of action of penicillamine is assumed to be direct removal of excess copper in the urine, but penicillamine may form nontoxic copper complexes in tissue that become unstable and toxic if the drug is discontinued.[20]

Children are initially treated with 250 mg/day and advanced by 250-mg increments until a dose of 1 gm is attained. Success of chelation is indicated by increased urinary copper output, which can reach 2 to 5 mg daily. The most common side effect of D-penicillamine is dose-dependent, reversible proteinuria, but bone marrow suppression, fever, rash, lymphadenopathy, Goodpasture's syndrome, and systemic lupus erythematosis have been reported.[5] A brief discontinuation of the therapy often allows reinstitution safely at a lower dose.[9]

Striking improvement is often seen in the liver function tests and neuropsychiatric manifestations, and the KF rings often disappear.[9] Less success is seen if hepatic fibrosis and portal hypertension have developed; D-penicillamine is of little use in fulminant hepatic failure,[5] as was seen in the case presented.

Patients unable to tolerate D-penicillamine can be effectively treated with another chelating agent, triethylenetetramine dihydrochloride (trientine).[19, 20] Anemia has been the only reported complication. More extensive experience with trientine may result in its use as first-choice drug therapy. Oral zinc, which blocks intestinal absorption of copper, has also been used,[21] but few data are available to assess its long-term efficacy.

The only known therapy for acute, fulminant liver failure in WD is liver transplantation. Transplantation has resulted in the apparent reversal of abnormal copper metabolism[22] and may be considered in patients whose disease is refractory to therapy or who cannot tolerate therapy.

The prognosis for patients with WD depends primarily on how early the diagnosis is made and therapy instituted.[9] Portal hypertension, hypoalbuminemia, prolonged PT, and markedly elevated bilirubin levels are poor prognostic signs for survival.

TABLE 40–2.
Laboratory Evaluation of Wilson Disease

Test	Abnormal Finding
Blood	
Hemoglobin, RBC smear, reticulocyte count	Hemolytic anemia
Ceruloplasmin	<22 mg/dl
Uric acid	Often elevated
ALT, AST, bilirubin	Often elevated
Albumin	Often decreased
PT	Can be prolonged
Copper	Variable, but often elevated
Urine	
24-hr copper	>64 mg/24 hr
Protein	Can be elevated
Glucose	Can be elevated
Amino acids	Can be elevated
Liver	
Copper	>250–300 μg/gm of dry wt

SUMMARY

Wilson disease is a rare inherited disorder of copper metabolism. Toxic accumulation of copper results in diffuse tissue injury affecting primarily the liver and CNS. The diagnosis should be considered in all cases of occult hepatic, neurologic, or psychiatric disease. Appropriate evaluation of asymptomatic family members and genetic counseling is imperative once the diagnosis has been established. Current drug therapy can arrest progressive tissue injury, frequently reverse incapacitating symptoms, and prevent onset of disease in asymptomatic patients.

REFERENCES

1. Walshe JM: Wilson's disease, the presenting symptoms. *Arch Dis Child* 1962; 37:253–256.
2. Slovis TL, Dubois RS, Rudgerman DO, et al: The varied manifestation of Wilson's disease. *J Pediatr* 1971; 78:578–584.
3. Danks DM: Hereditary disorders of copper metabolism in Wilson's disease and Menke's disease, in Stanbury JV, Wyngaarden JB, Fredrickson DS, et al (eds): *The Metabolic Basis of Inherited Disease,* ed 5. New York, McGraw-Hill Book Co, 1983; pp 1251–1263.
4. Bowcock AM, Farrer LA, Cavalli-Sporza LL, et al: Mapping the Wilson disease locus to a cluster of polymorphic markers on chromosome 13. *Am J Hum Genet* 1987; 41:27–35.
5. Gollan JL: Copper metabolism, Wilson's disease, and hepatic copper toxicosis, in Zakim D, Boyer TD (eds): *Hepatology: A Textbook of Liver Disease.* 1982, WB Saunders Co, Philadelphia, PA. pp 1138–1159.
6. Epstein O, Sherlock S: Is Wilson's disease caused by a controller gene mutation resulting in perpetuation of the fetal mode of copper metabolism in childhood? *Lancet* 1981; 1:303–305.
7. Scheinberg IH, Sternlieb J: The long term management of hepatolenticular degeneration. *Am J Med* 1960; 29:316 333.
8. Perman JA, Werlin SL, Grand RJ, et al: Laboratory measures of copper metabolism in the differentiation of chronic active hepatitis and Wilson disease in children. *J Pediatr* 1979; 94:564–568.
9. Deiss A, Lynche RE, Lu GR, et al: Long-term therapy of Wilson's disease. *Ann Intern Med* 1971; 75:57–65.
10. Deiss A, Lee GR, Cartwright GE: Hemolytic anemia in Wilson's disease. *Ann Intern Med* 1970; 73:413–418.
11. Scott J, Gollan JL, Samourian S, et al: Wilson's disease presenting as chronic active hepatitis. *Gastroenterology* 1978: 74:645–651.
12. McCullough AJ, Fleming CR, Thistle JL, et al: Diagnosis of Wilson's disease presenting as fulminant hepatic failure. *Gastroenterology* 1983; 84:161–167.
13. Werlin SL, Grand RJ, Perman JA, et al: Diagnostic dilemmas of Wilson's disease: Diagnosis and treatment. *Pediatrics* 1978; 62:47–51.
14. Dobyns WB, Goldstein NB, Gordon H: Clinical spectrum of Wilson's disease (hepatolenticular degeneration). *Mayo Clin Proc* 1979; 54:35–42.
15. Frommer D, Morris J, Sherlock S et al: Kayser-Fleisher-like rings in patients without Wilson's disease. *Gastroenterology* 1977; 72:1331–1335.

16. Goldstein NP, Ewert JC, Randall RV, et al: Psychiatric aspects of Wilson's disease (hepatolenticular degeneration): Results of psychometric tests during long term therapy. *Am J Psychiatr* 1968; 124:1555–1561.
17. Leu ML, Strickland GT, Gutman RA: Renal function in Wilson's disease: Response to penicillamine therapy. *Am J Med Sci* 1970; 260:381–398.
18. Sternlieb I: Diagnosis of Wilson's disease. *Gastroenterology* 1978; 74:787–793.
19. Walshe JM: Copper chelation in Wilson's disease. A comparison of penicillamine and triethylene tetramine. *Q J Med* 1973; 42:441–453.
20. Scheinberg IH, Jaffe ME, Sternlieb I: The use of trientine in preventing the effects of interrupting penicillamine therapy in Wilson's disease. *N Engl J Med* 1987; 317:209–213.
21. Brewer GJ, Hill GM, Prasad AS, et al: Oral zinc therapy for Wilson's disease. *Ann Intern Med* 1983; 99:314–320.
22. Beart RW Jr, Putman CW, Porter KA, et al: Liver transplantation for Wilson's disease. *Lancet* 1975; 2:176–177.

41 Portal Hypertension

Barry K. Wershil, M.D.

A 13-year-old boy was admitted for hematemesis and pancytopenia. He was well until 3 months prior to admission when he developed gastroenteritis along with several family members. This illness was followed by repeated episodes of upper respiratory tract congestion, cough, and occasional vomiting, which on one occasion was bloody. The hematemesis recurred two more times, and he was admitted to another hospital. He was noted to have an enlarged spleen and a hematocrit of 9.9%, mean corpuscular volume (MCV) of 57 μm³, platelet count of 44,000/mm³, and a white blood cell (WBC) count of 1,400/mm³ with 75% polymorphonuclear (PMN) leukocytes. The prothrombin time, partial thromboplastin time, and bleeding time were normal. The patient was transfused and referred to a hematologist for evaluation of pancytopenia.

On physical examination, the patient was slightly obese with stable vital signs. His skin revealed no stigmata of chronic liver disease such as spider angiomata or caput medusae, and he had no lymphadenopathy. His abdominal examination was remarkable for a normal liver size with a markedly enlarged spleen extending across the midline. No ascites was detected. Results of his neurologic exam and sensorium were normal.

Laboratory evaluation showed a WBC count of 1,300 (50% PMN leukocytes, 2% bands, 34% lymphocytes, 10% monocytes, and 3% eosinophils), platelet count of 59,000, and hematocrit 16.5% (MCV 67 μm³). The aspartate aminotransferase (AST), alanine aminotransferase (ALT), and bilirubin levels were normal; the serum protein level was 5.3 mg/dl and the albumin level 3.1 mg/dl. A bone marrow biopsy specimen showed a normal number of erythroid, lymphoid, and platelet precursors.

An abdominal ultrasound revealed normal liver size and echogenicity. In the region of the porta hepatis there was a mass of increased echogenicity comprised of many small tubular structures, a finding typical of cavernous transformation of the portal vein. Varices were seen in the region of the gastroesophageal junction. Finally, the spleen was noted to be massively enlarged. Endoscopy confirmed the presence of large esophageal and gastric varices.

Angiography identified a normal superior mesenteric artery, but in the venous phase, no portal vein was seen. Instead, a tangle of multiple sets of collateral vessels in the area of the porta was found (Fig 41-1).

Because of the upper gastrointestinal (GI) bleeding and the evidence of hypersplenism, a decision was made to perform a proximal splenorenal shunt.

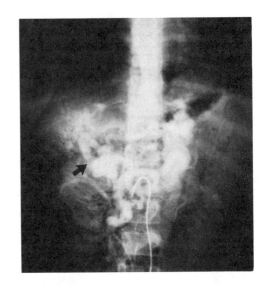

FIG 41–1.
Venous phase of superior mesenteric arteriogram demonstrating multiple collateral vessels in the area of the porta hepatis.

DISCUSSION

Portal hypertension in children can result from a variety of pathologic conditions involving either or both the hepatic vascular system and the liver. Portal hypertension in the pediatric population is uncommon, but the actual incidence is unknown. However, in pediatric tertiary care centers, portal hypertension is being seen more frequently, particularly as more children with complex liver diseases are surviving for longer periods of time.

Numerous causes of portal hypertension can be classified into three broad categories: (1) prehepatic, (2) intrahepatic, and (3) posthepatic (Table 41–1). The intrahepatic category can be further subdivided into presinusoidal, sinusoidal, and postsinusoidal causes. These categories are somewhat artificial since many causes of portal hypertension involve mixed classifications.[1] In children, the most common etiologies of portal hypertension are the prehepatic and intrahepatic causes.

Pathophysiology

Hepatic blood flow is supplied by the hepatic artery and the portal vein, with the liver receiving approximately 25% to 30% of the cardiac output. The hepatic artery supplies 20% to 30% of total hepatic blood flow, and the remaining 70% to 80% is supplied by the portal vein.[2] This blood flow is directed toward the liver sinusoids usually at a low pressure gradient across the liver (<5 mm Hg).

Pressure within a blood vessel is determined by the flow and resistance within that vessel. Increased resistance to blood flow appears to be the major factor in most cases of portal hypertension.[1] Techniques of measuring the portal pressure at different locations have been developed to localize the area of abnormal resistance.[3] The method considered most useful is the wedged hepatic venous pressure (WHVP). A venous catheter is advanced into a hepatic vein until occlusion (wedging) occurs or, if a balloon catheter is used, occlusion is achieved by balloon insufflation. The WHVP is an indirect measure of the pressure in the sinusoids and postsinusoidal areas. In pure prehepatic lesions, the WHVP is normal, whereas it is elevated in all types of sinusoidal, postsinusoidal, or posthepatic lesions.

As a consequence of increased portal pressure, collateral channels develop in an attempt to return blood to the systemic circulation. This gives rise to two of the major sequelae of portal hypertension, esophageal and gastric varices, and, if liver function is impaired, portal encephalopathy.

The single commonest cause of portal hypertension in children is prehepatic portal venous obstruction.[4] This can result from umbilical vein catheterization or omphalitis in the neonatal period, congenital abnormalities, or prior abdominal surgery; however, many cases have no definable cause.[4, 5]

Clinical Features

The specific signs and symptoms of portal hypertension depend on the etiology. The commonest presentation of prehepatic portal hypertension is GI bleeding and sple-

TABLE 41–1.
Causes of Portal Hypertension in Children

I.	Prehepatic
	A. Cavernous transformation of the portal vein
	B. Portal vein thrombosis
	C. Splenic arterio-venous fistula
	D. Tropical splenomegaly
	E. Splenic capillary hemangiomatosis
II.	Intrahepatic
	A. Presinusoidal (mixed)
	1. Idiopathic portal hypertension
	2. Congenital hepatic fibrosis
	3. Chronic active hepatitis
	4. Vinyl chloride toxicity
	5. Azathioprine?
	B. Sinusoidal (mixed)
	1. Cirrhosis
	2. Methotrexate
	C. Postsinusoidal
	1. Hypervitaminosis A
	2. Veno-occlusive disease
III.	Posthepatic
	A. Inferior vena cava web
	B. Constrictive pericarditis
	C. Severe heart failure
	D. Budd-Chiari syndrome

nomegaly.[5] In children, GI bleeding may be initiated by a minor, intercurrent infection or administration of aspirin.[6] There is no evidence that excessive exertion, swallowing large boluses of food, or gastroesophageal reflux initiate bleeding.[2]

Splenomegaly is almost always present while the liver is usually normal in size. The spleen may not be enlarged if the patient presents acutely with a massive bleeding episode. The spleen should again become palpable when the bleeding is controlled and fluid resuscitation is initiated. Ascites and portosystemic encephalopathy are unusual findings in prehepatic portal hypertension unless there is an additional insult such as septicemia or ischemia to the liver from bleeding.[2]

Intrahepatic causes of portal hypertension in children include congenital hepatic fibrosis and cirrhosis from biliary atresia, infectious hepatitis, α_1-antitrypsin deficiency, and Wilson disease. In most cases of cirrhosis, the spleen and liver are enlarged, and there is evidence of hepatic dysfunction. In addition to GI bleeding, ascites and portal encephalopathy are commonly seen but usually occur later in the course of the disease. Congenital hepatic fibrosis usually presents with GI bleeding, hepatosplenomegaly, and normal liver function, and it is commonly associated with renal abnormalities.[7]

Post-hepatic causes of portal hypertension are unusual in children. Budd-Chiari syndrome (thrombosis of the hepatic veins) can present in an acute or chronic form. Patients with acute Budd-Chiari syndrome are ill appearing, with abdominal pain, vomiting, hepatomegaly, ascites, and mild or no jaundice. The serum aminotransferase levels are usually markedly elevated. The more common chronic form of Budd-Chiari presents with ascites, hepatomegaly, and jaundice with normal or mildly elevated serum aminotransferase levels.

All three categories of portal hypertension can lead to the development of other clinical manifestations, including hemorrhoids from the formation of collateral vessels in the rectum and thrombocytopenia and leukopenia from hypersplenism.

Diagnosis

The evaluation of a patient with suspected portal hypertension should include determination of (1) the site of venous obstruction, (2) the portal pressure, (3) the presence of gastroesophageal varices, and (4) an evaluation for underlying liver disease.

Ultrasound should be performed initially in all patients, because it is a simple, noninvasive method of evaluating the portal venous system and the liver parenchyma. Ultrasound can determine the patency of the portal vein and the presence of collaterals such as esophageal varices. In one series of children with portal vein obstruction, ultrasound made the diagnosis in 36 out of 37 children.[4]

Portal venography is used for diagnostic purposes and to determine the site of obstruction. Splenoportography is a relatively safe and rapid method of determining the portal venous pressure. A needle is inserted into the splenic pulp, where pressure determination and contrast radiographs can be performed. All forms of portal hypertension will give an elevated intrasplenic pressure. Any abnormality in clotting is a contraindication to this procedure.

Transhepatic portal venography is more invasive and rarely necessary in patients suspected of having extrahepatic obstruction.[8] Angiography is indicated if the site of obstructed blood flow remains unclear or a surgical portosystemic shunt is considered. Most commonly, the celiac, hepatic, or superior mesenteric artery is selectively cannulated and injected with contrast. The portal system is visualized during the venous phase of the study; however, sometimes the technical quality may be unsatisfactory.[6]

Many of these radiographic methods will delineate collateral circulation, but upper endoscopy is a simpler, less invasive method of identifying clinically significant esophageal varices and should be performed in all cases of portal hypertension. In addition to identifying the presence of varices, endoscopy can help predict the risk of bleeding. In patients with alcoholic cirrhosis, large esophageal varices, not the degree of portal hypertension, correlated best with the risk of bleeding.[9]

Finally, a liver biopsy should be considered in patients with portal hypertension for diagnostic purposes. Prehepatic portal hypertension is associated with a normal liver and has a better prognosis than portal hypertension secondary to cirrhosis.[5]

Treatment

Although a great deal of information about the pathophysiology of portal hypertension has been gained over the last few years, many of the potential therapies remain unproved and controversial. Bleeding from esophageal varices is a major complication of portal hypertension and the major cause of mortality.[2] The approach to the management of acute upper GI hemorrhage is found in Chapter 4. This section will deal with the nonemergent therapy for esophageal varices. The major choices are sclerotherapy, portosystemic shunts, and propranolol therapy. No therapy has yet been proved to be clearly superior, and the choice of therapy should be guided by the experience and expertise of the physicians and facilities caring for the patient.[10]

Sclerotherapy has recently gained a prominent role in the treatment of variceal hemorrhage from both extrahepatic and intrahepatic portal hypertension.[11] Sclerotherapy is ideally performed after bleeding has been controlled by other methods, but sclerosis can also be attempted in emergent situations to control bleeding. Recent studies in adults have shown that endoscopic sclerotherapy performed within a few days of a bleeding episode significantly reduces the rate of rebleeding.[12–13] Multiple techniques and sclerosants have been used;[11] injections are usually repeated every 1 to 4 weeks until the varices are obliterated.

The incidence of complications of sclerotherapy in children appears to be relatively low.[14] The most frequent complications are chest pain and fever; however, more serious potential complications include esophageal erosions, stricture, and perforation.

Variceal hemorrhage can also be controlled surgically by portal venous decompression. The most commonly used shunts are the portocaval, mesocaval, and splenorenal shunts. Comprehensive discussions of the indications, surgical methods, and complications of portosystemic shunting are presented elsewhere.[15] Emergency shunting to control bleeding has a high mortality rate. Portosystemic shunts in children frequently occlude and run the risk of leading to portosystemic encephalopathy even with normal liver function,[16] although this has not been the experience in France.[17]

Bleeding episodes diminish with time in patients with prehepatic portal hypertension,[5] so that shunts in these patients should be avoided when possible. In patients with cirrhosis and liver failure in whom liver transplantation is a consideration, porto-systemic shunting may make that procedure technically difficult. For these reasons, in experienced hands, endoscopic sclerotherapy is preferred over surgical shunts for treating acute variceal hemorrhage in children.

Once a patient has been identified with portal hypertension and esophageal varices, the ideal course would be to institute a therapy that would prevent variceal bleeding. Unfortunately, both sclerotherapy and surgical shunting have been shown in several studies not to be effective prophylactic measures.[18]

Propranolol, a nonselective β-blocker, has been shown to significantly reduce the net portal venous pressure in patients with well-compensated alcoholic cirrhosis, but there was wide variation in individual response to the drug.[19] Several controlled trials of propranolol in patients with alcoholic cirrhosis and variceal bleeding have given conflicting results as to its efficacy;[2, 22] the reasons for these differences are not entirely clear. To date, the effectiveness of propranolol in children with portal hypertension has not been investigated. Propranolol may have untoward effects such as making resuscitation of a bleeding patient more difficult because of the β-blockade, and propranolol may induce encephalopathy.[2]

SUMMARY

Portal hypertension in children usually develops insidiously and may present with life-threatening variceal hemorrhaging. There are many causes of portal hypertension, but prehepatic and intrahepatic categories predominate in the pediatric population. The therapy for portal hypertension is directed toward treating the bleeding varices or performing a portosystemic shunt to reduce portal pressure. At the present time, these options are less than ideal, and it is hoped that future therapeutic modalities may effectively prevent the complications of portal hypertension.

REFERENCES

1. Groszman RJ, Atterbury CE: The pathophysiology of portal hypertension: A basis for classification. *Semin Liver Dis* 1982; 2:177–186.
2. Sherlock S: The portal venous system and portal hypertension, in Sherlock S (ed): *Diseases of the Liver and Biliary System*. Boston, Blackwell Scientific Publications, 1985, p 136.
3. Reynolds TB, Ito S, Iwatsuki S: Measurement of portal pressure and its clinical application: *Am J Med* 1970; 49:649–657.
4. Alvarez F, Bernard O, Brunell F, et al: Portal obstruction in children: I. Clinical investigation and hemorrhage risk. *J Pediatr* 1983; 103:696–702.
5. Webb LJ, Sherlock S: The aetiology, presentation, and natural history of extra-hepatic portal venous obstruction. *Q J Med* 1979; 48:627–639.
6. Sherlock S: Extrahepatic portal hypertension in adults. *Clin Gastroenterol* 1985; 14:1–20.

7. Alvarez F, Bernard O, Brunelle F, et al: Congenital hepatic fibrosis in children. *J Pediatr* 1981; 99:370–375.
8. Smith-Laing G, Camilo ME, Dick R, et al: Percutaneous transhepatic portography in the assessment of portal hypertension. Clinical correlation and comparison of radiographic techniques. *Gastroenterology* 1980; 78:197–205.
9. Lebrec D, De Fleury P, Rueff B, et al: Portal hypertension, size of esophageal varices, and risk of gastrointestinal bleeding in alcoholic cirrhosis. *Gastroenterology* 1980; 79:1139–1144.
10. Conn HO: Ideal treatment of portal hypertension in 1985. *Clin Gastroenterol* 1985; 14:259–288.
11. Mowat AP: Prevention of variceal bleeding. *J Pediatr Gastroenterol Nutr* 1986; 5:679–681.
12. Yassin YM, Sharif SM: Randomized control trial of injection sclerotherapy for bleeding oesophageal varices. An interim report. *Br J Surg* 1983; 70:20–22.
13. Copenhagen Oesophageal Varices Sclerotherapy Project. Sclerotherapy after 1st variceal haemorrhage in cirrhosis: A randomised multi-centre trial. *N Engl J Med* 1984; 311:1594–1600.
14. Proujansky R, Orenstein SR, Kocoshis SA: Risk factors for complications after variceal sclerotherapy in children. *Gastroenterology* 1988; 94:A360.
15. Henderson JM, Warren WD: Portal hypertension. *Curr Probl Surg* 1988; 3:155–223.
16. Hassall E, Benson L, Hart M, et al: Hepatic encephalopathy after portocaval shunt in a noncirrhotic child. *J Pediatr* 1984; 105:439–441.
17. Alvarez F, Bernard O, Brunelle F, et al: Portal obstruction in children: II. Results of surgical portosystemic shunts. *J Pediatr* 1983; 103:703–707.
18. Sauerbruch T, Wotzka R, Kopcke W, et al: Prophylactic sclerotherapy before the first episode of variceal hemorrhage in patients with cirrhosis. *N Engl J Med* 1988; 319:8–15.
19. Rector WG: Propranolol for portal hypertension: Evaluation of therapeutic response by direct measurement of portal vein pressure. *Arch Intern Med* 1985; 145:648–650.
20. Rector WG: Drug therapy for portal hypertension. *Ann Intern Med* 1986; 105:96–107.

42   Liver Transplantation in Children

Ronald E. Kleinman, M.D.

The patient was born following an uncomplicated full-term gestation. The delivery was uneventful, and he weighed 4.9 lb (2.2 kg) (small for gestational age) at birth. He was nourished on a commercial infant formula and at 4 months of age was noted to be jaundiced. An extensive examination for the cause of his jaundice revealed nonsyndromatic paucity of intrahepatic bile ducts. His subsequent course was marked by hepatosplenomegaly, ascites, rickets with multiple pathologic fractures, and marked growth and developmental delay. He was managed on a regimen of supplemental vitamins, diuretics, and intensive nutritional support. He had no history of gastrointestinal bleeding or encephalopathy. Because of persistent liver function abnormalities with severe failure to thrive, he underwent an orthotopic liver transplant at 2 years and 9 months of age. On the 12th postoperative day on cyclosporine and prednisone immunosuppression, he developed acute graft rejection, which was treated with increased doses of corticosteroids and a course of the monoclonal anti–T cell antibody OKT3. He was discharged in good condition 1 month after the transplant on a regimen of cyclosporine, azathiaprine, and prednisone. Following discharge he was in excellent health with a remarkable improvement in psychomotor development and marked increases in both length and weight. He had occasional upper respiratory tract infections but was otherwise healthy until 6 months following the liver transplant when he developed a persistently low-grade fever. A liver biopsy revealed only mild focal necrosis with no evidence of graft rejection. He was discharged from the hospital on the same immunosuppressive regimen but 2 days later developed watery diarrhea, temperature to 38.4°C, and vomiting. His diarrhea continued to increase in quantity over the next 6 days, and he was readmitted to the hospital 1 week after discharge with profuse, watery diarrhea, and dehydration. On admission to the hospital he was noted to have a 10% hyponatremic dehydration. Over the next 2 days he improved clinically and was afebrile, and cultures of blood, stool, and urine were negative. However, 48 hours after admission he became acutely febrile, cyanotic, and tachypneic with respirations of 80 per minute. A blood gas determination revealed a Pao_2 of 36 mm Hg, and a chest X-ray film showed bilateral diffuse alveolar infiltrates, greater on the right side. The patient was transferred to the intensive care unit and begun on oxacillin, gentamycin, and trimethoprim-sulfamethoxazole (Bactrim). Six hours after transfer to the intensive care unit he required intubation. His temperature was 40°C. An open lung biopsy was performed 4 days after admission, which showed *Pneumocystis carinii* pneumonia. Oxacillin and gentamycin were discontinued, and the patient was maintained solely on trimethoprim-sulfamethoxazole. His respiratory status remained stable for several days following the open lung biopsy and then slowly began to decline. Ten days after admission he required intensive ventilatory support and began to have wide fluctuations in blood pressure. Trimethoprim-sulfamethoxazole was discontinued, and pentamidine was started. Twenty-four hours later the patient suffered a respiratory arrest and could not be resuscitated. He died approximately 9 months after his liver transplant. The gross and microscopic examination of the patient's liver revealed no evidence of rejection. There was minimal or no recognizable inflammatory cell infiltrate in the portal tracts, and no inflammatory changes were seen in the major vessels or bile ducts in the hilum of the liver. There was diffuse fatty change and a few focal areas of cholestasis, consistent with the 3-week course of the terminal illness. Death was ascribed to severe, diffuse alveolar damage as a result of *P. carinii* infection.

DISCUSSION

This youngster's course provides an example of the remarkable benefits as well as dangers of liver transplantation in pediatric patients. For these patients with progressive compromise of hepatic function and the life-threatening consequences that follow, liver transplantation provides the only hope for survival and normal growth and development. The following discussion will review liver transplantation for infants and children with specific reference to this patient by describing the criteria for consideration for a liver transplant, the operative procedure, and the postoperative course.

Liver transplantation was attempted and performed successfully first in the 1960s.[1] Until recently most of these operations were done by Starzl in Pittsburgh and by Calne in Cambridge. Before 1979 the long-term (>2 years) survival was approximately 20% for all patients, including children.[1, 2] At the present time more than 1,000 pediatric patients have undergone orthotopic liver transplantation at more than 50 centers around the world. The most recent figures for long-term (>3 years) survival are 60% to 80% in pediatric patients.[1] Several factors are responsible for this impressive improvement in survival. Clearly, increased experience with the procedure and an awareness of the potential perioperative complications have played a major role in the improving survival. The increasing, but still insufficient, numbers of donor organs available for pediatric patients has also been a contributing factor, but major credit rests with the improved immunosuppression achieved with the introduction of cyclosporine into the immunosuppressive regimen.[3]

Consideration of Transplant

The patient presented here had a paucity of intrahepatic bile ducts, which led to progressive hepatic decompensation. The vast majority of pediatric patients have undergone orthotopic liver transplantation because of biliary atresia with failure of a portoenterostomy to correct the defect.[1, 2] The hepatic portoenterostomy first introduced by Kasai in 1959 has improved survival in patients with biliary atresia, but long-term survival is only 30% to 35% of all patients who undergo this procedure.[4] Thus, for the majority of patients with biliary atresia, death will occur before the age of 5 years unless the child undergoes liver transplantation. Survival for these patients is currently 60% to 80% following liver transplantation. In our own experience for those patients who weigh less than 26.5 lb (12 kg) at the time of operation, as in this case, the survival is closer to 60%. In patients with paucity of intrahepatic bile ducts, it is often difficult to determine the optimal time for liver transplantation or even if liver transplantation is indicated. Liver disease in these patients often stabilizes after the first years of life, particularly in those with syndromic paucity of intrahepatic ducts, which includes congenital heart disease, vertebral anomalies, hypogonadism, and opthalmalogic anomalies such as the posterior embryotoxin (see Chapter 34). Slow growth and development during this time may be part of the syndrome. Therefore, patients who have a paucity of intrahepatic ducts on liver biopsy must be examined carefully for concomittent congenital anomalies or dysmorphic features. Some patients, like this one, who had nonsyndromic paucity of intrahepatic ducts, have a progressive course with ultimate hepatic failure. For these patients and others with the early development of portal hypertension, liver transplant offers the hope of prolonged disease-free survival.

Patients with acute fulminant hepatic failure have been the recipients of orthotopic liver grafts, and although this procedure is much less successful in this setting, transplantation improves the chances for survival compared with standard medical therapy.[5] Patients who have an extrahepatic malignancy are also usually not candidates for liver transplantation. However, those patients who have hepatocellular carcinoma or hepatoblastoma entirely confined to the liver with no evidence of extrahepatic metastatic disease may be considered for transplantation. Of importance is the fact that biliary atresia and various metabolic diseases are occasionally complicated by unsuspected intrahepatic malignancies.[1]

Organ donation remains an important impediment in pediatric liver transplantation. Twenty percent to 30% of all potential pediatric recipients will die while waiting to obtain a liver.[1] The widespread publicity that liver transplantation has received in the past few years has improved the prospects for obtaining a liver sooner. Nevertheless, there is an acute and chronic shortage of livers for very small recipients. It is hoped that recent efforts that require physicians to ask families of potential donors to consider organ donation will increase the number of organs that become available. Recently a number of centers in the United States and in Europe have attempted to reduce a large liver from an adult or older child to a size appropriate for an infant.[6] This procedure has been performed successfully, although it is too early yet to tell what impact it will have on the overall availability of organs for very young infants.

Livers must come from donors who are hemodynamically stable and who are free of infection, vascular disease, and malignancy. Liver function tests from the donor must be normal or very near normal, and electrolytes must be in balance. When these criteria are present, a responsible physician notifies the regional organ bank, which then attempts to match patients first by priority and then by weight and blood type. Currently four categories of recipients exist. Patients listed as urgent priority means that they are unstable, rapidly decompensating, and in need of intensive

TABLE 42–1.

Criteria for Selection of Pediatric Liver Transplantation Patients

Progressive jaundice
Diminished hepatic synthetic function (prolongation of prothrombin time not correctable by vitamin K; hypoalbuminemia)
Symptomatic portal hypertension refractory to medical-surgical therapy (recurrent variceal bleeding; ascites)
Incapacitating hepatic encephalopathy
Intractable cholestasis
Growth failure despite exhaustive nutritional therapy
Inability to maintain a reasonable quality of life as a result of liver disease

*From Perlmutter et al.[1]

care. Priority 1 implies progression of disease with decompensating hepatic function requiring hospital care. Priority 2 patients require hospital care but are more stable, and priority 3 patients show evidence of progressive hepatic deterioration but are stable enough to remain at home. In general, infants and young children can receive livers from donors who are within 6.6 to 11 lb (3–5 kg) of their own weight.

Operative Procedure

The transplant team consists of two or three surgeons who travel to the potential donor to remove the organ. Careful removal of the liver is an essential part of the transplantation. At the time that the surgical team is notified that a liver is available, one team will go to the potential donor while the second team remains behind to begin the recipient hepatectomy. The recipient is notified, generally through a beeper system, that a liver has become available and must be at the hospital within 2 to 3 hours of being called. Recipient hepatectomy is begun as soon as one team of surgeons has left the hospital to harvest the donor liver. The recipient generally receives initial immunosuppression just before or at the time of the recipient hepatectomy.

Some mention of cost should be interjected at this point. From this discussion it should be quite clear that a large number of highly skilled people must be involved to ensure a successful transplant. The cost of evaluating the patient, procuring the donor organ, performing the transplant, and care during the posttransplant period ranges from $60,000 to more than $500,000 in our experience. Fortunately, these costs today are increasingly borne by third-party payers, although parents often find it necessary to raise some funds privately to, at the very least, support their own living expenses if the transplant is performed in a center far from their home.

Before discussing the operation itself, we should note that this child's condition satisfied several criteria that patients must have to be considered candidates for liver transplantation. Table 42–1 lists these criteria. Of great importance were the marked growth and developmental failure that the child displayed despite intensive therapy.

Patients who have advanced disease in organs outside of the liver, such as the heart, lungs, or kidneys, would be excluded from consideration for transplant. Other exclusion criteria include severe hypoxemia from right to left shunts, metastatic malignant disease, multiple life-threatening uncorrectable congenital anomalies, and, while it is present, sepsis.[1] As mentioned before, patients with acute hepatic failure may be considered for transplantation, although the mortality rate in this setting is exceedingly high.[5]

Prior surgery such as portoenterostomy and the presence of collateral vessels as a consequence of portal hypertension often complicate an already technically demanding procedure. As mentioned, the recipient liver is mobilized while the donor liver is being harvested. Because many pediatric patients will have anomalies of the vascular supply to the liver, angiography is often performed during the preoperative evaluation so that the surgeon can be prepared to deal with these anomalous vessels when performing the transplant. The recipient may be placed on venovenous bypass to avoid passive congestion of the kidneys and bowel during cross-clamping of the systemic and portal circulation during the operation.[1] The vascular supply to the diseased liver is not clamped until the team harvesting the donor liver has brought that liver into the operating room, where it undergoes final inspection and preparation for orthotopic placement into the recipient.

The vena cavae are the first vessels to be anastomosed, followed by the portal vein, and then the hepatic artery. The biliary reconstruction is performed last, and when possible, a duct-to-duct anastomosis is performed. For those recipients who have biliary atresia, the common bile duct is anastomosed to a Roux-en-Y limb.[2] A small feeding tube or T tube is placed in the common duct as an internal stent and is brought out through the anterior abdominal wall.[1, 2] Bile flow is often observed immediately after anastomosis of the bile duct in functioning donor livers.

The entire operation lasts between 7 and 24 hours. From 5 to more than 100 units of blood products may be used during the transplant operation. Current techniques of preservation allow up to 24 hours from the time that the blood supply to the donor liver is clamped to the time that the liver is reperfused in the recipient.[7] Although an attempt is made to match the donor and recipient major blood groups, transplants have been performed under conditions of ABO mismatch. In our own series and others, this does not appear to have affected the outcome of the procedure.[1]

Postoperative Course

Postoperative complications are common. Hypertension, infection and renal dysfunction, and primary graft nonfunction lead the list of complications.[8-10] Vascular thrombosis, bowel perforation and anastomotic leakage also occur. It is our impression that infants weighing less than 26.5 lb (12 kg) have, in general, a higher incidence of many of these complications.

The control of rejection is accomplished with a combination of immunosuppressive agents. The standard regimen includes the use of cyclosporine, initially intravenously and then orally as the patient recovers, together with a glucocorticoid such as prednisone.[11, 12] Cyclosporine, which was initially developed as an antibiotic, is completely insoluble in water and must be dissolved in an ethanol vehicle for intravenous use and in olive oil and ethanol for oral administration. It does not depress the bone marrow or cause leukopenia. Nephrotoxicity, hypertension, and hepatotoxicity are common side effects of this drug.[13] Less frequent toxicities include tremor, hirsutism, gum hypertrophy, and allergic reactions. As with many immunosuppressive agents, there appears to be a risk of developing malignancies during or following treatment with this drug, although at the present time this appears to be very small. Corticosteroids appear to produce a synergistic immunosuppressive effect with cyclosporine.

For those patients with chronic rejection or for those who do not tolerate usual doses of cyclosporine (2 to 6 mg/kg/day intravenously, 10–20 mg/kg/day orally), adjunctive immunosuppression is employed. Currently this is generally azathioprine. The control of acute rejection is usually accomplished by treatment with high-dose corticosteroids, which are tapered rapidly over a period of 7 to 10 days. Monoclonal antibody therapy to T-cell antigens has recently been employed to control acute rejection with very good success.[14]

The long-term management of patients includes the chronic use of immunosuppression, probably for the lifetime of the recipient. The threat of infection is constantly present, although patients appear to tolerate common pediatric infections quite well with increasing time on immunosuppression therapy. Every attempt should be made to fully immunize infants with standard vaccines prior to transplantation. Unfortunately, no safe, effective vaccine is currently available to prevent varicella, which may be a life-threatening event in the immunosuppressed patient. We currently recommend that once patients are immunosuppressed, they receive no live viral vaccines and that they be passively protected with immunoglobulin if exposed to life-threatening viral infections, such as varicella. Antiviral agents, when appropriate, should also be used in these patients.

This case demonstrates the potentially fatal effects of infection in patients who are chronically immunosuppressed. What appeared to be a common enteric and upper respiratory tract infection became rapidly fulminant in this youngster, and he died in spite of intensive antimicrobial and supportive therapy.

SUMMARY

This case report demonstrates that marked improvement in the quality of life can occur following liver transplantation. Liver function rapidly returns to normal following transplantation, and growth and development may accelerate dramatically. Improvements in surgical technique and advances in immunosuppression and organ preservation should, in the future, allow many more pediatric patients to be rescued from fatal hepatic decompensation. In spite of our best efforts at the present time, however, even those patients who appear to have had a successful transplantation and postoperative period continue to run the risks inherent in chronic immunosuppressive therapy

REFERENCES

1. Perlmutter D, Vacanti J, Donahoe P, et al: Liver transplantation in pediatric patients. *Adv Pediatr* 1985; 32:284–331.
2. Starzl TE, Iwatsuki S, Van Thiel DH, et al: Evolution of liver transplantation. *Hepatology* 1982; 2:614–636.
3. Starzl TE, Iwatsuki S, Malatack JJ, et al: Liver and kidney transplantation in children receiving cyclosporine A and steroids. *J Pediatr* 1982; 100:5:681–686.
4. Alagille D: Extrahepatic biliary atresia. *Hepatology* 1984; 4:7S–10S.
5. Peleman RR, Gavaler JS, Van Thield H, et al: Orthotopic liver transplantation for acute and subacute hepatic failure in adults. *Hepatology* 1987; 7:484–489.
6. Broelsch CE, Emond JC, Thistlethuwaite JR, et al: Liver transplantation with reduced size donor organs. *Transplantation* 1988; 45:519–523.
7. Kalayoglu M, Sollinger HW, Stratta RJ, et al: Extended preservation of the liver for clinical transplantation. *Lancet* 1988; 1:617–619.
8. Starzl TE, Iwatsuki S, Shaw BW, et al: Analysis of liver transplantation. *Hepatology* 1984; 4:47S–49S.
9. Vacanti JP, Lillehei CW, Jenkins RL, et al: Liver transplantation in children: The Boston Center experience in the first 30 months. *Transplant Proc* 1987; 14:3261–3266.
10. Ho M, Wajszczuk CP, Hardy A, et al: Infections in kidney, heart and liver transplant recipients on cyclosporine. *Transplant Proc* 1983; 15(suppl 1):2768–2772.
11. Starzl TE, Klintmalm GBG, Porter KA, et al: Liver transplantation with use of cyclosporine A and prednisone. *N Engl J Med* 1981; 305:5:266–269.
12. Dupont E, Wybran J, Toussaint C: Glucocorticosteroids and organ transplantation. *Transplantation* 1984; 34:4:331–335.
13. Stiller CR, Lampacis A, Keown PA, et al: Clinical considerations in cyclosporine treatment in the human. *Transplant Proc* 1983; 15:1886–1888.
14. Delmonico FL, Cosimi AB: Monoclonal antibody treatment of human allograft recipients. *Surg Gynecol Obstet* 1988; 166;89–98.

PART FOUR

The Pancreas

43   Pancreatitis

Barry K. Wershil, M.D.

A 5-year-old girl was admitted for evaluation of abdominal pain and a pancreatic mass. Five months prior to admission, she developed abdominal pain and vomiting and was found to have hyperamylasemia, which resolved with conservative management. Ten days prior to this admission, she developed abdominal pain and low-grade fever and was admitted to another hospital, where serum transaminase levels, amylase level, and blood counts were normal. She continued to have intense abdominal pain in the hospital but no vomiting. An abdominal ultrasound revealed a dilated pancreatic duct and a prominent head of the pancreas. An upper gastrointestinal (GI) radiologic series with small bowel follow through showed extrinsic compression of the second portion of the duodenum. There was no history of abdominal trauma, hypercholesterolemia, medications, or family history of pancreatitis.

On admission, she was a well-nourished girl who developed increasing abdominal discomfort over time and assumed a fetal position in bed. Her temperature, pulse, and respirations were normal. Results of the abdominal examination revealed the presence of bowel sounds and tenderness to palpation in both upper quadrants and epigastrium. There was no discoloration of the flanks.

Pertinent blood work included aspartate aminotransferase (AST) 86 mU/ml (normal <21 mU/ml), alanine aminotransferase (ALT) 68 mU/ml (normal <22 mU/ml), bilirubin 0.4 mg/dl total and 0 mg/dl direct, amylase 30 mU/ml (normal 20–110 mU/ml), and lipase 0.10 NaOH/ml (normal 0.2–1.5 NaOH/ml). An abdominal ultrasound revealed an enlarged head of the pancreas without dilatation of the ducts. An endoscopic retrograde cholangiopancreatogram (ERCP) was performed. It showed the common bile duct entering the duodenum along the minor pancreatic duct, which is consistent with pancreas divisum (Fig 43–1). In addition, the accessory duct was dilated with probable mild dilatation of the pancreatic duct.

Parenteral nutrition was begun, and the patient was given nothing by mouth. She continued to have pain and developed spiking temperatures to 40°C. Multiple blood cultures were negative, as were tests for presence of antinuclear antibody and rheumatoid factor. A computed axial tomographic (CT) scan demonstrated a diffusely enlarged and inhomogeneous pancreas; there was no evidence of a pancreatic abscess, but a single, small pseudocyst in the tail of the pancreas was identified. Broad-spectrum antibiotics and central hyperalimentation were administered for 3 weeks with general clinical improvement. A repeated CT scan showed slight enlargement of the pancreatic pseudocyst. The patient was taken to surgery, where a sphincteroplasty of the accessory and main ampulla was performed.

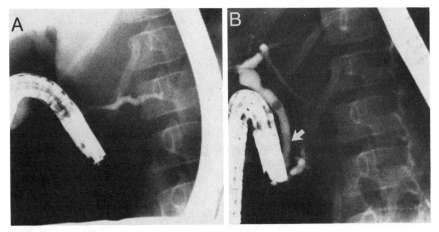

FIG 43–1.
Endoscopic retrograde cholangiopancreatogram. **A,** injection of duct of Santorini (minor papilla), which drains the majority of the pancreas. **B,** injection of duct of Wirsung with abrupt termination of dye. Note reflux into common bile duct *(arrow).*

DISCUSSION

Pancreatitis remains one of the more difficult diagnostic dilemmas faced by pediatricians, pediatric gastroenterologists, and surgeons. The variability of clinical symptoms, the obscurity caused by its anatomic location, and the inconsistency of the biochemical markers of pancreatic inflammation contribute to this diagnostic dilemma.

The precise incidence of pancreatitis in the pediatric age range is not known, but pancreatitis is not believed to be as uncommon as once believed.[1] This probably reflects better recognition and an increase in the use of therapeutic agents that may cause pancreatitis.

Pathophysiology

To understand the pathophysiology of pancreatic disease, one must understand the embryology and anatomy of this complex organ. The pancreas arises from two outgrowths, one from the dorsal aspect of the duodenum and a second from the common bile duct along the ventral portion of the duodenum.[2] During rotation of the gut, these ventral and dorsal anlage are brought together and eventually fuse, creating a single pancreas with the major duct supplied by the dorsal pancreas and the ventral duct fusing with the main duct. Pancreas divisum results when the dorsal and ventral pancreatic anlage fail to fuse.

The pancreas lies in a retroperitoneal position with the transverse mesocolon and stomach anteriorly, the vertebral column and aorta posteriorly, and the head fitting into the curve of the duodenum. The tail of the pancreas lies in close rela-

TABLE 43–1.
Important Causes of Pancreatitis in Children

Trauma
Drug-induced
 Azathioprine, hydrochlorothiazide, furosemide, sulfonamides, tetracycline, valproic acid
Infection
 Mumps, rubella, *Mycoplasma pneumoniae*, coxsackie B, hepatitis B, post-varicella
Anatomic
 Pancreas divisum (?), choledochal cyst, annular pancreas, duodenal or gastric
 duplication, choledocholithiasis
Metabolic
 Hyperlipoproteinemia types I, IV, and V, cystic fibrosis, hyperparathyroidism, refeeding
Vascular
 Hemolytic-uremic syndrome, systemic lupus erythematosus, Henoch-Schönlein purpura
Idiopathic

---

tionship to the spleen, left kidney, and left colic flexure. In general, the pancreas is fixed in this position with very little mobility.

The mechanisms that produce pancreatitis are still not completely understood, although many theories exist. A presently popular theory is that obstruction of the pancreatic duct by any mechanism (including inflammation, gallstones, or papillary spasm) can result in ductal disruption and extravasation of secretions into the pancreatic parenchyma.[3] Since most of the pancreatic enzymes are secreted in an inactive (zymogen) form, enzyme activation may occur within the pancreatic acinar cells via the coalescence of lysosomal and digestive enzymes within intracellular vacuoles.[3] At the present time, much more basic research remains to be done to completely explain the pathophysiology of pancreatitis.

The causes of pancreatitis in children and infants are varied (Table 43–1). Pancreatic trauma is a major cause of pancreatitis in the pediatric population,[1] and this is usually the result of blunt trauma to the epigastric region from bicycle handles, sledding, or child abuse.[4] In tertiary care centers, drug-related pancreatitis is another common etiology.[1] A long list of drugs from azathioprine to valproic acid have been implicated in the development of pancreatitis.[5] Less clearly implicated are drugs such as corticosteroids.[6] Infectious agents can also cause pancreatitis. Mild pancreatitis is not unusual in patients with systemic viral infections, and clinically significant pancreatitis can be seen with rubella or *Mycoplasma* infections and in up to 10% of children with mumps.[7]

Anatomic lesions or malformations of the biliary or pancreatic ducts and ductal obstruction secondary to abnormalities like annular pancreas or intestinal duplication can all result in pancreatic inflammation. The direct relation between pancreas divisum and pancreatitis is still debated.[8, 9] Pancreas divisum is a common lesion occurring in 3% to 6% of individuals in autopsy and endoscopic studies,[9] and the incidence of pancreatitis in patients with pancreas divisum may be no higher than in patients without the abnormality.[8]

Other causes of pancreatitis include metabolic disorders such as hyperlipopro-teinemia types I, IV, and V, cystic fibrosis, and hyperparathyroidism. Vasculitic disorders, hereditary pancreatitis, and unusual causes such as refeeding pancreatitis should also be considered.

Clinical Features

Clinically, pancreatitis often presents in an insidious fashion, although it can, in severe cases, present like an abdominal emergency with shock and a rigid abdomen. Most frequently, patients have left upper quadrant, flank, or epigastric pain. The pain may radiate to the shoulder. Evidence for a sympathetic pleural effusion should always be sought. Nausea and vomiting are frequently associated with the pain. In severe cases, children may be likely to assume a fetal position or hyperextend the neck and back. Unusual clinical findings include Turner's sign (ecchymoses on the abdomen and flanks) and Cullen's sign (bluish umbilicus), which are indicative of hemorrhagic pancreatitis.

Diagnosis

There is no clinical or laboratory finding diagnostic of pancreatitis. The diagnosis is based on historic and physical examination clues, and the results of indirect tests and must always be considered a working, not a final, diagnosis.[10] The serum amylase determination is still the most commonly used test to support the diagnosis of pancreatitis. However, elevations of serum amylase levels may result from a number of disease processes unrelated to the pancreas (Table 43–2). In contrast, even severe pancreatitis can occur in the face of a normal serum amylase value, especially if it is obtained a few days after the onset of symptoms.[11] Because the serum amylase level may rise and fall rapidly in acute pancreatitis, a random urinary amylase value (normal <750 international units (IU)/L) may be useful if the patient presents a few day after the onset of symptoms.[10] The serum lipase determination is no more specific for pancreatitis than the serum amylase determination and often parallels it but usually persists longer.[12] The amylase-to-creatinine clearance ratio initially held promise as a diagnostic test, but recent studies have indicated that it is a nonspecific indicator of tubuloproteinuria and the severity of acute illness.[13] The ratio cannot be used when

TABLE 43–2.

Causes of Hyperamylasemia

Pancreatic disease
Nonpancreatic disorders
Salivary gland lesion (e.g., mumps), renal insufficiency, macroamylasemia   /
Complex disorders
Biliary tract disease, perforated peptic ulcer, intestinal obstruction, ectopic pregnancy, mesenteric infarction, acute appendicitis, peritonitis, diabetic ke-toacidosis, burn trauma, cerebral trauma

TABLE 43–3.
Diagnostic Tests

Laboratory Tests	Radiology
Serum amylase	Chest and abdominal plain films
Serum lipase	Ultrasound of gallbladder and pancreas
Complete blood cell count	CT scan of the pancreas*
Blood chemistries (electrolyte values, BUN level, creatinine clearance, calcium concentration, serum aminotransferase levels)	Upper GI series*
	ERCP*
Serum triglyceride levels	
Sweat test*	
Urine amylase level*	
Peritoneal lavage analysis*	

*When indicated

the serum amylase level is normal, and a number of nonpancreatic diseases can give a false positive result.[14]

The other laboratory tests useful for the evaluation of suspected pancreatitis are listed in Table 43–3. Serum lipid values are obtained to assess hypertriglyceridemia as a possible etiologic factor. Some laboratory tests have been shown to have prognostic significance, such as hypocalcemia (<8 mg/dl), which may be a sign of severe pancreatitis and pancreatic necrosis.[10, 15] Increased mortality is associated with decreased hematocrit without obvious blood loss (hemorrhagic pancreatitis), an elevated white blood cell count (>16,000/mm^3), increased blood urea nitrogen (BUN) level (>30 mg/dl) or creatinine level (>2 mg/dl), a decreased albumin level (<3.0 mg/dl), or the development of arterial hypoxemia.[10, 15] In some instances where the diagnosis remains uncertain and the patient is extremely ill, analysis of peritoneal lavage fluid may be diagnostic and have prognostic significance.[16]

A variety of radiologic tests may also be helpful in assessing the patient with suspected acute pancreatitis (see Table 43–3). Plain radiographs may demonstrate an air-filled, distended small intestinal loop called a *sentinel loop*, which occurs with extensive abdominal inflammation.[14] Likewise, colonic spasm can occur with pancreatic inflammation resulting in the *colon cut-off sign*. Extraluminal gas bubbles suggest the formation of an abscess. Contrast studies of the upper GI tract may show displacement of the stomach, widening of the duodenal C loop, or mucosal changes such as thumbprinting or gastric antral erosions.

The CT scan and ultrasonography are extremely useful in identifying complications of pancreatitis but may be normal or show nonspecific findings early in the disease.[14] Ultrasound is also the test of choice to look for gallstones or a choledochal cyst. Endoscopic retrograde cholangiopancreatography (ERCP) allows visualization of the pancreatic and biliary ductal system. It is particularly useful in evaluating patients with recurrent pancreatitis in whom a ductal anamoly is suspected.[17]

Outcome

The sequelae of acute pancreatitis can be divided into three categories. The first includes inflammatory masses such as phlegmons (solid mass of indurated pancreas), pseudocysts, and pancreatic abscesses. Pancreatic pseudocysts, the commonest of these masses, is discussed in detail in Chapter 44.

The second category of complications arising from acute pancreatitis are problems occurring in contiguous organs. As already mentioned, inflammatory masses in the pancreas can affect the liver, biliary tree, stomach, duodenum, and colon. Gastrointestinal bleeding can occur through contiguous inflammation and mucosal erosions or by variceal formation.[19] Pleural effusions can occur with or without the formation of a pancreaticopleural fistula, and finding a high amylase level in thorocentesis fluid is highly suggestive of pancreatic origin. Inflammation of the pancreas can involve the kidney causing hematuria, acute tubular necrosis, and renal failure, whereas splenic involvement can result in splenic infarction, splenic artery hemorrhage, and splenic vein thrombosis.[19]

The final category of complications are systemic problems arising from pancreatitis. These include shock, congestive heart failure, acute respiratory distress syndrome, coagulation abnormalities, osteolytic lesions from fat necrosis, and CNS problems.[19]

Treatment

The goals of therapy in acute pancreatitis are twofold. Supportive therapy is aimed at maintaining circulating volume, acid-base and electrolyte status, adequate ventilation, and control of pain. The second aim is minimizing pancreatic activity to decrease the inflammatory process. The methods to achieve the first goal include intensive supportive care with meticulous monitoring of cardiovascular, pulmonary, renal, and metabolic status.[1] Pain control should be obtained with nonopiate medications since opiates effect the sphincter of Oddi.

The second goal is more controversial because no measures beyond general support and fasting have been conclusively shown to influence the course of acute pancreatitis.[14] Fasting is recommended because it decreases pancreatic secretions and removal of acid diminishes secretin release, a potent stimulus for pancreatic secretion.[20] Nasogastric suctioning is also often instituted but has not been proved to be of benefit compared with fasting.[21] However, nasogastric suctioning may be appropriate particularly in patients with vomiting and abdominal distension. Administration of H_2 antagonists to inhibit acid production and the use of proteolytic enzyme inhibitors have no proved efficacy.[22, 23] Glucagon and prophylactic antibiotics have no place in the treatment of acute pancreatitis.

The mortality rate for pancreatitis has remained relatively unchanged despite medical advances and aggressive therapy. The majority of deaths occur in patients with severe disease at presentation or those who rapidly develop severe disease.[14, 19] Patients who develop complications such as rupture of a pseudocyst or abscess formation are also at increased risk of death.[10, 14, 19] The etiology of the pancreatitis does not seem to effect outcome.[24]

SUMMARY

Acute pancreatitis has a varied spectrum of presentations in the pediatric population from nonspecific abdominal pain to fulminant shock. Accurate diagnosis requires a high index of suspicion. No one test is sufficient to make the diagnosis, so the clinician must rely on a careful history and physical examination as well as a complete laboratory and radiographic evaluation. Once the diagnosis is established, therapy is supportive until the inflammatory process has resolved. Complications of acute pancreatitis are a major cause of mortality and should be considered in any patient whose condition does not improve.

REFERENCES

1. Hillemier C, Gryboski JD: Acute pancreatitis in infants and children. *Yale J Biol Med* 1984; 57:149–159.
2. Hollinshead WH: *Textbook of Anatomy*, ed 3. New York, Harper & Row, Publishers, 1974, pp 557–674.
3. Steer ML, Meldolesi J: The cell biology of experimental pancreatitis. *N Engl J Med* 1987; 316:144–150.
4. Pena SDJ, Medovy H: Child abuse and traumatic pseudocyst of the pancreas. *J Pediatr* 1973; 83:1026–1028.
5. Mallory A, Kern F: Drug-induced pancreatitis: A critical review. *Gastroenterology* 1980; 78:813–820.
6. Steinber WA, Lewis JH: Steroid-induced pancreatitis: Does it really exist? *Gastroenterology* 1981; 81:799–808.
7. Rosenblum JL, Keating JP; Pancreatitis, in Feigin RD, Cherry JD (eds): *Textbook of Pediatric Infectious Diseases*. Philadelphia, WB Saunders Co, 1981, p 541.
8. Delhaye M, Engelholm L, Cremer M: Pancreas divisum: Congenital anatomic variant or anomaly? *Gastroenterology* 1985; 89:951–958.
9. Sugawa C, Walt AJ, Nunez DC, Masuyama H: Pancreas Divisum: Is it a normal anatomic variant? *Am J Surg* 1987; 153.62–67.
10. Moossa AR: Diagnostic tests and procedures in acute pancreatitis. *N Engl J Med* 1984; 311:639–643.
11. Jordan SC, Ament ME: Pancreatitis in children and adolescents. *J Pediatr* 1977; 91:211–216.
12. Song H, Tietz NW, Tan C: Usefulness of serum lipase, esterase, and amylase estimation in the diagnosis of pancreatitis—a comparison. *Clin Chem* 1970; 16:264–268.
13. McMahon MJ, Playforth MJ, Rashid SA, et al: The amylase-to-creatinine clearance ratio—a non-specific response to acute illness? *Br J Surg* 1982; 69:29–32.
14. Soergel KH: Acute pancreatitis, in Sleisenger MH, Fordtran JS (eds): *Gastrointestinal Disease: Pathophysiology, Diagnosis, Management*, ed 3. Philadelphia, WB Saunders Co, 1983, p 1462.
15. Jacobs ML, Daggett WM, Civetta JM, et al: Acute pancreatitis: Analysis of factors influencing survival. *Ann Surg* 1977; 185:43–51.
16. Corfield AP, Williamson RCN, McMahon MJ, et al: Prediction of severity in acute pancreatitis: Prospective comparison of three prognostic indices. *Lancet* 1985; 2:403–407.

17. Blustein PK, Gaskin K, Filler R, et al: Endoscopic retrograde cholangiopancreatography in pancreatitis in children and adolescents. *Pediatrics* 1981; 68:387–393.

18. Yale CE, Crummy AB: Splenic vein thrombosis and bleeding esophageal varices. *JAMA* 1971; 217:317–320.

19. Banks PA: Complications of acute pancreatitis, in Banks PA (ed): *Pancreatitis.* New York, Plenum Publishing Corp, 1979, p 131.

20. Johnson LR: Pancreatic secretion, in Johnson LR (ed): *Gastrointestinal Physiology.* St Louis, CV Mosby Co, 1981, p 77.

21. Fuller RK, Loveland JP, Frankel MH: An evaluation of the efficacy of nasogastric suction treatment in alcoholic pancreatitis. *Am J Gastroenterol* 1981; 75:349–353.

22. Goff JS, Reinberg LE, Brugge WR: A randomized trial comparing cimetidine to nasogastric suction in acute pancreatitis. *Dig Dis Sci* 1982; 27:1085–1088.

23. Medical Research Council Multicentre Trial: Morbidity of acute pancreatitis: The effect of aprotonin and glucagon. *Gut* 1980; 21:334–338.

24. Bank S, Wise L, Gerstan M: Risk factors in acute pancreatitis. *Am J Gastroenterol* 1983; 78:637–640.

44 Pancreatic Pseudocyst

Stephen C. Hardy, M.D.

John D. Snyder, M.D.

A previously well 3-year-old boy presented with a history of intermittent severe abdominal pain. His bouts of pain occurred every few weeks and were so severe as to wake him from sleep and cause him to double over with pain. The painful episodes usually lasted about 8 hours and then spontaneously resolved. There was some anorexia and weight loss, but no vomiting, diarrhea or fever.

He was initially thought to have constipation, and he was treated unsuccessfully with mineral oil and enemas. Six months later he presented with a 3-week course of continuous pain of waxing and waning intensity. The physical examination at this time did not reveal any abnormalities. The serum amylase level was 400 mU/ml (normal range 20 to 110 mU/ml). At that time an abdominal ultrasound was performed, revealing a homogeneous solid mass in the pancreas. This was confirmed by a CT scan. An upper gastrointestinal (GI) series showed some widening at the duodenal loop but was otherwise normal. Other laboratory test results showed a lipase level of 10.2 NaOH/ml (normal 0.2 to 1.5 NaOH/ml), a calcium level of 10.5 mg/dl, and a normal white blood cell (WBC) count and hematocrit. A lipid profile was also normal.

Additional questioning revealed that as an infant he had a history of intermittent periods of irritability at about the same frequency as the abdominal pain. He weighed 7.7 lb (3.5 kg) at birth and grew well until the ninth month and then fell to the fifth percentile on the growth curve, where he remained until the time of presentation. There was no history of recent trauma, new medications, or unusual infections. Family history was negative for cystic fibrosis, hepatitis, and hyperlipidemia.

A repeated ultrasound revealed a pancreatic cyst (Fig 44–1). He was followed with weekly outpatient abdominal ultrasonography for 2 months. The cystic structure persisted, and the patient was taken to the operating room for exploration. A darkly colored cystic lesion was found in the region of the pancreatic head. An internal drainage procedure was performed without complications. There were no postoperative complications, and the patients' symptoms subsequently resolved.

DISCUSSION

The term pancreatic pseudocyst is applied to a collection of fluid arising from inflammatory processes of the pancreas. The term pseudocyst is used because these

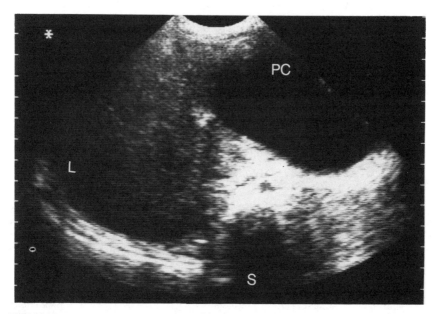

FIG 44–1.
Abdominal ultrasound (cross-sectional view) showing the large pancreatic pseudocyst *(PC),* liver *(L),* and spine *(S).*

cystic lesions are not lined with epithelial cells as "true" cysts are but are lined with granulation and fibrous connective tissue. These cysts are commonly solitary but can be multiple. They can be massive but are usually 5 to 10 cm in diameter.[1] The pseudocyst may be anywhere within the pancreas itself but usually forms adjacent to the pancreas, commonly near the tail.[2] Often there is no communication with the pancreatic ductal system.[1, 2]

Contents of the cysts vary somewhat with the cause of the pseudocyst and its age. Surgeons report cyst volume of 50 to 5,000 ml although 500 ml is the average.[3] The cystic fluid is often clear but can be cloudy if infected. The amylase concentration of cyst fluid averages 500 to 20,000 IU/L, but levels greater than 1,000,000 IU/L have been reported.[1, 2]

Bacterial cultures of cyst fluid are positive approximately 25% of the time when cultures are obtained. The actual incidence of infection is probably lower since most surgeons culture cystic fluid only when clinical evidence for infection is present. Common bacterial pathogens include *Escherichia coli, Enterococcus*, and *Staphylococcus*. Culture results reveal polymicrobial infections with anaerobic involvement in up to 50% of cases.[4, 5]

Pathophysiology

Pancreatic pseudocysts are commonly associated with pancreatitis, and any cause of pancreatitis or pancreatic inflammation can cause a pseudocyst. The epidemiology of pseudocysts follows that of pancreatitis. The most common causes of pseudocysts in adults are alcoholism, biliary tract disease, and trauma. In contrast, most childhood cases of pancreatitis are caused by trauma, drug toxicity, or viral infections or are idiopathic.[6] These causes have in common the ability to injure the pancreatic acinar cell and the ability to activate pancreatic enzymes. These two processes seem to be necessary to form a pseudocyst.[7, 8]

The pancreas is protected from its own destructive enzymes because these enzymes are produced and stored in precursor form. These precursors are activated in the gut lumen by proteases and lipases. The best studied example of this process is trypsin, which is stored in its proenzyme state as trypsinogen, and is activated to trypsin by enterokinase in the small bowel. Trypsin activates more trypsinogen as well as other proenzymes.

Severe pancreatic injury occurs in pancreatitis when these precursor enzymes are activated in the pancreas itself, causing pancreatic autodigestion.[8] Trypsin, chymotrypsin, elastin, kalliekrein, and lipases all act to cause proteolysis, edema, necrosis, and often hemorrhage.

Pancreatic pseudocysts are collections of the debris of this destruction. The collections may occur in the pancreas itself or in peripancreatic tissue such as the lesser sac. Pancreatic duct disruption is common in the setting of pseudocyst, and the disrupted ducts can empty their contents into the cysts and then seal off.[7] It appears that growth and possibly rupture of pseudocysts occur when these ducts do not seal off and continue to empty fluid into the cyst.[7]

Clinical Features

Pseudocysts usually occur as a complication of pancreatitis. In approximately one half of the cases a pseudocyst presents within 3 to 6 weeks after onset of pancreatitis and is called an *acute pseudocyst*.[9] In other cases it may occur months to years after an acute attack of clinical pancreatitis. There is no history of antecedent pancreatitis in 5% of cases.[10] When the history of pancreatitis is distant, or nonexistent, the term *chronic pseudocyst* is used.[9, 11] The grouping of pseudocysts into acute and chronic has therapeutic significance and will be discussed later.

The most common presenting complaint is abdominal pain, which is present in 85% to 100% of cases[10] (Table 44–1). Other symptoms include nausea and vomiting, weight loss, fever, and jaundice.[10] If the pseudocyst ruptures or erodes into a major vessel, the presenting complaint can be that of acute abdomen or GI hemorrhage.

The physical examination reveals abdominal tenderness and often a palpable mass[7] (Table 44–1). Results of laboratory tests show an increased amylase level in 50% to 70% of cases. An elevated WBC count (11,000–22,000/mm^3) is also common. Less common laboratory abnormalities include prolonged prothrombin time, increased alkaline phosphatase level, and increased serum calcium level.[11]

Plain radiographs of the chest can show pleural effusions, an elevated hemidiaphragm, or atelectasis but is often normal. Plain films of the abdomen can often be abnormal, showing signs of acute pancreatitis such as the sentinel loop of a localized ileus, or signs of chronic pancreatitis, such as pancreatic calcifications.[7] Signs of the pseudocyst itself may include loss of iliopsosas shadows or displacement of a renal shadow, both signs of retroperitoneal inflammation. The pseudocyst may cause a mass effect on the stomach, colon, or small bowel.

Once formed, most pseudocysts persist or continue to grow, often resulting in severe complications. Studies have shown, however, that many pseudocysts spontaneously resolve, and there has been much controversy over the frequency of spontaneous resolution. Studies have shown resolution rates as low as 6% and as high as 30%.[7, 11–13] This disparity may be explained in part by the common practice of grouping all pancreatic pseudocysts into one group instead of separating them into acute and chronic groups. Acute pseudocysts have a much higher rate of resolution; chronic pseudocysts almost never resolve spontaneously.

Studies suggest that unresolved, untreated pancreatic pseudocysts have a high rate of complications and that the rate of complications increases over time if no intervention is performed.[12] The most common major complications include rupture, hemorrhage, and abscess formation. All of the major complications carry a mortality rate of 20% to 80%.[7]

Rupture is usually spontaneous and may occur when intracystic pressure increases from hemorrhage or from increasing cystic contents. Blunt trauma can cause pseudocyst rupture, and even mild pressure such as a physical exam has been known to cause cyst rupture. The rupture may be intraperitoneal, or it may occur into a contiguous part of the gastrointestinal tract. The presentation of a ruptured pseudocyst is that of an acute abdomen and is not usually suspected (unless the patient is known to have a pseudocyst) until the diagnosis is made at laparotomy. When the rupture occurs into a hollow viscus, the presentation may be that of upper GI hemorrhage, or the mass representing the pseudocyst may simply disappear.

Hemorrhage occurs when the pseudocyst erodes into a major vessel. First a

TABLE 44–1.

Clinical Findings and Laboratory Features of Pancreatic Pseudocysts*

	% of Cases
Clinical Findings	
Abdominal pain	85–100
Nausea and vomiting	40–70
Palpable mass	30–50
Weight loss	10–40
Pleural effusion	10–30
Fever	5–20
Jaundice	5–20
Laboratory results	
Elevated amylase level	50–70
Leukocytosis	30–50
Elevated alkaline phosphatase level	27–57
Elevated prothrombin time	11–15

*Adapted from Kane and Guenter,[7] Ephgrave and Hunt,[10] and Bradley et al.[11]

pseudoaneurysm may occur. This pseudoaneurysm can then rupture into the peritoneum or into a hollow viscus and cause shock or acute GI hemorrhage.[7]

The cause of most pancreatic abscesses is not clear. Some are suspected to be iatrogenic and follow percutaneous biopsy or endoscopic retrograde cholangiopancreatography (ERCP).[8] The flora of abscess is usually polymicrobial, with enteric gram-negative organisms and anaerobes predominating.[4]

Other complications of pancreatic pseudocyst occur less frequently and include pancreatic ascites, pancreatic pleural effusions, biliary obstruction, GI obstruction, and portal vein obstruction.[7, 8]

Studies show that spontaneous resolution of pseudocysts usually occurs within the first 3 weeks after diagnosis and almost always within the first 6 weeks of diagnosis.[12, 13] Resolution almost never occurs after 6 weeks. Complications can occur anytime but occur with increasing frequency as the pseudocyst ages. Serious complications have been reported to occur in up to 20% of patients during the first 4 to 6 weeks after diagnosis and in 50% of patients after 6 weeks.[12]

All large studies of pancreatic pseudocysts to date have been done on adults. A large number of these adults have pseudocysts related to alcoholism. Because of poor reliability in these patient populations, follow-up and compliance have been poor. The applicability of the data collected on these adult populations to pseudocysts in children is tenuous at best.

Diagnosis

The clinical presentation, laboratory examination, and plain film findings of pancreatic pseudocyst are so nonspecific that the diagnosis is easily missed unless there is clear association with recent pancreatitis. The diagnosis of pseudocyst is usually made or confirmed by abdominal sonography or by computed tomography (CT) scanning.

The sensitivity and specificity of abdominal ultrasound for detection of pancreatic pseudocyst is approximately 90%.[12, 14, 15] In patients where a pseudocyst is suspected, abdominal sonography is the procedure of choice because it is very accurate, is readily available, is less expensive than CT scanning, and does not expose the patient to radiation.[7] Ultrasonography is also a sensitive test for associated biliary disease. Because patients often have serial imaging studies to follow the growth or regression of a pseudocyst, the lack of radiation becomes more important.

In certain settings however, ultrasonography is not the best imaging technique. The pancreas may not be easily imaged by sonography in a very obese patient or in a patient with a large amount of bowel gas. In these settings, CT scanning is necessary. The CT scan has been shown to be as sensitive and specific as abdominal sonography.[15, 16] The CT scan generally shows more detail than ultrasound and can give a good estimate of the thickness of the cyst wall, which may be useful when timing surgery (see later discussion of management).

The differential diagnosis of a cystic lesion in the pancreas (imaged by ultrasound or CT) includes pancreatic pseudocyst, pancreatic cystic neoplasia (benign or malignant), retention or congenital cyst, and very rare entities such as a large ovarian cyst.[7] Of all of these, pancreatic pseudocysts are by far the commonest. Often it is not possible to make the final diagnosis until biopsy of the cyst wall and examination of cyst contents are both completed.

Treatment

The cornerstone for treatment of pancreatic pseudocysts is surgical drainage. However, there is controversy regarding the timing of surgery and the operation of choice. In general, the choice of operation is determined by the condition of the patient, the location of the pseudocyst, and the maturity of the pseudocyst.

In some patients (10% to 15%)[12] the pancreatic pseudocyst presents with a major complication such as rupture, hemorrhage, or sepsis. These complications have a high mortality rate and must be treated as surgical emergencies. Most of these patients have external drainage procedures.

External drainage is performed by placing a catheter into the cyst and draining the cyst through the abdominal wall into an external, but closed, system. This procedure is both rapid and relatively easy to do and can be used for an unstable patient and is required in the setting of pancreatic abscess.[4] Unfortunately, this procedure has a high rate of complications (50% to 80%), including recurrence of the pseudocyst, infection, pancreatitis, hemorrhage, fluid loss, fistula formation, and skin irritation.[8] The mortality of external drainage is approximately 23%, but this high mortality probably reflects the often critically ill condition of the patient rather than the risky nature of the procedure itself.[7]

Internal drainage is the operation of choice when feasible. Its success is related to the stability of the patient, the location of the cyst, and the thickness of the cyst wall. Connection to the stomach (cystogastrostomy) or to the proximal jejunum (cystojejunostomy) are the commonest procedures. Complications of internal drainage occur at a lower rate (20% to 30%) than that of external drainage. Common complications include abscess, recurrence of the cyst, pancreatitis, and hemorrhage.[8]

Resection of the cyst is occasionally the best procedure, especially if the cyst is small and superficial.[8] Distal pancreatectomy can be performed when the cyst is localized to the pancreatic tail.

Percutaneous pseudocyst aspiration, under ultrasound guidance, has recently been reported as a possible alternative to surgery.[7] The percutaneous catheter may be left for chronic drainage. This less invasive procedure may represent an alternative to surgery. More experience needs to be accumulated before it can be seriously considered as an option.

The management of a stable pseudocyst, free of complications at the time of presentation, is a chronic process. The natural history of pseudocysts suggests that the rate of potentially fatal complications is so high that it is not safe to observe a patient with a pseudocyst indefinitely. However, several arguments can be made for a 4- to 6-week waiting period before surgery.

First, as mentioned earlier, a significant number of pseudocysts will spontaneously resolve. Spontaneous resolution, if it occurs, virtually always does so within 6 weeks of diagnosis.[11, 12] The pseudocysts most likely to resolve are those previously termed acute pseudocysts, that is, those cysts clearly associated with a recent bout of pancreatitis (regardless of cause).

Second, a short waiting period gives a newly formed pseudocyst time to develop a thick (>3.0 mm) cyst wall.[11] This is important because cysts with thick walls are more easily drained internally. Pseudocysts with thin walls usually require external drainage, which has a higher morbidity rate. A chronic pseudocyst does not need this maturation time.

Third, although severe complications may occur at any time, complications occur at a much lower rate during the first several months after diagnosis. Observation during this limited period of time is not as risky as indefinite observation.

For these reasons, in the setting of a stable, acute pancreatic pseudocyst (which represents the most common presentation of pseudocyst), a period of 4 to 6 weeks to allow either spontaneous resolution or cyst wall maturation is appropriate. In most cases, the patient should be observed in the hospital. During the observation period, the patient should be reevaluated regularly with follow-up ultrasound or CT scan. Signs of severe complications should be carefully monitored during this period of observation. Specific signs of complications include temperature greater than 39°C, WBC count greater than 15,000/mm³, hypotension, change in abdominal mass size, increase in abdominal tenderness, and drop in hematocrit.[7] Urgent surgery is indicated in the setting of any serious complication and is associated with considerable morbidity.[10]

In patients presenting with a chronic pseudocyst or a pseudocyst without apparent relation to a recent pancreatitis, a waiting period is probably not beneficial and may be hazardous.[8–11] In these patients, an abdominal CT scan may be performed to document maturity of the cyst wall.

The choice of surgery, as previously mentioned, is dictated by the clinical setting and nature of the cyst. Some surgeons require ERCP prior to surgery in certain settings. The ERCP may be of benefit in demonstrating an underlying pancreatic abnormality or biliary disease such as common bile duct stones. It may also be helpful preoperatively in the setting of a pseudocyst with ascites and can demonstrate a site of leakage from the pseudocyst to the peritoneal cavity and thus influence the surgical procedure.[8]

The long term postsurgical prognosis for pancreatic pseudocyst varies according to its underlying cause. Most morbidity and mortality of the pancreatic pseudocyst is related to the initial presentation and preoperative or postoperative complications. Once surgery has been successfully completed and the pseudocyst permanently drained, the prognosis can be excellent.

REFERENCES

1. Aranha GV, Prinz RA, Freeark RJ, et al: Evaluation of therapeutic options of pancreatic pseudocysts. *Arch Surg* 1982; 117:717–721.
2. Shatney CH, Lillehei RC: Surgical treatment of pancreatic pseudocysts: Analysis of 119 cases. *Ann Surg* 1979; 189:386–394.
3. Frey CF: Pancreatic pseudocyst—operative strategy. *Ann Surg* 1978; 188:652–662.
4. Warshaw AL, Gongliang J: Improved survival in 45 patients with pancreatic abscess. *Ann Surg* 1985; 119:408–417.
5. Owens BJ, Hamit HF: Pancreatic abscess and pseudocyst. *Arch Surg* 1977; 112:42–45.

6. Silverman A, Roy CC: in *Pediatric Clinical Gastroenterology*, ed 3. St Louis, CV Mosby Co, 1983, pp 844–845.
7. Kane MG, Guenter JK: Pancreatic pseudocyst. *Adv Intern Med* 1984; 29:271–300.
8. Martin EW, Catalano P, Cooperman M, et al: Surgical decision-making in the treatment of pancreatic pseudocysts. *Am J Surg* 1979; 138:821–824.
9. Crass AC, Way LW: Acute and chronic pancreatic pseudocysts are different. *Am J Surg* 1981; 142:660–663.
10. Ephgrave K, Hunt JL: Presentation of pancreatic pseudocysts: Implications for timing of surgical intervention. *Am J Surg* 1979; 151:749–753.
11. Bradley EL, Gonzalez AC, Clements JL: Acute pancreatic pseudocysts: Incidence and implications. *Ann Surg* 1976; 184:734–737.
12. Bradley EL, Clements JL, Gonzalez AC: The natural history of pancreatic pseudocysts: A unified concept of management. *Am J Surg* 1979; 137:135–141.
13. Sankaran S, Walt AJ: The natural and unnatural history of pancreatic pseudocysts. *Br J Surg* 1975; 62:37–44.
14. Gonzalez AC, Bradley EL, Clements JL: Pseudocyst formation in acute pancreatitis: Ultrasonographic evaluation of 99 cases. *AJR* 1976; 127:315–317.
15. Kressel HY, Margulis AR, Goodling GW, et al: CT scanning and ultrasound in the evaluation of pancreatic pseudocysts: A preliminary comparison. *Radiology* 1978; 126:153–157.
16. Ferrucci JT, Wittenberg J, Black EB, et al: Computed body tomography in chronic pancreatitis. *Radiology* 1979; 130:175–182.

Systemic Conditions Affecting the Gastrointestinal Tract

45 Pediatric Acquired Immunodeficiency Syndrome and its Gastrointestinal Manifestations

S. R. Martin M.D., F.R.C.P.(C)

A 3-year-old boy was admitted with fever and respiratory distress. He was born full term to a 28-year-old woman after an uncomplicated pregnancy. At 5 months of age he was hospitalized for gastroenteritis with dehydration, vomiting, and weight loss. He received intravenous (IV) hydration and was discharged after resolution of the illness.

At 7 months of age, he was readmitted with diarrhea, otitis media, and signs and symptoms of bronchiolitis. He had shown no weight gain over the previous 2 months and had fallen to the 10th percentile for weight, but remained at the 95th percentile for height. Physical examination at that time was remarkable for a palpable liver, enlarged spleen, and cervical, axillary, and inguinal lymphadenopathy.

Investigations included several stool examinations for ova and parasites, stool cultures, 72-hour fecal fat determination, and 1-hour serum D-xylose test, results of which were all normal. Repeated sweat electrolyte levels were normal, and results of the radioallergosorbent test (RAST) for milk proteins were negative. Evaluation of his hepatosplenomegaly included TORCH (toxoplasmosis, rubella, cytomegalovirus [CMV], and herpes simplex virus [HSV]) which indicated prior infection with CMV and HSV and current infection with Epstein-Barr virus (EBV), titers rising from 1:60 to 1:1,280 over 2 weeks. A liver-spleen scan showed homogeneous uptake and enlargement of the liver and the spleen. Screening tests for immune function included a normal white blood cell (WBC) count with mild eosinophilia (absolute count 650/mm^3), normal T-cell number and function, normal B-cell numbers, and antibody responses to immunization. Immunoglobulin levels were normal with the exception of IgG, which was elevated at 2,440 mg/dl. He returned home on caloric supplements, with a diagnosis of EBV infection.

Over the next 2 years he showed little weight gain and experienced recurrent otitis media, upper respiratory tract infections, including at least one documented pneumonia, and recurrent skin infections. During this time his mother died after a brief but severe illness caused by *Candida* sepsis. Subsequent investigation revealed her to have been human immunodeficiency virus (HIV) antibody positive. His father and two siblings were also found to be positive, and the father admitted to frequent abuse of IV drugs.

At 30 months of age the patient was admitted for further evaluation of recurrent fevers and failure to thrive with diarrhea. His immune status had deteriorated; his WBC count was 3,100/mm³, with an absolute neutrophil count of 620/mm³. T-cell numbers were reduced to 21% of total, with T4 and T8 subset levels of 7% and 9%, respectively. No reaction was observed on in vitro testing with tetanus or *Candida*. His IgG level was normal at 900 mg/dl, and his IgA level was elevated at 300 mg/dl. The HIV antibody was positive by enzyme-linked immunosorbent assay (ELISA) and confirmed by the Western blot immunoelectrophoresis technique; p24, p55, and gp45 bands were present, representing the most commonly found viral core proteins in patients with acquired immunodeficiency syndrome (AIDS). His stools contained *Giardia* cysts, and he was treated with oral metronidazole (Flagyl). His diarrhea improved a little.

Four months later he was admitted with increasing fatigue, fevers, and new onset of anorexia. A blood *Candida* antigen was positive. On esophagoscopy the esophagus was inflamed, with white plaques and ulcerations visible. Results of brushings and biopsies confirmed invasive candidiasis, and he was treated with IV amphotericin.

He developed respiratory distress, and arterial blood gas analysis showed moderate hypoxia (Po_2 68, Pco_2 34). Chest x-ray film showed increased bilateral interstitial pneumonitis. An open lung biopsy specimen revealed *Pneumocystis carinii* on silver stain. Trimethoprim-sulfamethoxazole therapy begun preoperatively was continued but was withdrawn after 10 doses due to a severe skin eruption. Pentamidine was substituted, but his condition deteriorated. He became progressively more hypoxic despite maximal ventilatory support and died the following day.

DISCUSSION

Since 1981, more than 84,000 cases of AIDS have been reported to the Centers for Disease Control (CDC), Atlanta, and 86% of those diagnosed prior to January 1985 have died.[1] More than 1,300 pediatric cases have been reported, and, to date, 55% of these have died. These statistics probably underestimate the true extent of the disease since they include only cases of full-blown AIDS reported to the CDC, whose criteria are relatively strict. Moreover, these data reflect only the situation in the United States; in Europe, similar trends are seen, although they are 2 to 3 years behind the U.S. experience.[2] In central Africa the disease has become a major public health problem.[2, 3]

In the United States, most cases of AIDS occur in white adult men, and the majority (92%) are homosexuals, bisexuals, or IV drug abusers.[1] Women constitute only 9% of adult cases, with most being IV drug abusers or partners of men at high risk for AIDS. Of the pediatric cases, 83% of these children are less than 5 years of age, with a racial distribution almost identical to that of adult women (black 52%, white 24%, hispanic 23%).[1]

This underscores the fact that 78% of pediatric cases are children born to parents with or at high risk for AIDS. The remainder are accounted for by hemophiliacs

(6%), children (mostly neonates) who received blood transfusions (13%), and a small number (4%) whose source of infection has yet to be identified.[1]

The natural history of AIDS in children is not well characterized, since most of the published data concern the adult male homosexual population. Data from transfusion related cases, where the time of infection is more precisely known, show a 1- to 2-month interval from infection to the development of seropositivity.[2] During this period, virus may be excreted and probably accounts for reports of transmission from seronegative blood donors.[2, 3] Initial data indicate that 5% to 20% of HIV-infected persons will go on to develop AIDS.[4, 5] Longitudinal cohort studies and statistical estimates show that 5% to 34% of seropositive individuals will develop AIDS within 3 years.[6]

Since it is likely that the proportion of AIDS cases accounted for by hemophiliacs and recipients of blood transfusions will decline following the routine use of blood screening, the most important group of pediatric cases to consider is that of infants acquiring infection from their parents. Much evidence has accumulated to suggest that infection occurs in utero as well as during the birth process.[7] The early onset in infants (5.5 months after birth) compared with adults (2–4 years after injection) suggests an in utero infection, although immunologic immaturity in early infancy and the innoculum relative to body size may be important factors.[7] The HIV antibody has been found in cord blood and thymus tissue, and HIV has been cultured from brain tissue of abortuses.[7, 8] Finally an AIDS-related dysmorphic syndrome has been described, although other maternal factors such as drug ingestion and poor nutrition during pregnancy must be considered.[9]

CLINICAL FEATURES

Due to the variable clinical presentation of AIDS, the case definition put forward by the CDC in 1982 and amended in 1985 because of the availability of HIV antibody testing is particularly complex.[10] In children especially, congenital infections and primary immunodeficiencies must be considered (Table 45–1). Clinically, most infants with AIDS fail to thrive, have hepatosplenomegaly, and have chronic interstitial pneumonitis. Adenopathy is common, as is chronic or recurrent diarrhea.[4, 7, 11] Children are more prone than adults to bacterial infections as a result of a more prominent B cell defect.[12] They may also develop pulmonary lymphoid hyperplasia (PLH), a diffuse alveolar septal and peribronchial lymphocytic infiltration, uncommon in adults and in children less than 5 years of age. Other associated conditions include developmental delay, encephalopathy, thrombocytopenia, chronic parotid swelling, and eczematoid rash.[4, 7, 11]

GASTROINTESTINAL MANIFESTATIONS

Many of the gastrointestinal (GI) complications of AIDS are related to the numerous opportunistic infections that occur in these patients and may affect the GI tract at

TABLE 45–1.

Differential Diagnosis of Congenital Acquired Immunodeficiency Syndrome

I. Primary immunodeficiency syndromes
   A. Predominant defect in humoral immunity—agammaglobulinemia (Bruton's), hypogammaglobulinemia, selective immunoglobulin deficiencies, common variable immunodeficiency
   B. Predominant defect in cell-mediated immunity—severe combined immunodeficiency including Nezelof's, adenosine deaminase and nucleoside phosphorylase deficiencies
   C. Immunodeficiency associated with other defects—Wiskott-Aldrich syndrome, DiGeorge syndrome, ataxia telangiectasia, graft-vs.-host disease
II. Secondary immunodeficiency
   A. Congenital infection—TORCH infections, EBV
   B. Malnutrition
   C. Following immunosupressive medication
   D. Malignancy

TABLE 45–2.

Gastrointestinal Manifestations in Acquired Immunodeficiency Syndrome

Presentation	Etiology
Oroesophageal	*Candida albicans*, HSV, CMV, *Cryptosporidium*, reflux esophagitis
Gastritis	CMV
Enteritis	CMV, adenovirus, *Mycobacterium avium-intracellulare*, *Salmonella*, *Shigella*, *Campylobacter*, *Mycobacterium tuberculosis*, *Clostridium difficile*, *Giardia*, *Cryptosporidium*, *Isospora belli*, *Microsporidia*, *Strongyloides stercoralis*, *Entamoeba histolytica*. Idiopathic: malabsorption, secretory diarrhea
Proctitis(rare in children)	HSV, CMV, *Neisseria gonorrhoeae*, *Chlamydia*, *Treponema pallidum*
Hepatosplenomegaly(80%–90%)	Idiopathic, EBV, CMV, Hepatitis B, *M. avium-intracellulare*
Malignancy	Kaposi's sarcoma, lymphoma

different sites (Table 45–2). These infectious agents may sometimes also affect the normal population. However, in AIDS the infections tend to be more severe, difficult to eradicate, and more often will relapse.

The most common oral infection is candidiasis, although HSV may also frequently be implicated. Both agents may also cause esophagitis. In contrast to normal hosts, thrush is difficult to treat in patients with AIDS and is generally believed to accompany esophagitis in these patients.

Esophagitis is usually accompanied by odynophagia, dysphagia, or both. In addition to *Candida* and HSV, CMV has been implicated, and one case of *Cryptosporidium* esophagitis has been reported.[13]

Although severe esophagitis can be seen on barium swallow, this method of detection is not as sensitive or as specific as endoscopy with biopsy.[14] Esophagoscopy has also been recommended in follow-up of *Candida* esophagitis since clearing of oral lesions and relief of symptoms has not correlated well with resolution of esophageal lesions.[14]

Nystatin is often ineffective in these patients other than to suppress growth of *Candida* chronically. Acute treatment is more successful with ketoconazole orally or with IV amphotericin.[14] Herpex simplex virus may be treated with acyclovir. No effective therapy currently exists for CMV, although several investigational drugs are being evaluated clinically.

Chronic or recurrent diarrhea occurs in 40% to 60% of children and 50% to 60% of adults who develop AIDS.[4, 7, 11] In Africa, it may affect up to 80% of patients, probably related to the high general prevalence of enteric infections in that region.

Cytomegalovirus may cause lesions throughout the GI tract. Usually the lesions are ulcerating, and typical intracellular inclusions may be seen on biopsy.[14, 15] Adenovirus has been isolated from AIDS patients with diarrhea, usually strains with serotypes greater than 29.

Diarrhea due to the common bacterial pathogens, including *Salmonella, Shigella,* and *Campylobacter*, has been reported. These organisms seem to be more invasive, and prolonged bacteremia requiring lengthy treatment is not uncommon.[14, 16] *M. avium-intracellulare* is a rare enteric pathogen in infants but may cause enteritis in patients with AIDS.[14, 17] Infections seem to originate in the lungs and GI tract, and the presentation is usually with diarrhea, malabsorption of fat, and enlargement of mesenteric lymph nodes. In adults, infection is often disseminated and is found also in the intestine, biliary tract, liver, bone marrow, lung, brain, and lymph nodes. Results of the intestinal biopsy appear similar to, and have been confused with, Whipple's disease, although the latter is not a disease of children. Moreover, the bacillus of *M. avium-intracellulare* is acid fast and remains intact within the macrophages of the lamina propria. No effective therapy is yet available.

Mycobacterium tuberculosis may be associated with enteritis, although in children in North America today this is very rare. *Clostridium difficile*–associated diarrhea may affect the AIDS patient, especially in cases where recurrent bacterial infection leads to frequent use of antibiotics.[14, 17]

Giardiasis, as in other immunodeficiency states, is a common enteric pathogen and may be associated with diarrhea, fat malabsorption, and weight loss.[4, 18] It can also be found in specimens from stool examinations or in duodenal aspirates and biopsy specimens.

The coccidian organisms *Cryptosporidium* and *I. belli* also present with diarrhea, often very watery and in large volume; abdominal cramps and fever are common.[19] Eosinophilia is seen in up to 50% of cases of isosporiasis due to the more invasive nature of its larger oval sporocysts.[19] Detection in the stool is often difficult and requires examination of duodenal fluid and biopsy specimens. Treatment of *Cryptosporidium* is unsatisfactory, although some have reported limited success with spiramycin. Isosporiasis has been successfully treated with trimethoprim-sulfamethoxozole.

A related coccidian, *Microsporidia*, has been found in AIDS patients with diarrhea, although a causative role remains to be established. This organism can be detected only by electron microscopy.[20] Other less common organisms are *S. stercoralis* and *E. histolytica*, both potentially treatable infections. Although *Candida* is easily isolated from the stool of AIDS patients, it is rare for it to cause diarrhea. Similarly, other fungal agents tend not to affect the GI tract.

Several reports of prolonged diarrhea and weight loss in the absence of infection have been published, comprising 75% of the patients in one study.[21] These patients may have fat malabsorption and protein-losing enteropathy and generally have abnormal D-xylose absorption.[17, 21] Preliminary prospective data from patients followed at Children's Hospital show an abnormal 1-hour serum D-xylose test result in five of eight patients tested, independent of the presence of diarrhea or weight loss. Some patients have had secretory diarrhea. Biopsy changes tend to be nonspecific: partial villous atrophy, crypt hyperplasia, increased intraepithelial lymphocytes and plasma cells in the jejunum, mast cell infiltration of the lamina propria, and focal crypt cell degeneration in the rectum have been reported.[20]

One study has demonstrated a decrease in intestinal mucosal total T cells, especially T helper cells, with an increase in T suppressor cells in homosexual AIDS patients compared with healthy heterosexual and homosexual controls. This was associated with normal histologic findings.[21]

Colitis, including proctitis, may be caused by many of the bacterial and viral pathogens previously mentioned. Cytomegalovirus, in particular, may be frankly hemorrhagic and may induce a vasculitis of the intestine, progressing to thrombosis, ischemia, or perforation.

Isolated proctitis is unusual in children and is likely to be seen only in adolescent homosexuals. Herpes simplex virus, CMV, and the more common diseases *Chlamydia, T. pallidum,* and *N. gonorrhoeae* may be found.

Hepatomegaly with or without associated splenomegaly is one of the most consistent physical findings in children with HIV infection. This is frequently associated with elevated transaminase levels, though elevation of the bilirubin and alkaline phosphatase levels is less common.[4, 23] Hepatic function, in general, tends to be well preserved. The population at risk for AIDS is in most instances also at risk for hepatitis B and toxic effects of medications, which must be taken into account when the source of liver dysfunction is evaluated. Infections such as CMV and EBV are well recognized. In addition, *Cryptococcus* may infect the liver, usually being found in the sinusoids, though the inflammatory response is minimal. *Mycobacterium avium-intracellulare* has been noted to involve the liver in up to 57% of patients with disseminated disease. Kaposi's sarcoma, associated with elevated alkaline phosphatase levels, has been reported in 14% of patients, usually with skin and visceral involvement. One case report of primary lymphoma has been published.

Liver biopsy has not been performed routinely in patients with liver dysfunction and AIDS. In the few reported cases, the usual finding is that of nonspecific changes similar to chronic active hepatitis.[23, 24] Periportal and lobular lymphocytic infiltrates have been observed, with predominantly cytotoxic/suppressor (T8) cells.[24] Biopsy is, perhaps, most useful in the diagnosis of infection not demonstrated by any other means or prior to the use of potentially hepatotoxic experimental medications.

Malignancy is rare in children, occurring in 1% of patients less than 15 years old with AIDS.[1] The youngest reported AIDS victim is age 7 months.[25] In children, it is most commonly found in the lymph nodes, whereas in adults it may affect the oropharynx, stomach, small bowel, colon, liver, and spleen. Of those with skin involvement, 50% have visceral lesions. Gastrointestinal evaluation may include barium studies, which may show polypoid mucosal lesions. Endoscopy may demonstrate flat, bluish lesions not detectable radiographically.

Patients are usually asymptomatic with intestinal involvement, although diarrhea, obstruction, or bleeding may all occur.

Intestinal lymphoma is rare in the normal population and is similarly rare in AIDS patients. It is usually advanced at presentation and frequently the B cell type.

NUTRITIONAL ISSUES

No published data outlining the nutritional deficiencies occurring in children with AIDS exist. Prenatally, maternal disease and malnutrition may affect the developing fetus, and many infants are born small for gestational age. From early life, these children are at risk for malnutrition because of frequent severe infections, especially pneumonias and esophagitis, which result in poor intake during periods of illness. Intermittent or chronic diarrhea with malabsorption are also frequent, further compromising their absorption of nutrients.

In selected cases oral supplementation is useful. However, compliance can be a major problem, and the child's ability to take adequate supplementation is often suboptimal.

Enteral feeding, especially using overnight nasogastric feedings, has been successful in maintaining weight gain in some AIDS patients. However, persistent diarrhea, presumably from diminished absorptive capacity of many etiologies, often precludes use of this route.

Contrary to the opinion of some who believe that total parenteral nutrition (TPN) does not appear to be useful,[7] our early experience shows a good response to parenteral nutrition. Some patients have shown gains in height and weight with intravenous nutrition that was not achieved with equivalent caloric intake by enteral tube feeding, suggesting that the major limiting factor for nutrition is in the intestine. Total parenteral nutrition may allow these children to maintain their weight despite frequent illness. Because of the adverse effect of malnutrition on immunologic function and, thus, susceptibility to infection, aggressive nutritional therapy in AIDS patients would thus seem warranted.

However, TPN is not without its risks, and the capabilities and reliabilities of the parents must be assessed on a case by case basis. Our current experience suggests that the incidence of catheter-related complications in children with AIDS is not greater than other children requiring long-term central catheters.

SUMMARY

Evaluation of the child with AIDS and GI symptoms is outlined in Table 45–3. Initially, an aggressive search should be made for a potentially treatable infection.

Nutritional status should be determined, and, especially if no infectious etiology is found, investigation for specific nutrient malabsorption should be undertaken. This may allow a more rational nutritional therapy to be made. At present, there remains much to be learned about the effects of AIDS in children, especially how it affects life expectancy and the quality of life. Currently, other than for some select infections, treatment is largely supportive and will remain so until effective vaccines and antiviral therapies are found.

TABLE 45–3.
Evaluation of the Child With Acquired Immunodeficiency Syndrome and Gastrointestinal Symptoms

---

   I. Nutritional status—to set intake goals and monitor effect of nutritional therapy
      A. Anthropometrics
          1. Height, weight, head circumference
          2. Triceps skin fold
          3. Midarm circumference
      B. Intake
          1. 3-day diary
      C. Laboratory
          1. Serum albumin
          2. Transferrin, prealbumin
          3. Hemoglobin, red blood cell morphology
          4. Serum iron, plasma zinc
  II. Infections—cultures and procedures determined by presenting symptoms
      A. Stool
          1. Culture and sensitivity 3 times, ova and parasites 3 times
          2. *C. difficile* toxin
          3. Virology
             a. Rapid antigen (rotavirus)
             b. Electron microscopy
             c. Viral culture
      B. Endoscopy*
          1. Esophageal brushings; biopsy
          2. Duodenal aspirate for ova and parasites, culture and sensitivity; biopsy
          3. Rectal culture and sensitivity; biopsy
 III. Malabsorption—should be sought to help guide optimal nutritional therapy
      A. Fat
          1. Qualitative, 72 hr fecal fat
      B. Carbohydrate
          1. Stool pH, reducing substance
          2. Lactose breath hydrogen
          3. D-Xylose 1-hr serum level
      C. Protein
          1. Stool α_1-antitrypsin excretion
      D. Biopsy
          1. Small intestine morphology

*Endoscopic biopsies may be cultured or examined by light and electron microscopy for pathogens.

REFERENCES

1. Centers for Disease Control: AIDS Weekly Surveillance Report. Atlanta, CDC, Jan 30, 1989.
2. Salahuddin SZ, Groopman JE, Markam PD, et al: HTLVIII in symptom free, seronegative persons. *Lancet* 1984; 2:1418–1420.
3. Fischer MC: Transfusion associated acquired immunodeficiency syndrome: What is the risk? *Pediatrics* 1987; 79:157–160.
4. Barbour SD: Acquired immunodeficiency of childhood. *Pediatr Clin North Am* 1987; 34:247–268.
5. Taylor JMG, Schwartz K, Detels R: The time from infection with HIV to the onset of AIDS. *J Infect Dis* 1986; 154:694–697.
6. Polk BF, Fox R, Brookmeyer R, et al: Predictors of the acquired immunodeficiency syndrome developing in a cohort of seropositive homosexual men. *N Engl J Med* 1987; 316:61–66.
7. Rubinstein A: AIDS. *Curr Probl Pediatr* 1986; 7:361–409.
8. Srecher S, Soumenkoff G, Puissant F, et al: Vertical transmission of HIV in a 20 week old fetus. *Lancet* 1986; 2:288.
9. Marion RW, Wiznia AA, Hutcheon G, et al: Fetal AIDS syndrome score. Correlation between severity of dysmorphism and age at diagnosis of immunodeficiency. *Am J Dis Child* 1987; 141:429–431.
10. Revision of the case definition of acquired immunodeficiency syndrome for national reporting—United States. *MMWR* 1985; 34:373–375.
11. Rogers MF: AIDS in children: A review of clinical, epidemiologic and public health aspects. *Pediatr Infect Dis* 1985; 4:230–236.
12. Pahwa S, Fikrig S, Menez R, et al: Pediatric acquired immunodeficiency syndrome: Demonstration of B-lymphocyte defects in-vitro. *Diagn Immunol* 1986; 4:24–30.
13. Kazlow PG, Shah K, Benkov KJ, et al: Esophageal cryptosporidiosis in a child with acquired immune deficiency syndrome. *Gastroenterology* 1986; 91:1301–1303.
14. Rogers VD, Kagnoff MF: Gastrointestinal manifestations of AIDS. *Western J Med* 1987; 146:57–67.
15. Meiselman MS, Cello JP, Margaretten W: Cytomegalovirus colitis: Report of the clinical, endoscopic and pathological findings in two patients with acquired immunodeficiency syndrome. *Gastroenterology* 1985; 88:171–175.
16. Glaser JB, Morton-Klute L, Berger SR, et al: Recurrent *Salmonella typhimurium* bacteremia associated with the acquired immunodeficiency syndrome. *Ann Intern Med* 1985; 102:189–193.
17. Kotler DP, Goetz HP, Lange M, et al: Enteropathy associated with the Acquired immunodeficiency syndrome. *Ann Intern Med* 1984; 101:421–428.
18. Hoskins LC, Winawer SJ, Broitman SA, et al: Clinical giardiasis and intestinal malabsorption. *Gastroenterology* 1967; 53:265–279.
19. Dehovitz JA, Pape JW, Boncy M, et al: Clinical manifestations and therapy of *Isospora belli* infection in patients with the acquired immunodeficiency syndrome. *N Engl J Med* 1986; 315:87–90.
20. Dobbins WO, Weinstein WM: Electron microscopy of the intestine and rectum in AIDS. *Gastroenterology* 1985; 88:738–749.
21. Gillin JS, Shike M, Alcock N, et al: Malabsorption and mucosal abnormalities of the small intestine in AIDS. *Ann Intern Med* 1985; 102:619–622.
22. Rogers VD, Fassett R, Kagnoff MF: Abnormalities in intestinal mucosal T cells in homosexual populations including those with the lymphadenopathy syndrome and AIDS. *Gastroenterology* 1986; 90:552–558.

23. Duffy LF, Daum F, Kahn E, et al: Hepatitis in children with acquired immune deficiency syndrome. *Gastroenterology* 1986; 90:173–181.
24. Lebovics E, Thung SN, Shaffner F, et al: The liver in acquired immunodeficiency syndrome: A clinical and histologic study. *Hepatology* 1985; 5:293–298.
25. Buck BE, Scott GB, Valdes-Dapena M, et al: Kaposi sarcoma in two infants with acquired immunodeficiency syndrome *J Pediatr* 1983; 103:911–913.

46 Henoch-Schönlein Purpura

Richard A. Schreiber M.D.C.M., F.R.C.P.(C.)

A 5-year-old boy was admitted to the hospital because of persistent vomiting. He had been in his usual state of good health until 5 days prior to admission when he slipped and fell in a brook and was found to have a tender right hemiscrotum with mild scrotal ecchymosis. An ultrasound and Doppler study of the scrotum showed no damage except peritesticular fluid; urinalysis was normal. One day prior to admission he developed episodes of vomiting associated with abdominal pain. He denied fever, weight loss, change in bowel habits, hematemesis, melena, hematochezia, abdominal trauma, headache, dizziness, change in vision, rash, joint pain, tainted food ingestion, drug use, or allergies. There was no family history of gastrointestinal (GI) disease.

On physical examination he appeared slightly dehydrated. The vital signs were stable, and he was afebrile and anicteric. Results of his head, ear, eye, nose, and throat, pulmonary, and cardiovascular examinations were normal. There was no adenopathy. The abdomen was diffusely tender, especially in the epigastric region. No guarding, rebound, masses, or hepatosplenomegaly were found; the stool was heme negative. Results of the scrotal examination were now normal without evidence for tenderness or swelling.

The hematocrit was 35%, and values for the white blood cell (WBC) count and differential, platelet count, prothrombin time, partial thromboplastin time, erythrocyte sedimentation rate, serum electrolyte, BUN, creatinine, and amylase levels were all normal. A urinalysis, including microscopic analysis, was unremarkable. The urine-specific gravity was 1.025. An abdominal radiograph was normal.

He was hospitalized for observation and fluid support; by day 3 the vomitus became bilious, and an upper GI x-ray series demonstrated narrowed segments of the duodenum (Fig 46–1). An abdominal ultrasound and computed tomography (CT) scan indicated a possible intramural lesion but no involvement of the mesenteric nodes. An upper endoscopy showed an inflamed duodenum; biopsy results confirmed duodenitis. A nasogastric tube was inserted, and antacid therapy and peripheral parenteral nutrition were started. He continued to have abdominal pain and large nasogastric drainage. After 10 days of observation, he underwent exploratory laparotomy. At operation, the duodenum appeared normal, and multiple intestinal and local mesenteric node biopsy specimens were negative for an infiltrative lesion.

Two days postoperatively he developed proteinuria and hematuria. The following morning a palpable purpuric rash appeared on his lower extremities associated with bilateral ankle and knee swelling. His blood pressure remained normal, as did the

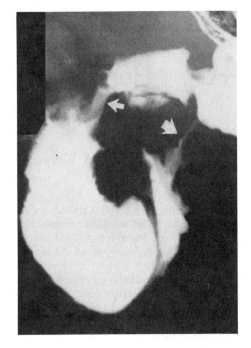

FIG 46–1.
Upper GI radiogram showing
narrowing of the second and fourth
portions of the duodenum *(arrows).*

BUN and creatinine levels. The serum immunoglobulin A (IgA) level was elevated. A clinical diagnosis of Henoch-Schönlein purpura (HSP) was made. During the next week his symptoms of abdominal and joint pain improved without drug therapy, and he was discharged home in good condition.

DISCUSSION

Henoch-Schönlein purpura is a syndrome whose diagnosis is based on a constellation of clinical and laboratory signs and symptoms (Table 46–1); there are no definitive diagnostic tests.[1] The major clinical features include a purpuric rash, arthritis, nephritis, and GI symptoms. Other less common manifestations include scrotal and testicular swelling,[2] CNS vascular insults,[1] and, more rarely, pulmonary[3] and cardiovascular involvement.[4]

Schönlein in 1837 first described the relationship between the joint symptoms and purpura.[5] In 1874, Henoch described the GI symptoms of this condition, and in 1889 Schönlein added the observation of the final component of the syndrome, renal disease.[6] Because of the chronology of their contributions, some refer to this syndrome as the Schönlein-Henoch syndrome. Other names include anaphylactoid purpura, allergic purpura, and allergic vasculitis.

Henoch-Schönlein purpura is a disorder primarily of childhood although cases in adults have been reported.[6] In a classical review of 131 cases of HSP in children by Allen and Diamond, the median age of onset was 4 years, with a range from 6 months to 16 years.[7] More than 75% of cases occurred in the under 7 years age group, with one third of cases having their onset in the 2 to 3 years age range. No cases were reported in children less than 6 months of age.

Pathophysiology

The etiology of this condition remains obscure. Many physicians have observed an antecedent respiratory tract infection occurring about 2 weeks prior to the onset of disease, but no single agent has been isolated. Historically, HSP was thought to have an allergic basis, but no specific allergen has been identified. The consistent finding of an elevated serum IgA level and deposition of IgA in affected tissues has led to the concept that HSP is an immune mediated disease.[8]

The classical purpuric rash results from a leucocytoclastic vasculitis.[9] Immunofluorescent studies can demonstrate deposition of IgA in the venules of the affected skin regions.

Clinical Features

Appearance of cutaneous lesions is central to the diagnosis of HSP (see Table 46–1). Initially the rash may be urticarial rather than purpuric, particularly in the younger infant who may also have subcutaneous edema of the scalp, eyes, hands, and feet.[1] Typically the purpuric rash is distributed on the buttocks and legs. Occasionally other areas such as the face and upper extremities may be involved, but the trunk is usually spared. As evidenced by the case presented, other manifestations of HSP may preceed the onset of the rash. In one case report, the rash appeared as late as 2 weeks after the onset of other symptoms.[10]

Renal disease occurs in about 40% of all patients with HSP. In less than 5% of cases the renal abnormalities will appear prior to the rash or other symptoms. The spectrum of renal involvement can range from microscopic hematuria to acute nephritis, the nephrotic syndrome and chronic renal failure.[11] Patients with severe renal

TABLE 46–1.
Manifestations of Henoch-Schönlein Purpura*

Manifestations	Incidence,%
Rash	100
Gastrointestinal	80
Rheumatologic	70
Renal	40
Scrotal, testicular	10
Neurologic	6
Pulmonary, cardiovascular	<5

*Adapted from Barratt and Drummond.[1]

disease tend to be older and have more pronounced skin and GI manifestations; their prognosis is poorer. The vast majority of children have minimal renal involvement and ultimately do well without sequelae.

Arthritis is seen in at least two thirds of cases and in one review, joint swelling was the second commonest feature of HSP.[1] Large joints such as the knees and ankles are most often involved, but swelling of the wrists and fingers may also occur. As witnessed by the patient presented, arthritis is transient rather than migratory, usually lasts for several days, and resolves completely without deformity.

The GI manifestations of HSP are seen in up to 80% of cases. In a review by Feldt and Stickler of 139 childhood cases of HSP, 65% had complaints of either abdominal pain or GI bleeding.[12] In 10% of these cases the abdominal symptoms preceded the onset of purpura or arthritis. The period of isolated GI symptomatology varied from 1 to 17 days, with an average of 5 days.[12] Thus, HSP should be included in the differential diagnosis of bloody diarrhea of infancy and should also be considered in the child who presents with an acute abdomen.

Diagnosis

The onset of severe abdominal symptoms in HSP, mimicking an acute abdomen prior to the appearance of the characteristic rash, has been known to create a diagnostic dilemma. A similar problem occurred with this case. This patient had an undiagnosed intramural lesion of his small intestine. The differential diagnosis included an intramural hematoma secondary to trauma, an infiltrative process such as intestinal lymphoma or leiomyoma, or an inflammatory lesion. The history of previous injury to his scrotum was attributed to his falling into a brook. Acute scrotal swelling occurs in about 10% of males with HSP, but scrotal manifestations have not been known to occur before the rash appears.[1] Because of the possibility of an infiltrative lesion and with no other stigmata of HSP present, he was taken for explorative laparotomy. No lesion was found. Clearly, when the abdominal symptoms precede the cutaneous lesions, HSP can mimic many other acute abdominal conditions.

No single test or study is available to confirm the diagnosis of HSP. Radiographic assessments are often obtained and may provide some suggestive findings. In one series of 22 patients with HSP, 17 had small bowel mucosal abnormalities detected by a barium swallow examination.[13] Duodenal and jejunal involvement predominated with findings ranging from thumbprinting to intussusception. Crohn's ileitis can have radiographic features similar to HSP. Features such as pseudotumor or strictures have also been described.[14]

Endoscopic evaluation can also provide evidence suggestive of HSP. Findings include erythematous patches similar to those seen in this case report, but petechial and purpuric lesions of the duodenal mucosa have also been described.[15] Other important laboratory features include an elevated serum IgA level, a normal serum C3 value, a moderate leukocytosis, and a normal platelet count.[1] Factor XIII activity has been shown to be a marker for prognosis.[16] Levels below 50% activity are correlated with disease complications, whereas normalization of this level coincides with recovery.

Treatment

The treatment of HSP is supportive. Careful observation for intestinal hemorrhage and attention to fluid and electrolyte balance, particularly for those patients with nephropathy, is indicated. Expectant management for the complication of intussusception is warranted.

The role for steroid therapy remains controversial.[1] There is no prospective controlled study that demonstrates the efficacy of steroids in HSP. A recent study suggested that steroids tended to hasten the resolution of symptoms if given early in the course of the disease, but did not alter the final outcome.[17] Most experts agree that if steroids are to be used, it is for the GI manifestations and not for the renal or joint complications.[1]

In the majority of cases the prognosis is excellent, although the GI complications, including abdominal pain and intestinal blood loss, can lead to significant morbidity. The long-term prognosis depends on the degree of renal involvement. Children with prominent renal manifestations should be followed regularly since complications such as renal failure and hypertension can occur as late as 10 years after onset.[18]

SUMMARY

Henoch-Schönlein purpura is a disease of unknown etiology whose diagnosis is based on a constellation of clinical and laboratory signs and symptoms (see Table 46–1). The classic purpuric rash is central to the diagnosis; GI, musculoskeletal, and renal symptoms may also be seen. Treatment is supportive, although steroids are often used for the GI symptoms despite the lack of controlled clinical trials to prove their efficacy. Most children recover completely, as did the child presented here.

REFERENCES

1. Barratt TM, Drummond KN: The vasculitis syndromes: Henoch-Schönlein syndrome or anaphylactic purpura, in Kelley VC (ed): *Practice of Pediatrics,* vol 8. New York, Harper & Row, 1980, pp 1-12.
2. O'Regan S, Robitaille P: Orchitis mimicking testicular torsion in Henoch-Schönlein purpura. *J Urol* 1981; 126:834–835.
3. Scitinder K, Gregario C: Fatal pulmonary Henoch-Schönlein syndrome. *Chest* 1982; 82:654–656.
4. Abdel-Hadi O, Hartley RB, Greenstone MA, et al: Myocardial infarction—a rare complication in Henoch-Schönlein purpura. *Postgrad Med J* 1981; 57:390–392.
5. Schonlein JL: *Allgemeine und specielle Pathologie und Therapie,* ed 3. Herisau, Lit Compt, 1837, Vol 2, p 48.
6. Cream JJ, Grumpel JM, Peachey RDG: Schönlein-Henoch purpura in the adult. *Q J Med* 1970; 39:461–484.
7. Allen DM, Diamond LK, et al: Anaphylactoid purpura in children. *Am J Dis Child* 1960; 99:147–168.

8. Morichau-Beauchant M, Touchard G, Maire P, et al: Jejunal IgA and C3 deposition in adult Henoch-Schönlein purpura with severe intestinal manifestations. *Gastroenterology* 1982; 82:1438–1442.
9. Fauci AS, Haynes BF, Katz P: The spectrum of vasculitis: Clinical pathologic, immunologic and therapeutic considerations. *Ann Intern Med* 1978; 89:660–676.
10. Katz A: Henoch Schonlein purpura. *N Engl J Med* 1980; 302:853–858.
11. Meadow SR, Glascow EF, White HR, et al: Schönlein-Henoch nephritis. *Q J Med* 1972; 41:241–258.
12. Feldt RW, Stickler GB: The gastrointestinal manifestations of anaphylactoid purpura in children. *Proc Mayo Clin* 1962; 137:465–483.
13. Glasier CM, Siegel MJ, et al: Henoch-Schönlein syndrome in children: Gastrointestinal manifestations. *AJR* 1981; 136:1081–1085.
14. Lombard KA, Shah PC, Thrasher TV, et al: Ileal stricture as a late complication of Henoch-Schönlein purpura. *Pediatrics* 1986; 77:396–398.
15. Goldman LP, Listenberg RL: Henoch-Schönlein purpura gastrointestinal manifestations with endoscopic correlation. *Am J Gastroenterol* 1981; 75:357–360.
16. Dalens B, Travade P, Labbe A, et al: Diagnostic and prognostic value of fibrin stabilizing factor in Schönlein-Henoch syndrome. *Arch Dis Child* 1983; 58:12–14.
17. Rosenblum ND, Winter HS: Steroid effects on the course of abdominal pain in children with Henoch-Schönlein purpura. *Pediatrics* 1987; 79:1018–1021.
18. Counahan R, Winterborn MH, White RHR, et al: Prognosis of Henoch-Schönlein nephritis in children. *Br Med J* 1977; 2:11–14.

47 Hemolytic-Uremic Syndrome

Cheryl J. Bunker, M.D.

A 3.5-year-old formerly healthy girl was admitted to the hospital with diarrhea, vomiting, somnolence, and hypotension.

She was well until the evening 3 days prior to admission when she began to have diarrhea, which persisted. Two days before admission she complained of intermittent epigastric pain; that evening she began to vomit, and her stools changed to a currant-jelly appearance. The following morning she was taken to her pediatrician, who prescribed trimethoprim-sulfamethoxazole. The patient, however, could not tolerate her antibiotic, and her symptoms continued. On the day of admission the patient was found to be somnolent and disoriented with cool extremities and was brought to the emergency room. She had not had fever, chills, or recent immunizations.

On arrival the patient was an acutely ill-appearing, well-developed child with a blood pressure of 50 mm Hg systolic and a pulse of 210 with a regular rate. Her temperature was 39.1°C rectally. Results of skin, head, neck, heart, and lung examinations were normal. Her abdomen was soft with normal bowel sounds. She was mildly tender to palpation to the right of her umbilicus in the midclavicular line but had no masses or organomegaly. Rectal examination revealed heme-positive currant-jelly–appearing stool with mucus present. Her extremities were cool but otherwise unremarkable. The neurologic examination was nonfocal.

Laboratory values on admission included a white blood cell (WBC) count of 25,300/mm^3 with 65% neutrophils, 9% bands, and 20% lymphocytes; hematocrit 37.3%, and platelet count 137,000/mm^3. Her peripheral smear revealed occasional ovalocytes, burr cells, teardrop forms, and bizarre forms. The serum electrolyte levels were normal except for a bicarbonate of 17 mEq/l. The BUN level was 69 mg/dl, with a creatinine level of 1.8 mg/dl. An arterial blood gas on room air revealed pH of 7.37, Po$_2$ of 128, Pco$_2$ of 20, and bicarbonate 12 mEq/l. The prothrombin time was elevated at 15.6 seconds. Liver function test results revealed aspartate aminotransferase (AST) 56 mU/ml, alanine aminotransferase (ALT) 33 mU/ml, total bilirubin level 0.3 mg/dl, alkaline phosphatase level 68 mU/ml lactic dehydrogenase 293 mU/ml total protein level 3.4 gm/dl, and albumin level 1.7 gm/dl. Amylase level was 219 mU/ml calcium 7.6 mg/dl and phosphorus 4.2 mg/dl. The urinalysis revealed a specific gravity of 1.015, pH 5, 2 + protein, red blood cells (RBCs) too numerous to count, 4 to 6 white blood cells (WBCs) per high-power field (HPF), a small amount of bacteria and moderate uric acid crystals. The urine sodium level

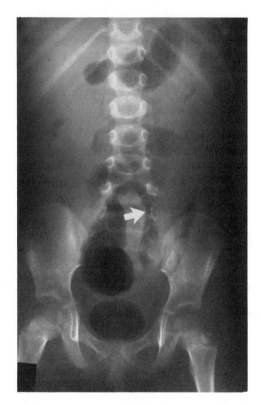

FIG 47–1.
Upright abdominal film demonstrating "thumbprinting."

was 32 mmol/L, and urine potassium level was 26 mmol/L. The stool smear revealed no polymorphonuclear leukocytes. Stool, blood, and urine cultures were sent, and all returned later with no growth. A nasogastric tube was passed, and a heme-positive aspirate was obtained. Admission chest x-ray film was normal. Admission x-ray examination of the kidneys, ureter, and bladder and upright abdominal films demonstrated a nonspecific bowel gas pattern and thumbprinting (Fig 47–1).

In the emergency room the patient was stabilized with intravenous (IV) fluids through a central venous catheter and was treated with IV ampicillin and chloramphenicol. She was admitted to the hospital.

By the fourth hospital day her gastrointestinal (GI) symptoms had resolved, although her stools remained heme positive. The BUN level, however, had risen to 109 mg/dl; creatinine level was 6.2 mg/dl, and amylase level was 692 units/ml. In addition, her urine output dropped to 0.3 ml/kg/hour. A renal ultrasound revealed increased echogenicity consistent with bilateral parenchymal injury and a small amount of ascites. Hemodialysis was begun, and her antibiotics were changed to ceftriaxone.

She required two transfusions of packed RBCs when her hematocrit fell below

20%, but she otherwise did well, and her renal function gradually improved. After 2 weeks of hemodialysis, the patient was discharged.

Two weeks after discharge her hematocrit had remained stable and the BUN and creatinine levels had fallen to 28 and 0.6 mg/dl, respectively. By 3 months after discharge her hematocrit had risen to 32%, BUN and creatinine levels were 15 and 0.5 mg/dl, respectively, and she had returned to her normal state of good health.

DISCUSSION

Hemolytic-uremic syndrome (HUS) is an acute disorder characterized by renal failure, microangiopathic hemolytic anemia, and thrombocytopenia. It is a disease of primarily infancy and early childhood, and it represents the commonest cause of acute renal failure in this age group.[1] Although the vast majority of HUS cases are children less than 4 years of age, adults, especially postpartum women, women taking oral contraceptives, and patients receiving chemotherapy (particularly mitomycin) may also be affected.[2-6] Familial and hereditary presentations have also been described.[7] Cases of HUS occur predominantly in the summer months and are equally divided among males and females.[8]

Pathophysiology

Hemolytic-uremic syndrome is a syndrome, not a disease, and so is likely caused by a variety of agents.[1, 4] The pathogenesis is unknown but appears to be related to endothelial damage of primarily glomerular capillaries and renal arterioles, with occasional involvement of vessels in other organs as well. A currently popular hypothesis speculates that a variety of infectious agents may damage the renal vascular endothelium and initiate the coagulation cascade. This, in turn, traps platelets in the kidney and causes mechanical fragmentation of erythrocytes, thus producing acute renal failure.[1, 2, 4, 5, 9, 10] Damage to organs other than the kidney also appears to be due to microangiopathic injury. Characteristic vascular lesions have been found in brain, lung, heart, pancreas, thyroid, thymus, intestine, adrenals, lymphoid tissue, and bladder from affected patients.[11, 12] Infectious agents that have been associated with HUS include *Escherichia coli*, *Shigella*, *Salmonella*, and several viruses: influenza, coxsackie, echo, myxovirus, and Epstein-Barr.[2, 5, 8, 13] *E. coli* serotype 0157:H7 is the most frequently isolated single pathogen.[14]

Clinical Features

Clinically, patients uniformly present with the history of a prodromal illness that usually includes diarrhea, vomiting, or both; rarely, the antecedent illness is upper respiratory in nature.[1, 9] The diarrhea is bloody in approximately one half of the cases.[9] These signs and symptoms generally precede the development of anemia and renal disease by about 1 week. The full clinical presentation may include pallor, lethargy, anorexia, irritability, abdominal pain, fever, bloody diarrhea, decreased urinary output, bruising or purpura, and, occasionally, seizures.[3, 9, 10]

As with our patient, the laboratory evaluation reveals hematuria and proteinuria as well as severe anemia with a hematocrit of less than 25%. All cases demonstrate evidence of microangiopathy, with schistocytes and burr cells present on blood smears.[9] Thrombocytopenia is commonly found and occasionally may reach 20,000/mm^3.[9] Azotemia with BUN level more than 100 mg/dl is manifest in 75% of cases.[9] Uric acid levels are frequently elevated.[9] Aminotransferases are typically abnormal with up to 4- and 10-fold elevations of ALT and AST levels, respectively.[10] The prothrombin time is often prolonged, and the albumin level is depressed. Brisk hemolysis may result in hyperbilirubinemia.[10]

Radiographic findings on plain abdominal films or barium enemas may be normal or may demonstrate nonspecific findings of mucosal irregularity, dilatation, and "thumbprinting."[15, 16] These findings are well demonstrated in the radiograph from this patient (see Fig 47–1). Endoscopic procedures are not usually required in the evaluation of patients with HUS and can increase the risk of perforation.

The clinical course of HUS often includes oliguria or anuria, which usually persists for 1 to 3 weeks.[9] Dialysis is required in approximately one half of the patients.[9] At presentation the nature of the renal disease may initially be an enigma, the oliguria seemingly the result of decreased circulating blood volume secondary to the prodromal diarrhea. In patients with renal insufficiency solely on the basis of volume depletion, a brisk response to fluid replacement occurs with an appropriate lowering of BUN and creatinine levels. However, the intrinsic renal damage in HUS will not improve with fluid replacement alone, resulting in persistent oliguria with BUN and creatinine levels that continue to rise.[1]

The clinical course of HUS also may include the development of hypertension, anemia, and seizures.[9, 11] Hypertension, which is a common finding early in the disease course, rarely becomes a chronic problem. The microangiopathic anemia is often severe enough in the acute stages of the illness to require one or more blood transfusions. Generalized seizure activity that is manifest in 40% of patients acutely seldom becomes a chronic problem.[9, 11] However, the rare development of coma and the attendant cortical insult and atrophy carry a much graver prognosis.[9, 11]

The interpretation of gastrointestinal symptoms in HUS can be confusing and misdiagnosis can lead to inappropriate and potentially hazardous therapy. The prodromal GI symptoms, for example, may mimic surgically correctable diseases such as intusseception or appendicitis. In such cases, if characteristic ischemic changes are demonstrated by barium enema and the diagnosis of a surgical condition concurrent with HUS is in doubt, it is best to opt for conservative management since the ischemic lesions in this early stage usually spontaneously resolve. In the later stages of the illness, lingering or progressive GI complaints may still represent self-limited ischemia, but at this point the astute clinician must be on guard for the development of bowel infarction, perforation, gangrenous colitis, pseudomembranous enterocolitis, or toxic megacolon. Although these complications are rare, they have all been reported and can be disastrous if their diagnosis is delayed.[10–13, 17, 18] Occasionally stricture formation has been documented following the ischemic injury of HUS. Some clinicians therefore advocate screening for strictures with a barium enema within 2 months of the acute episode in all patients who experience severe colitis with HUS.[12, 15]

Diagnosis

The diagnosis of HUS rests on a combination of clinical and laboratory findings, including the history of a prodromal illness, followed by the development of acute renal failure, microangiopathic anemia, and thrombocytopenia. The differential diagnosis early in the illness in those patients presenting as this patient did includes gastroenteritis, infectious colitis, appendicitis, inflammatory bowel disease, and intestinal obstruction such as intussusception.[13, 18] (See Table 47–1 for a list of the differential diagnoses.) When the characteristic laboratory findings of microangiopathic hemolytic anemia, thrombocytopenia, and acute renal failure become evident, the differential diagnosis shifts to other vasculitic possibilities. Henoch-Schönlein purpura (HSP), for example, is an important disease to consider because it also may present with abdominal pain, purpura, and nephritis following a flulike illness.[16] In HSP, however, the platelet count is normal, anemia is generally not present, and renal insufficiency, when manifest, occurs 4 to 8 weeks into the disease course.[16] Systemic lupus erythematosis also may present with thrombocytopenia, nephritis, and hemolytic anemia, but lupus patients are generally older and their anemia, when hemolytic, is more typically Coombs' positive and not microangiopathic.[1] Thrombotic, thrombocytopenic purpura (TTP) bears remarkable similarity to HUS and is believed by some observers to be part of a continuum of the same pathogenetic process, differing primarily in the extent and distribution of the vascular changes.[1, 2] Thrombocytopenic purpura is generally an illness of adults and essentially always includes neurologic symptoms in addition to renal insufficiency, microangiopathic hemolytic anemia, and thrombocytopenia. In addition, the prognosis for patients with TTP is usually far graver than for HUS.[2, 18] Disseminated intravascular coagulopathy can also cause a clinical picture resembling HUS. However, the fibrinogen level is often elevated in HUS (as opposed to depressed in DIC), and the prothrombin time and partial thromboplastin time are frequently normal. The hemolysis of HUS also tends to be more severe than that of DIC.[1, 5, 11]

TABLE 47–1.
Differential Diagnosis of Hemolytic Uremic Syndrome

Gastroenteritis
Infectious colitis
Appendicitis
Inflammatory bowel disease
Intestinal obstruction
Intussusception
Volvulus
Vasculitis
HSP
TTP
DIC

Treatment

Treatment for HUS is supportive and is focused primarily on managing the acute renal failure by providing adequate nutrition, maintaining electrolyte balance, avoiding circulatory overload, and employing hemodialysis in the more severely affected individuals. Transfusions are usually administered when the hematocrit falls below 20%. The GI manifestations generally resolve spontaneously. No controlled trials of the use of steroids, anticoagulants, thrombolytic therapy, plasmapheresis, or exchange transfusions have been published, and anecdotal reports have not yet identified an ideal therapeutic regimen. The best results have been reported for those patients who received prompt, aggressive supportive care.[1, 2, 4, 9-11]

The prognosis is good in most cases of HUS, although the mortality rate approximates 10%.[10] Recovery is usually complete, and long-term sequellae are rare.[10] Persistent hypertension, mild renal insufficiency, or chronic neurologic sequellae such as seizures, cortical blindness, or psychomotor retardation are seen in 5% to 10%.[5, 9, 17] The atypical form of HUS, however, such as those related to chemotherapy, familial occurrence, or those that follow a respiratory rather than a GI illness, often carry a poorer prognosis.[1, 4, 15] Recurrences of HUS are extremely rare.[9]

SUMMARY

The key to successful management of HUS is the recognition of the presenting signs and symptoms as manifest by the patient in this case study, with the early institution of aggressive supportive care. Hemolytic uremic syndrome should be considered in any patient who presents with pallor, lethargy, anorexia, irritability, seizures, abdominal pain fever, bloody diarrhea, decreased urinary output, bruising or purpura, and who has a history of a prodromal illness, including diarrhea, vomiting, or both. In such a patient it is imperative to obtain renal function tests, a complete blood cell count with examination of the peripheral blood smear, an abdominal flat plate to assess the bowel gas pattern and possible thumbprinting, and a urinalysis to rule out proteinuria. If any of these tests suggest possible HUS, the patient should be admitted to a hospital for close observation and supportive care. If HUS is diagnosed early and proper supportive care is provided, the great majority of affected individuals will enjoy a full and complete recovery without sequelae.

REFERENCES

1. Scully RE, Galdabini JJ, McNeely BU: Case records of the Massachusetts General Hospital. *N Engl J Med* 1981; 304:715–722.
2. Brynes JJ, Moake JL: Thrombotic thrombocytopenic purpura and the haemolytic-uremic syndrome: Evolving concepts of pathogenesis and therapy. *Clin Haematol* 1986; 15:413–442.
3. Fong JS, deChadarevian JP, Kaplan BS: Hemolytic-uremic syndrome. Current concepts and management. *Pediatr Clin North Am* 1982; 29:835–856.

4. Kaplan BS, Drummond KN: The hemolytic-uremic syndrome is a syndrome. *N Engl J Med* 1978; 298:964–966.
5. Karmali MA, Petric M, Lim C, et al: The association between idiopathic hemolytic uremic syndrome and infection by verotoxin-producing *E. coli. J Infect Dis* 1985; 151:775–782.
6. Verweij J, van der Burg ME, Pinedo HM: Mitomycin C–induced hemolytic uremic syndrome. Six case reports and review of the literature on renal, pulmonary and cardiac side effects of the drug. *Radiother Oncol* 1987; 8:33–41.
7. Kaplan BS, Chesney RW, Drummond KN: Hemolytic-uremic syndrome in families. *N Engl J Med* 1975; 292:1090–1093.
8. Gully PR. Haemolytic-uraemic syndrome: Epidemiology and report of an outbreak. *J R Soc Health* 1984; 104:214–217.
9. Brasher C, Seigler RL: The hemolytic-uremic syndrome. *West J Med* 1981; 134:193–197.
10. Whitington PF, Friedman AL, Chesney RW: Gastrointestinal disease in the hemolytic-uremic syndrome. *Gastroenterology* 1979; 76:728–733.
11. Upadhyaya K, Barwick K, Fishaut M, et al: The importance of nonrenal involvement in hemolytic-uremic syndrome. *Pediatrics* 1980; 65:115–120.
12. Van Stiegmann G, Lilly JR: Surgical lesions of the colon in the hemolytic-uremic syndrome. *Surgery* 1979; 85:357–359.
13. Kendall PA, Reid I, Wright JE, et al: Gangrenous colitis in the haemolytic-uremic syndrome. *Med J Aust* 1984; 140:543–544.
14. Neill MA, Tarr PI, Clausen CR, et al: *Escherichia coli* 0157:H7 as the predominant pathogen associated with the hemolytic uremic syndrome: A prospective study in the Pacific Northwest. *Pediatrics* 1987; 80:37–45.
15. Kawanami T, Bowen A, Girdany BR: Enterocolitis: Prodrome of the hemolytic-uremic syndrome. *Radiology* 1984; 151:91–92.
16. Scully RE, Galdabini JJ, McNeely BU: Case records of the Massachusetts General Hospital. *N Engl J Med* 1980; 302:853–858.
17. Schwartz DL, Becker JM, So HB, et al: Segmental colonic gangrene: A surgical emergency in the hemolytic-uremic syndrome. *Pediatrics* 1978; 62:54–56.
18. Sun CJ, Hill JL, Combs JW: Hemolytic-uremic syndrome: Initial presentation mimicking intestinal intussusception. *Pediatr Pathol* 1983; 1:415–422.

48   Munchausen Syndrome by Proxy

Samuel Nurko, M.D.

A 20-month-old girl was noted to pass bright red blood per rectum for 3 weeks prior to admission. This was not associated with diarrhea, pain, or passage of stools. According to the mother, the child passed a teaspoonful of bright red blood and was taken to another institution, where she was found to be afebrile and to have a normal physical examination, including the rectal examination, which showed no fissures, hemorrhoids, or stool on guaiac test. The mother brought the diaper containing about 5 ml of blood. The child's hematocrit was 38%, and after a Meckel's scan and a barium enema study were normal, she was discharged. One week later she was again noted by the mother to pass bright red blood per rectum. She returned to the same hospital, where her physical examination was unremarkable, and no stool was present on rectal examination. The diaper again contained 5 ml of blood. The child was discharged but came that night to the Children's Hospital emergency room with a history of having had one episode of vomiting bright red blood. A nasogastric tube was passed and revealed a clear guaiac-positive gastric aspirate without bright red blood or coffee ground material. Her vital signs were stable, and her physical examination was normal, including the rectal examination that showed guaiac-negative stool. Her hematocrit was 38%, mean corpuscular volume 89, and reticulocyte count 0.3%, and the prothrombin and partial thromboplastin times were normal. The mother brought a piece of clothing that had emesis and blood mixed on it. The child was admitted to the hospital. The child came from an intact family in which the father was a teacher and the mother had been a medical technician until the child was born.

The child's evaluation included a normal upper endoscopy, and normal ear, nose, and throat examination results. On her third hospital day she had another episode of bright red blood in her diaper. Results of her physical examination were normal, including a careful examination of her vaginal area. A rectal examination revealed bright red blood without any stool. A colonoscopy to the cecum was later performed, and the mucosa was normal; however, fresh blood was found in the distal rectum. Her repeated hematocrit was 37%.

Throughout the hospitalization, the mother was always in the hospital, was very helpful and pleasant, and maintained a very good relationship with the nursing staff. The day following the colonoscopy the child had another episode in which bright red blood was found by the mother in the diaper. Results of a careful examination at that time were normal, including a rectal examination that showed guaiac-negative stool. The diaper was sent to the blood bank for blood typing, which proved to be type B positive blood. The child's blood type was A positive. The mother was then confronted with this fact, and at first showed surprise and denied any wrongdoing. However, later she admitted to having used her own blood to produce all of the previous episodes. The child was later taken into custody by protective agencies and was placed in temporary foster care.

DISCUSSION

Individuals suffering from Munchausen syndrome purposely and needlessly subject themselves to potentially painful and life-threatening procedures and treatments.[1] The label of Munchausen syndrome by proxy may be applied to anyone who persistently fabricates symptoms on behalf of another, causing that person to be regarded as ill.[2] Deliberate parental involvement of their progeny in this syndrome is a disturbing form of child abuse.[3]

The fabrication of clinical symptoms undermines the very foundation of clinical assessment. Physicians depend on a precise medical history to guide their clinical decisions. Medical education emphasizes the importance of listening to patients carefully,[3] and the physician's belief in the veracity of the patient's story is the cornerstone of clinical medicine.[4] Physicians often undertake a specific plan of evaluation and investigation when certain signs and symptoms are reported by the patient,[5] and this expected response is anticipated by the patient who has planned the deception.[3] In Munchausen syndrome by proxy it is the parents' deceit that leads to injury, usually caused by the physician in pursuit of the diagnosis.[6] Naish has described this predicament succinctly: "The essential feature of all these deceptive and manipulative situations is that you have a patient presenting a problem, demanding a solution, and you have a doctor who sees his role as that of a scientific technician.''[6] Physicians develop reflexive ways of reacting to a symptom or a sign by proceeding to certain investigations or treatment and feel pressured to find an organic cause to explain the difficulties encountered by patients.[5]

Clinical Features

Munchausen syndrome by proxy is a rare disorder, although it is one that should be considered when any of the signs mentioned in Table 48–1 are present. A large number of presentations have been reported for Munchausen syndrome by proxy,[2, 3, 6, 7] and almost every organ system has been implicated. The symptoms may vary from those of relatively benign upper respiratory tract infections to life-threatening cardiorespiratory arrests.[8] The presentation may involve only maternal accounts of the events (e.g., seizures),[3] but may also involve tampering with urine (adding sugar, stones, or blood), stool (adding blood), or central venous lines or the injection of substances into the child to cause sepsis.[7]

TABLE 48–1.

Warning Signs of Munchausen Syndrome by Proxy*

1.	Unexplained illness, usually prolonged, and so extraordinary that experienced physicians frequently state that they "have never seen anything like this before."
2.	Symptoms and signs that are incongruent or implausible.
3.	Symptoms and signs that occur only when the parent is present.
4.	Treatments that are ineffective.
5.	History of multiple allergies to food and drugs
6.	Parent who is usually not as worried by the child's illness as the medical staff.
7.	Parents who never leave the bedside, prompting even the staff to remark that they are "ideal parents."
8.	Parents who are usually at ease with and have a good relationship with the medical staff.
9.	Parents with previous medical or nursing experience.
10.	Parents with a previous history of Munchausen syndrome or with a family history of sudden infant death or family members with multiple and varied serious medical disorders.

*Adapted from Meadow.[13]

Episodes of bleeding are commonly reported. In one recent report, 12 of 19 patients presented with a history of bleeding, including hematuria, hematemesis, hemoptysis, and hematochezia.[5] Neurologic problems, glycosuria, fevers, and fecalent vomiting were also reported.[5]

The gastrointestinal (GI) tract is a common site for factitious complaints that can range from intractable diarrhea secondary to laxative abuse[9–11] to GI bleeding,[6] as in this case. In most instances in which GI bleeding was a presenting sign, an exogenous source of blood (usually the parent's) was added to the child's feces, diaper, or perirectal area.[12] There is one case report in which a mother phlebotomized her child through an indwelling Broviac line and placed the child's blood in the diaper area.[7]

Diagnosis

The severity of the presenting signs and symptoms often leads to patients being subjected to multiple and often invasive studies. The realization that a child's prolonged illness may have been fabricated tends to come slowly. The first step in diagnosis is suspicion. The warning signs that should alert the physician to the presence of this syndrome were noted in Table 48–1. As can be seen in the table, the case under discussion has many of these characteristics. The mother had worked as a medical technician, she never left the child's beside, and she made very good friends with the nurses. The child's symptoms were inconsistent with the physicial findings, and the symptoms never occurred when the mother was absent.

In 95% of all reported cases the mother has been found to be the guilty party.[3, 13] Fathers usually keep a low profile and are often described as unable to cope with the child's problems.[3, 5, 8, 13] They can, however, be extremely helpful and usually cooperate once the situation has been made clear to them.[3]

The reasons for a parent knowingly fabricating a story that leads to painful and potentially harmful evaluation of the child are unknown.[5] Most mothers have undergone extensive psychiatric evaluation; the test results are usually normal, and no diagnosable psychiatric disorder is found.[6, 13] Part of the problem in selecting a diagnosis may be the difficulty of defining normal and abnormal personality.[6]

Several hypotheses have been suggested to explain the parent's behavior. The first is that the fabricated illness may express the parent's sense of illness and need for attention and help.[14] Another possibility is that the child's "illness" seems to bring a closer relationship between the parents or to provide a welcome distraction from personal and home difficulties.[14] Interestingly, most mothers involved seem caring and loving and exhibit no cruelty or negligence.[5] In those mothers in whom detailed early experiences and family life have been obtained, no history of deprivation or institutional life has been found.[5]

When the diagnosis of Munchausen syndrome by proxy is suspected, every effort should be made to establish it with certainty. This can prove dangerous at times, especially when the symptoms produced can be life-threatening to the child.[5, 8] Meadow has recommended a series of steps to follow to try to establish the diagnosis.[5, 13] First, review the history to decide which events are likely to be real and which are fabricated. Second, look for a temporal association between illness events and the presence of the parent (most often the mother). Then, check the details of the personal, social, and family history that the parent has given. Make contact with other family members, particularly with the spouse. Discuss the illness episodes within the family with the primary care provider. A motive for the behavior should be sought. If the child is in the hospital, all the charts and records should be protected so that they will not be altered by the parent. At the time of unexplained events, any pertinent samples should be retained and analyzed for evidence of possible tampering. If bleeding is a symptom, the blood should be checked to determine that it is human and whether it is the same blood type as the child's. It may become necessary to establish very close surveillance of the parent, and video equipment has been used to document the abuse.[8, 11] The parent may need to be kept from visiting for a period of time in the hope that the symptoms or signs will subside. Finally, the necessary social service departments should be involved.[5, 13]

Management

Once the diagnosis has been made, management centers on the primary goal of protecting the child from any further abuse,[14] and the plan of action is similar to that adopted for other cases of child abuse.[5] The first step is to confront the parent with the evidence.[13] This is usually best accomplished by explaining to the parent that his or her actions have been uncovered and that the caretakers want to help the child and parent.[13] At this time there is usually denial, although tacit admissions are sometimes made. This can be a dangerous time, and attempted suicide has been described.[13] The long-term therapeutic aim is to stop the abuse and protect the child. To accomplish this, parents must be made to understand the consequences of their actions, and optimally, to become motivated to seek continued treatment and help.[13, 14] Social service and child protection agencies play a central role in finding a safe environment for the child.[3, 5, 13] Their input is essential for deciding whether the child should be removed from the family.

SUMMARY

This case is a reminder that when the history, physical findings, and laboratory evaluation present a confusing and conflicting picture, Maunchausen syndrome by proxy should be considered. This case also emphasizes the need to objectively document the presence of potentially serious signs and symptoms before embarking on an extensive evaluation that includes invasive testing of an otherwise well-appearing child.

REFERENCES

1. Asher R: Munchausen's syndrome. *Lancet* 1951; 1:339–341.
2. Meadow R: Munchausen syndrome by proxy—the hinterland of child abuse. *Lancet* 1977; 2:343–354.
3. Guandolo VL: Munchausen syndrome by proxy: An outpatient challenge. *Pediatrics* 1985; 75:526–530.
4. Clarke E, Melnick SC: The Munchausen syndrome or the problem of hospital hoboes. *Am J Med* 1958; 25:6–12.
5. Meadow R: Munchausen syndrome by proxy. *Arch Dis Child* 1982; 57:92–98.
6. Naish JM: Problems of deception in medical practice. *Lancet* 1979; 2:139–142.
7. Malatak JS; Munchausen syndrome by proxy: Complications of central venous catheter. *Pediatrics* 1985; 75:523–525.
8. Rosen CL: Two siblings with recurrent cardio respiratory arrest: Munchausen syndrome by proxy or child abuse. *Pediatrics* 1983; 71:715–720.
9. Ackerman NB, Strobell CT: Polle syndrome: Chronic diarrhea in Munchausen's child. *Gastroenterology* 1981; 81:1140–1142.
10. Fleisher D, Ament ME: Diarrhea, red diapers and child abuse. *Clin Pediatr* 1977; 17:820–824.
11. Epstein MA, Markowitz RL, Gallo DM, et al: Munchausen syndrome by proxy: Considerations in diagnosis and confirmation by video surveillance. *Pediatrics* 1987; 80:220–224.
12. Kurlandesky L, Lukoff JY, Zinkham WH, et al: Munchausen syndrome by proxy: Definition of factitious bleeding in an infant by 51Cr labeling of erythrocytes. *Pediatrics* 1979; 63:228–231.
13. Meadow R: Management of Munchausen syndrome by proxy. *Arch Dis Child* 1985; 60:385–393.
14. Waller DA: Obstacles to the treatment of Munchausen by proxy syndrome. *J Am Acad Child Psychiatry* 1983; 22:80–85.

49 Failure to Thrive

Daniel M. Epstein, M.D.
William G. Bithoney, M.D.

An 8-month-old girl presented with poor growth of 3 months' duration. She was the full-term, 6.6-lb (3-kg) product of a pregnancy complicated only by maternal alcohol ingestion until the pregnancy was discovered. Adequate prenatal care and uneventful delivery preceded an easy postnatal adjustment. The child was breast-fed exclusively until 4 months, with feedings lasting 5 to 6 minutes on each side. By 5 months, the child's weight had dropped to the 5th percentile (length and head circumference were at the 25th percentile), and weight gain over the next 3 months was minimal. Beginning at age 6 months, she had the first of three ear infections. Spitting up was noted with increasing frequency at 7 months. Developmentally, the child appeared normal. She spent several hours daily adeptly using a walker.

The mother was 24 years old, single, middle class, with 2 years of college. When her pregnancy was discovered, she was told to leave home, and shortly after the birth of the child, the mother and infant went to a shelter. The father of the child was not available for emotional support, and the parental relationship dissolved. The mother and child remained at the shelter for 4 months, when they were able to obtain an apartment. The maternal and family histories were strongly positive for affective illness, and the mother indicated she was depressed. Despite this, she appeared very concerned and caring when dealing with her child.

Physical examination of the infant was unremarkable. She was comfortable in her mother's arms but anxious when put down. Though observant of other people, she became distressed if people came too close. A feeding observation showed lack of eye contact between mother and child. Feeding occurred only when the child was distracted from the feeding event, allowing her mother to slip the food, unnoticed, into her mouth.

Outpatient efforts to begin weaning and to modify feeding behaviors were unsuccessful. The child would not take a bottle, and she became increasingly apathetic and sad appearing. Concerns over dehydration emerged. The child was admitted to the hospital with a diagnosis of reactive attachment disorder secondary to maternal depression. Because of the child's apathy, supplemental tube feedings were initiated at night. Treatment focused on nutritional support and emotional stimulation of the child, institution of an age-appropriate feeding program, support for the mother, and treatment of the mother's depression. A primary nurse was responsible for feeding the child, and appropriate developmental stimulation was provided. Finger foods were introduced through a program of oral desensitization, and weaning from breast to bottle occurred. The mother began taking antidepressant medication, and efforts at family reunification were met with some success. After 3 weeks and a weight gain of 12 oz (18 gm)/day, the mother resumed successful oral feeding of the child.

DISCUSSION

Failure to attain or maintain normal physical growth, or failure to thrive (FTT), may result from disturbances in any area of a child's functioning, including physiologic, psychologic, or social realms.[1, 2] Failure to thrive is common and may occur in as many as 10% of both rural and inner city populations.[3, 4] Although FTT is the admitting diagnosis for 1% to 5% of pediatric hospital admissions,[5] in reality, it is not a diagnosis but merely a symptom of unmet caloric needs caused by a variety of conditions. Every child with FTT has either not taken, not been offered, or not retained adequate calories to sustain growth.[2]

Traditionally, FTT was divided into organic and nonorganic categories, with organic FTT associated with medical illness and nonorganic FTT diagnosed by excluding organic causes. However, since malnutrition is a chronic disease state, cases of nonorganic FTT contain at least one organic feature that can contribute to accompanying behavioral and hormonal changes.[6] Similarly, children with organic FTT are at risk for developing interactional difficulties, often around feeding.[7] These observations have led to the creation of a category known as mixed FTT, routinely used to describe children with medical as well as interactional problems.[8]

Recent studies have demonstrated that the preponderance of inpatient[5, 9] and the overwhelming majority of outpatient[3] cases of FTT fit the nonorganic classification. An efficient workup must aim at making a positive rather than an exclusionary diagnosis for the underlying causative condition. This can be accomplished by evaluating the child, family, and environment for the presence of risk factors in all areas simultaneously.

RISK FACTORS

Risk factors may be associated with the child, the parents or family, interactions between child and caretakers, or with the surrounding environment (Table 49–1).

Factors related to the child include temperament, minor congenital anomalies, prematurity, and chronic medical illness. Infants and children with FTT are often described as sickly, immature, and passive, with an unpredictable, inconsistent, and ambiguous communication style.[2] Problems with emotional lability and oppositionality make them difficult children. These temperamental characteristics are also seen in children with multiple congenital anomalies and prenatal malnutrition, two conditions that carry significant risk for FTT.[10, 11] Organic problems such as fetal alcohol syndrome and intrauterine growth retardation also put a child at risk for FTT. More than 90% of children with fetal alcohol syndrome show prenatal and postnatal growth failure, and more than one third of small for gestational age infants remain below the fifth percentile at age 4 years.[12]

TABLE 49-1.
Risk Factors for Failure to Thrive

Child
    Temperament
    Prematurity
    Congenital anomalies
    Chronic illness
Parents
    Maternal social isolation or depression
    Father unavailable
    Marital tension
    Poor maternal nurturing as a child
Interactional
    Irregularly scheduled meals
    Report of feeding problems
    Lack of eye or physical contact
    Predominantly negative affect
    Poor interpretation of child's cues
    Inappropriate level of stimulation
Environmental
    Increased stress
    High family density
    Losses
    Poverty

Extreme prematurity resulting in very low birth weight (<3.3 lb [1.5 kg]) is associated with later growth deficiency even when measurements are corrected for gestational age.[13] Prematurity itself is not a risk factor for FTT since infants who suffer no prenatal, perinatal, or postnatal complications have normal growth potential.[12] However, premature infants are at greater risk for perinatal insults that can affect their ultimate growth.

Chronic illness increases the risk for developing FTT. Cystic fibrosis or chronic diarrhea, for example, can have profound effects on appetite, the ability to ingest, retain, or utilize food, and the need for additional energy supplies to meet altered metabolic requirements.

Factors arising in the parents include social isolation, depression, and a tendency to become overwhelmed by events.[2, 14] An unavailable father (often present but not supportive), increased marital tension, and a maternal history of being poorly nurtured as a child are additional risk factors.[4] In the case presented, all of these features were present, marking this area as a major one for treatment.

A history of small, irregularly scheduled meals is an important interactional risk factor for FTT. Feeding problems are documented both by report and observation[7] and often include inappropriate caretaker responses to the child's behavioral cues, with too much or too little stimulation offered.[7] Nonfeeding interactions, including harsh discipline, understimulation, and interactions characterized by caretaker unresponsiveness are risk factors for child maltreatment in general and FTT in particular.[15] These infants may prefer interactions with inanimate objects or with caretakers at a safe distance.[16] Again, in our case example, feeding interactions were devoid of nurturing. Feeding and nonfeeding interactions were passive and not developmentally appropriate (too much time in walker or being held, no finger feeding, etc.).

Environmental risk factors include stress, marital dissatisfaction, higher family density, and poverty. These are commoner in situations where FTT exists.[10, 14]

DIAGNOSIS

The diagnosis of FTT is based on anthropometric evaluation and comparison with standard (National Center for Health Statistics) growth charts. Any child whose weight is consistently below the fifth percentile for age or whose weight is less than 80% of the ideal weight for age should be evaluated for FTT.[5] Most clinicians consider a child who has crossed more than two standard deviations on NCHS charts over a period of 6 months to be at risk for FTT. When weight and length are below the fifth percentile, assessment of mean parental height assists in identifying the child with constitutional short statures.[17] Children born prematurely should have their weights, lengths, and head circumference adjusted for degree of prematurity: weight should be corrected until age 24 months; height until 40 months; and head size until 18 months.[2] For a given age, a child's height can be plotted against mean parental height.[17]

Comparison of the patient's *weight for height* is always important when making a diagnosis of FTT. Weight for height below the fifth percentile indicates acute, ongoing malnutrition. Other useful measurements for quantitating relative malnutrition are weight and height age, the age at which the patient's weight (or height) would be at the 50th percentile. When the weight age and height age are similar but both decreased, and especially when head circumference is also affected, severe stunting from chronic malnutrition is likely.

When *weight for length* measurements near the 50th percentile accompany weight and length measurements below the 5th percentile, interpretations can be misleading. Although these findings can be seen with severe stunting, such a picture is more commonly found with congenital short stature, constitutional delay of growth and adolescence, or an underlying endocrine abnormality, such as growth hormone deficit.

A complete history, physical examination, and careful interactional observation will suggest the underlying etiology for FTT in virtually all cases.[5] It is best to begin the search for underlying pathology by seeking risk factors in both organic and nonorganic realms simultaneously.

A medical history, including, prenatal, developmental, and nutritional components, should be obtained. A history of prior or present family illness, including psychiatric illness, abuse, accidents, or neglect, should also be ascertained. Identified risk factors such as prematurity or low birth weight do not rule out pathology in other areas. A review of systems will usually guide the clinician to the presence of chronic disease. Gastrointestinal, urologic, and endocrinologic conditions are commonest, and particular attention to the presence of vomiting, diarrhea, bulky stools, polyuria or polydypsia, and rumination is warranted.[1, 5]

The importance of a careful, complete nutritional evaluation cannot be over-emphasized. A 3-day diet history and a feeding observation are vital to obtain early in the assessment. Attention to the quality and quantity of the diet is important, and comparison with requirements for normal and catch up growth should be made.[18] Collaboration with a nutritionist or dietician, if available, can be extremely helpful.

A complete physical examination should document dysmorphic features, temperamental characteristics, and signs of possible neglect or trauma. Infants with severe malnutrition can show abnormalities of posture and tone. Delays in language acquisition and gross motor skills are present in as many as 50% of children with FTT, and their detection has bearing on later treatment.[2]

Laboratory testing is useful only when guided by historic or physical findings, and comprehensive screens are seldom helpful or cost effective.[9, 19] Retrospective studies have demonstrated limited usefulness of laboratory testing in children with FTT.[1, 5, 9] A prospective study of laboratory data in 100 outpatient children with FTT confirmed that no laboratory test was ever useful unless there was a clear indication for doing that test by either history or physical examination.[20] Routine laboratory testing should be limited to the following (Table 49–2).

A social history will outline family functioning. Ascertaining the parents' understanding of the locus of dysfunction is crucial to alliance formation. Where social risk factors directly influence the child's safety or future growth and development, social service support may become mandatory.

Observation of feeding and nonfeeding interactions forms the basis for diagnosis and treatment in many situations. Quality of interaction, degree of eye and physical contact, and degree of pleasure should be noted. Abnormal separation patterns and depression may be present.

Infants who develop FTT in their first 2 months of life often demonstrate disorders of self-regulation. Attachment disorders usually manifest during ages 2 to 6 months, and children who develop FTT after 8 months of age often have problems

TABLE 49–2.
Routine Laboratory Tests in Failure to Thrive*

Complete blood cell count
Urinalysis
Urine culture
Urine for reducing substances
BUN or creatinine
Tuberculin test
Free erythrocyte protoporphyrin/lead
Stool for pH, reducing substances, occult blood, ova, and parasite†
Sweat test†
Chest x-ray film†

*Modified from Bithoney and Rathbun.[2]
†Indicated if history is suggestive, (e.g., stool ova and parasites for recent immigrant children).

with separation or individuation, resulting in oppositional behavior around feeding.[21]

Diagnostic workups for FTT often bog down during the social and interactional assessment. Parents and practitioners are often reluctant to explore sensitive areas of family relationships or dysfunction, and concrete information may be collected slowly. The assistance of a mental health professional may facilitate this process. Visiting nurses can make home evaluations, both of environment and of feeding and nonfeeding interactions in the home setting.

Once established, FTT can be self-perpetuating. Malnutrition is associated with iron deficiency, a tendency toward increased lead absorption from the environment, and some deterioration of immunologic function.[10, 22] Increased whole blood lead levels and decreased iron stores are each associated with poor appetite and cognitive and behavioral difficulties. Frequent infections can lead to decreased appetite and intake but also to increased metabolic needs or nutrient losses (i.e., from diarrhea). This has been dubbed the *infection-malnutrition cycle.*[23]

TREATMENT

Treatment of FTT involves elucidating the factors perpetuating the symptom. Malnutrition, accompanying physical illnesses, developmental delay, caretaker-infant interactions, social issues, and so forth should be noted and concrete, individualized strategies developed for every identified factor.

Undernutrition can promote developmental, behavioral, feeding, and immunologic compromises.[10, 22] A plan for nutritional rehabilitation should be instituted immediately, including both dietary recommendations and strategies to encourage child and family compliance. Clear descriptions of the amounts and types of foods should be given to the parents. Food fortification by concentration and by the addition of high caloric–density supplements is the first step. Nonfat dry milk can be added to whole milk, and polycose, a glucose polymer, can be added to many other beverages and foods. Fortified milk shakes made with instant breakfast products and ice cream are often successful in providing supplemental calories. Liquids with low nutritional value (apple juice) should be eliminated and replaced with milk or milk substitutes. The addition of fats will not only make the diet higher in calories but often more palatable as well. The formation and implementation of such recommendations are greatly facilitated by collaboration with a dietician.[18]

Infant stimulation programs are appropriate for most children with FTT. With understimulation, appropriate day-care placement is often warranted. Physical or occupational therapists are rarely viewed negatively by parents, even in the home setting. They can provide services to FTT children while helping to integrate parents into the treatment program.[2]

Parental support and a nonjudgmental, nonaccusatory professional relationship are needed.[4] Strategies for treating interactional disturbances have been described[21] and must be tailored to the specific child-parent system. Videotaping feeding and nonfeeding interactions and supportively reviewing these with parents are effective tools for inaugurating changes in family feeding dynamics.

Disorders of homeostasis occurring early in infancy often involve infant temperamental difficulties or oral and motor problems. Professionals, skilled in understanding such a child's cues, can provide interactional modeling for parents.

Problems with attachment can be difficult to treat in an outpatient setting, because both parent and child need considerable assistance. Nutritional, developmental, and especially emotional support for the infant can be provided by a primary nurse. At the same time, successful efforts at teaching the parents appropriate interactional skills will permit transferring the infant's feeding responsibilities back to the parents.

When FTT begins after the age of 6 to 8 months, it is usually the result of oppositional behaviors around eating. Meals become affect-laden experiences for the family, and behavioral patterns become entrenched. The child often dictates what, when, and how he or she will eat. General recommendations for this common presentation of FTT include regularly scheduled meals and planned snacks (no grazing), limitation of meal times (maximum 20–30 minutes), encouragement of self-feeding, maintenance of a neutral affect by the caregiver during feeding, avoiding use of food as a reward, and meal termination if the child throws food or becomes disruptive.[21]

Hospitalization is necessary when outpatient treatment has failed or if there are significant risks to the child's safety. Severe protein-calorie malnutrition, when actual weight is less than 60% of ideal weight, is an indication for admission.[2] When infants are listless and anorectic secondary to the effects of malnutrition, supplemental tube feedings during sleep may stimulate appetite and hasten recovery if combined with an overall interactional and behavioral program.[2, 22] Severe neglect or the presence of abuse mitigates hospitalization for social stabilization. Admission is also required when diagnostic or treatment efforts have been unsuccessful.

OUTCOME

The few long-term follow-up studies of children with FTT suggest that eventual catch-up weight gain occurs, and the majority of children reach weights above the fifth percentile.[7, 24] The outlook for cognitive and behavioral development is much less optimistic. When children require hospitalization for FTT, long-term studies indicate that cognitive impairment, disturbances of language acquisition and usage, and behavioral difficulties occur in more than one half of children followed for 3 years or more.[2, 24, 25]

Clearly, an aggressive and comprehensive approach to diagnosing and treating children with the symptom of FTT is warranted. Success will depend on the development of a close, ongoing relationship with the child and family. In difficult cases, a pediatrician is well advised to enlist the aid of a coordinated team of health care professionals, including nutritionists, psychologists, and social workers.

SUMMARY

Failure to thrive is a symptom of unmet caloric needs. Underlying etiologies must be sought and usually include some interactional or environmental factors, often augmented by undernutrition. Efficient diagnostic workups examine multiple areas simultaneously, because FTT can result from pathology in any area of a child's functioning. Treatment can be facilitated by a multidisciplinary team of professionals.

REFERENCES

1. Hannaway P: Failure to thrive: A study of 100 infants and children. *Clin Pediatr* 1970; 9:96–99.
2. Bithoney WG, Rathbun J: Failure to thrive, in Levine M, Carey W, Crocker A, et al (eds): *Developmental-Behavioral Pediatrics.* Philadelphia, WB Saunders Co, 1983, pp 557–572.
3. Mitchell WG, Gorrell RW, Greenberg RA: Failure to thrive: A study in a primary care setting. *Pediatrics* 1980; 65:971–977.
4. Altemeier WA III, O'Connor SM, Sherrod KB, et al: Prospective study of antecedents for nonorganic failure to thrive. *J Pediatr* 1985; 106:360–365.
5. Berwick D: Non-organic failure-to-thrive. *Pediatr Rev* 1980; 1:265–270.
6. Pollit E, Thomson C: Protein caloric malnutrition and behavior: A view from psychology, in Wurtman RJ, Wurtman JJ (eds): Determinants of the nutrients to the brain. New York, Raven Press, 1977, pp 261–306.
7. Chatoor I, et al: Non-organic failure to thrive: A developmental perspective. *Pediatr Ann* 1984; 13:829–843.
8. Homer C, Ludwig S: Categorization of etiology of failure to thrive. *Am J Dis Child* 1981; 135:848–851.
9. Sills RH: Failure to thrive, the role of clinical and laboratory evaluation. *Am J Dis Child* 1978; 132:967–969.
10. Bithoney WG, Dubowitz H: Organic concomitants of nonorganic failure to thrive: Implications for research, in Drotar D (ed): *Failure to Thrive.* New York, Plenum Publishing Corp, 1985, pp 47–68.
11. Brazelton TB: Nutrition during early infancy, in Suskind RM (ed): *Testbook of Pediatric Nutrition.* New York, Raven Press, 1981, pp 271–284.
12. Fitzhardinge PM, Steven PM: The small-for-date infant: I. Later growth patterns. *Pediatrics* 1972; 49:671–681.
13. Kimble KJ, et al: Growth to age 3 years among very low-birth-weight sequelae-free survivors of modern neonatal intensive care. *J Pediatr* 1982; 100:622–624.
14. Kotelchuck M, Newberger EH: Failure to thrive: A controlled study of familial characteristics. *J Am Acad Child Psychiatry* 1983; 22:322–328.
15. Bradley RH, Casey PM: A transactional model of failure to thrive: A look at misclassified cases, in Drotar D (ed): *Failure to Thrive.* New York, Plenum Publishing Corp, 1985, pp 107–118.
16. Rosenn DW, Loeb LS, Jura MB: Differentiation of organic from non-organic failure to thrive syndrome in infancy. *Pediatrics* 1980; 66:698–704.
17. Himes JH, Roche AF, Thissen D, et al: Parent-specific adjustments for evaluation of recumbent length and stature of children. *Pediatrics* 1985; 75:304–313.
18. Peterson KE, Washington J, Rathbun JM: Team management of failure to thrive. *J Am Diet Assoc* 1984; 84:810–815.
19. Goldbloom RB: Growth failure in infancy. *Pediatr Rev* 1987; 9:57–61.
20. Bithoney WG: Unpublished data, 1987.
21. Chatoor I, Dickson L, Schaefer S, et al: A developmental classification of feeding disorders associated with failure to thrive: Diagnosis and treatment, in Drotar D (ed): *Failure to Thrive,* New York, Plenum Publishing Corp, 1985, pp 235–258.

22. Frank DA: Biologic risks in "nonorganic" failure to thrive: Diagnostic and therapeutic implications, in Drotar D (ed): *Failure to Thrive*. New York, Plenum Publishing Corp, 1985, pp 17–26.
23. Scrimshaw NS: Significance of the interactions of nutrition and infection in children, in Suskind RM (ed): *Textbook of Pediatric Nutrition,* New York, Raven Publishing Corp, 1981, pp 229–240.
24. Oates RK, Peacock A, Forrest D: Long-term effects of nonorganic failure to thrive. *Pediatrics.* 1985; 75:36–40.
25. Singer LT, Fagan JF: Cognitive development in the failure to thrive infant: A three-year longitudinal study. *J Pediatr Psychol* 1984; 9:363–382.

50 Nutritional Assessment

Kristy Hendricks, R.D., D.Sc.

A 13-month-old girl was referred for evaluation of diarrhea and failure to thrive. She had been the 7.6-lb (3.4-kg) product of a normal, full-term pregnancy, labor, and delivery and enjoyed good health for the first 3 months of life. However, at 4 months of age her bowel movements became more frequent, foul smelling, and loose. Weight gain slowed after 7 months, and irritability became noticeable. The patient had been breast-fed for the first month of life, then was fed cow's milk formula until 4 months of age, soy formula from 4 to 9 months, and whole cow's milk from 9 months to the time of evaluation. Cereals were begun at 2 months of age, and fruits, vegetables, and juices were added at 3 months of age. Wide dietary variety was achieved by age 6 months. A 24-hour recall and 3-day food record revealed an average intake of 600 calories/day (range 350–1,200 calories/day) and an average intake of 10 gm of protein, 18 gm of fat, and 100 gm of carbohydrate. The diet was remarkable for a low intake of dairy products and other protein-rich foods and a high consumption of juice and grains. Dietary intake was limited by the severity of the diarrhea. None of a large number of dietary manipulations caused improvement in the diarrhea.

On physical examination, the child appeared cranky and chronically ill. Her weight was 15.4 lb (7.0 kg) (<5%), height 70 cm (<5%), with weight for height at the 5th percentile and her head circumference at the 25th percentile for age. The physical examination was remarkable for a distended abdomen without tenderness or organomegaly, prominent gluteal atrophy, and edema of her legs. Anthropometric measurements showed decreased tricep skinfold thickness and arm muscle circumference with wasting of both fat and muscle mass. The radiographic bone age was 9 months. By use of the Gomez criteria for malnutrition (Table 50–1), the patient's weight for age was 70% of the standard (50th percentile for age), corresponding to moderate malnutrition.

Results of the laboratory evaluation included normal hemoglobin value, absolute lymphocyte count, electrolyte concentrations, BUN level, calcium level, phosphorus level, prothrombin time, partial thromboplastin time, urinalysis, stool cultures, evaluation for ova and parasites, and qualitative stool fat analysis. The albumin level was low (2.5 mg/dl), a D-xylose test result was abnormal, and results of her small bowel biopsy showed a flat mucosa with crypt hyperplasia and mild chronic inflammatory infiltration. A diagnosis of gluten-sensitive enteropathy (celiac disease) was made, and the child started on an elemental infant formula with supplemental vitamins and minerals. The diarrhea resolved, and the weight stabilized over the following week when the patient was advanced to a gluten- and lactose-free diet in addition

TABLE 50–1.

Classification of Malnutrition, Percentiles

Reference	Normal	Mild	Moderate	Severe
Gomez et al.[1] (weight for age)	>90	90–75	75–61	<60
Jelliffe[2] (weight for age)	110–90	90–81	80–61	<60
McLaren & Read[3] (weight for height)	110–90	90–85	85–75	<75

to the formula. The patient had excellent weight gain, growth, and normalization of her albumin levels over the subsequent 2 months. Dietary evaluation showed good adherence to the gluten restriction and an estimated intake of 1,200 calories/day. At that time a lactose tolerance test was normal, and the elemental formula was replaced by milk.

DISCUSSION

Evaluation of nutritional status has several important goals, including the detection of acute and chronic malnutrition, assessment of specific nutrient deficiencies, development of recommendations for treatment, and appropriate intervention for individuals identified as being at risk. A combination of anthropometric, clinical, biochemical, and dietary measures are used to provide a comprehensive assessment of nutritional status. In each area of evaluation, the individual is compared to an established norm that provides a basis for objective recommendations and ongoing evaluation of nutritional therapy. Selection of standards appropriate to the population, accurate technique and equipment for measurement, and perceptive interviewing skills are important components. Historic data in each area of nutritional assessment can be extremely important in making specific short- and long-term recommendations for nutritional intervention.

Basic guidelines for screening for nutritional problems and methods to proceed with a more extensive and costly workup are outlined in Table 50–2. For a more detailed discussion of standards and techniques used for nutritional assessment, the following references are recommended.[4–6]

Anthropometric Evaluation

Physical growth from conception to maturity is a simple but effective means of evaluating nutritional status. Anthropometric measures repeated over time provide excellent objective data on overall health and well-being of the individual. Routine screening should include weight, height, weight/height, and head circumference. National Center for Health Statistics (NCHS) growth charts are the most representative of these measurements in infants, children, and adolescents in the United States. All measurements were done between 1962 and 1974 by the U.S. Public Health

TABLE 50–2.
Nutritional Assessment Guidelines*

	Anthropometric	Clinical	Biochemical	Dietary
Initial screening	Weight, length, weight/length, head circumferance	History and physical examination, sexual maturation	Hematocrit, hemoglobin level, cholesterol level	Typical pattern of intake, supplements
Intermediate	Tricep skinfold thickness, arm circumference	More extensive examination (teeth, gums, eyes, skin, hair, etc.)	Mean corpuscular volume, albumin level, total protein level, total lymphocyte count	Assessment of feeding skills, 24-hour dietary recall, food records
In-depth evaluation	Bone age, height velocity, prediction of mature height	More extensive examination, classification of malnutrition	Skin testing, specific vitamin, mineral or trace element levels	Observation in hospital

*From Walker WA, Hendricks KM: *Manual of Pediatric Nutrition*. Philadelphia, WB Saunders Co, 1985, pp 3–49. Used by permission.

Service on large samples of children throughout the United States and represent the most comprehensive measures available for comparison.[7]

Weight is a good index of acute nutritional status, with the standard being the 50th percentile for sex and age; values below the 5th percentile or above the 95th percentile indicate possible weight deficit or excess, respectively. These measurements must be considered in relation to the growth patterns of the child's family.

Height may be more affected by chronic undernutrition and provides the clinician with objective data on past nutritional status. Again, the standard is the 50th percentile for sex and age, with values below the 5th percentile indicating possible growth failure and chronic undernutrition. Weight for height more accurately assesses body build and can be used to distinguish wasting from dwarfism. Measurements near the 50th percentile indicate appropriate weight for height. The further the deviation from this value, the more overnourished or undernourished the individual. Head circumference is influenced by nutritional status for approximately the first 3 years of life. Effects lag behind those seen on weight and height, with measurements below the 5th percentile indicating possible chronic undernutrition in fetal life and infancy.

An in-depth evaluation of body composition should include skinfold thickness and arm circumference measures. Skinfold thickness provides an estimation of total body fat and, used in combination with arm circumference, can determine muscle and fat mass through use of a simple nomogram calculation. These measures are especially useful in identifying those individuals who may be overweight but not overfat (as with highly athletic individuals) and those who are overfat but not overweight (as with the normal weight individual with a high percentage of body fat). Standards compiled by Franchismo are based on the NCHS measurements.[6, 8]

Growth velocity, bone age, evaluation of sexual development, and prediction of mature height can be used to distinguish nutritional dwarfism from constitutional short stature. Growth velocity evaluates change in the rate of growth over time and is a more sensitive way of assessing slowed growth. Tanner growth velocity charts are recommended for evaluation of growth velocity.[10] Bone age, or the radiographic evaluation of epiphyseal closure, measures skeletal maturity and potential for catch-up growth. Skeletal maturation generally correlates with sexual maturation, and the Tanner stages of sexual development.[11, 12] Although variability exists as to the ages at which sexual development and increased growth velocity occur, the sequence is fairly uniform. Skeletal and sexual development are generally retarded in conditions where growth is slowed and may be caused by primary or secondary malnutrition. Prediction of mature height may be helpful in determining constitutional short stature. Fel's parent-specific standards for height are based on mean parental height and are age and sex specific.[11]

Clinical Assessment

Clinical signs of severe malnutrition are easily detected in most cases. A thorough physical examination for specific clinical signs of nutrient deficiencies is important in patients known to be at risk because of disease or social situation. These signs include abnormalities of skeletal development, eye lesions, skin, hair, and mucous membrane changes.[4] Validation generally requires confirmation by other biochemical, dietary, or anthropometric data. Malnutrition has most commonly been classified as low weight for height or low weight for age. In some cases of chronic undernutrition, severely slowed growth may be the only clinical sign. This is referred to as nutritional dwarfism, because height has been stunted but weight may be appropriate for height. The various classifications for malnutrition are outlined in Table 50–1.[1-3]

Overt malnutrition is usually categorized as either marasmus or kwashiorkor. Marasmus is secondary to severe deprivation of both calories and protein and is characterized by severe weight loss in combination with wasting of subcutaneous fat and muscle. Kwashiorkor is a disease of primarily protein deficiency, and edema accompanies muscle wasting, often masking weight loss. In both conditions, indifference, apathy, irritability, and fatigue are present.

Biochemical Evaluation

Biochemical evaluation of nutritional status is useful in identifying individuals with subclinical nutrient deficiencies or in confirming deficiencies suspected by anthropometric, clinical, or dietary assessment. Early biochemical detection provides for early intervention of nutrient deficiencies before the severe clinical effects are apparent. It is important to keep in mind that biochemical tests differ in reproducibility and that diseases may effect blood levels of many nutrients. Routine biochemical screening should include measures of hematologic status (hematocrit, hemoglobin) and protein status (albumin, total protein). Some clinicians believe routine screening of blood cholesterol is important for possible nutritional intervention. Evidence for the effect of malnutrition on immune function indicates that both total lymphocyte count and delayed hypersensitivity (skin testing) are depressed.[5, 6] Both can be useful measures in evaluation of nutritional status and response to nutritional therapy. More specific tests for vitamin, mineral, and trace elements deficiencies are available. Such tests are often complex and expensive. Their use should be reserved for individual cases with a high degree of risk or clinical suspicion of deficiency.

Dietary Evaluation

Accurate dietary evaluation plays an important role in comprehensive nutritional assessment. Determination of quality and quantity of food intake, nutrient composition of the diet, and the various factors that affect past and present intake can be assessed by a variety of dietary methods (typical pattern, 24-hour recall, food diaries). Each methodology has certain limitations, and the difficulty in quantifying actual intake is well documented.[13-15] In many cases, it is helpful to use two different methods to evaluate intake, particularly in young children whose intake is inconsistent from day to day. Extreme cases may require observation in the hospital to document intake accurately. A pattern of normal intake for young children ages 2 to 5 years is summarized in Table 50–3.[16]

The Recommended Dietary Allowances (RDAs) are the most appropriate general standards used to evaluate nutrient intake. They are designed for maintenance of

TABLE 50–3.

Recommendations for Normal Feeding in Childhood*

Food Group	2–3 yr	4–5 yr
Milk, including fortified whole or skin milk, yogurt, cheese, ice cream, custard, pudding, buttermilk: *3–4 servings/day*	1 serving = 6 oz ($^3/_4$ c) milk or equivalent	1 serving = 8 oz (1 c) milk or equivalent
Meat, fish, poultry, legumes, nuts, eggs (recommended for eggs, 2–3/wk): *2 or more servings/day*	1 serving = 1–2 oz meat, poultry, or fish; 1 egg; 2 tbsp peanut butter; $^1/_2$ c legumes	1 serving = 2 $^1/_2$–3 oz meat, fish, or poultry; 1 egg; 3 tbs peanut butter; $^1/_2$–$^3/_4$ c legumes
Cereals and bread, whole grain or enriched bread, muffins, cereal, rice, noodles, rolls, pasta: *3 or more servings/day*	1 serving = $^1/_2$ slice bead or roll; $^1/_3$–$^1/_2$ c cereal, macaroni, spaghetti, noodles, or rice	1 serving = 1 slice bread or roll, $^1/_2$–$^3/_4$ c cereal or pasta
Fruits and vegetables including fresh, frozen, dried or canned fruits, vegetables or their juices: *3 or more servings/day,* including one good source of vitamin C daily, one good source of vitamin A 3 times/week	1 serving = $^1/_3$–$^1/_2$ c juice; $^1/_4$ c fresh, frozen, or canned fruit or vegetable; 2 tbs dried fruit	1 serving = $^1/_2$ c juice, $^1/_3$ c fruit or vegetable
Fats, oils, and simple sugars	Used as needed as an extra energy source	Used as needed as an extra energy source

*Adapted from Walker and Hendricks.[4]

good nutrition in a healthy population and are meant to be applied to population groups. Thus, in certain individuals more precise methods for estimating energy and nutrient requirements are needed. In such cases the following references are recommended.[4, 5] Energy and protein requirements based on the RDAs are summarized in Table 50–4. Recommended intakes of macronutrients and micronutrients are discussed in detail and summarized in the RDAs.[17]

SUMMARY

The nutritional assessment is an essential part of the evaluation of most gastrointestinal disease. The evaluation includes anthropometric, clinical, biochemical, and dietary components. Basic guidelines for nutritional assessment are included in Table 50–2.

TABLE 50–4.

Estimated Nutrient Needs

Age, yr	Calories	(per kg)	Protein	(per kg)
0–0.5		(115)		(2.2)
0.5–1.0		(105)		(2.0)
1–3	1,300	(100)	23	(1.8)
4–6	1,700	(85)	30	(1.5)
7–10	2,400	(85)	34	(1.2)
Boys				
11–14	2,700	(60)	45	(1.0)
15–18	2,800	(42)	56	(.85)
Girls				
11–14	2,200	(48)	46	(1.0)
15–18	2,100	(38)	46	(.85)

REFERENCES

1. Gomez F, Glavan R, Cravioto J, et al: Malnutrition in infancy and childhood with special reference to Kwashiorkor. *Adv Pediatr* 1955; 3:131–169.
2. Jelliffe D: The assessment of nutritional status of the community. Geneva, Switzerland, World Health Organization Monograph, 1966, vol 53, pp 32–45, 135–168, 185–212.
3. McLaren DS, Read WWC: Weight/length classification of nutritional status. *Lancet* 1975; 2:219–221.
4. Walker WA, Hendricks KM: *Manual of Pediatric Nutrition*. Philadelphia, WB Saunders Co, 1985, pp 3–49.
5. Roberts SLW: *Nutrition Assessment Manual*. Iowa City, Iowa, University of Iowa Hospitals and Clinics, 1977, pp 1–50.
6. Christakis G: Nutritional assessment in health programs. *Am J Public Health* 1973; 63(suppl):1–82.
7. Hamill PVV, Drizd TA, Johnson CL, et al: *NCHS Growth Charts*. Rockville, Md, Monthly Vital Statistics Report (HBA)76-1120, vol 25, no 3 (suppl) 1976.
8. Frisancho AR: New norms of upper limb fat and muscle areas for assessment of nutritional status. *Am J Clin Nutr* 1981; 34:2540–2545.
9. Gurney JM, Jelliffe DB: Arm anthropometry in nutritional assessment: Nomogram for rapid calculation of muscle circumference and cross-sectional muscle and fat areas. *Am J Clin Nutr* 1973; 26:912–915.
10. Tanner JM, Whitehouse RH, Fakaistti M: Standards from birth to maturity for height, weight, and height velocity and weight velocity: British children, 1965. *Arch Dis Child* 1966; 41:454–457.
11. Garn SM, Rothman CG: Interaction of nutrition and genetics in the timing of growth and development. *Pediatr Clin North Am* 1966; 13:353–379.
12. Gardner LI (ed): *Endocrine and Genetic Diseases of Childhood and Adolescence*. ed 2. Philadelphia, WB Saunders Co, 1975, pp 14–64, 99–103.
13. Carter RL, Sharbaugh CO, Stapell CA: Reliability and validity of the 24-hour recall. *J Am Diet Assoc* 1981; 79:542–547.
14. Karvetti RL, Knuts LR; Agreement between dietary interviews. *J Am Diet Assoc* 1981; 79:654–660.

15. Stunkard AJ, Waxman M: Accuracy of self-reports of food intake. *J Am Diet Assoc* 1981; 79:547–551.

16. American Academy of Pediatrics Committee on Nutrition: *Pediatric Nutrition Handbook.* Evanston, Ill, American Academy of Pediatrics, 1979, pp 28–52.

17. National Research Council, Food and Nutrition Board Dietary Allowances Committee: *Recommended Dietary Allowances*, ed 9. Washington DC, National Academy of Sciences, 1980, pp 1–15, 23, 186.

Index

in portal hypertension diagnosis, 274
Upper GI contrast study
  in inflammatory bowel disease diagnosis, 56
  in malrotation diagnosis, 116
  in peptic ulcer disease diagnosis, 35

V

Vaccine, hepatitis B, in hepatitis B prevention, 240
Vancomycin for pseudomembranous colitis, 146, 148
Vasopressin infusion for upper GI bleeding, 29
Venography, portal, in portal hypertension diagnosis, 274–275
Vertebral defects in Alagille syndrome, 228
Vitamin B_{12} deficiency in inflammatory bowel disease, 60
Vomiting

induction of, for acetaminophen overdose, 225
nonbilious, in pyloric stenosis, 41

W

Wedged hepatic venous pressure (WHVP)
  in portal hypertension, 273
Weight in nutritional assessment, 345
Wilson disease, 264–269
  autoimmune chronic active hepatitis differentiated from, 247
  clinical features of, 265–266
  diagnosis of, 266–267
  pathophysiology of, 265
  treatment of, 267–268

Z

Zinc deficiency in inflammatory bowel disease, 60–61